Systemic Approaches in Bioinformatics and Computational Systems Biology:

Recent Advances

Paola Lecca
The Microsoft Research – University of Trento, Centre for Computational and Systems Biology, Italy

Dan Tulpan
National Research Council of Canada, Canada

Kanagasabai Rajaraman
Institute for Infocomm Research, Singapore

A volume in the Advances in Bioinformatics and Biomedical Engineering (ABBE) Book Series

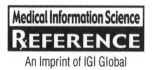

Medical Information Science
REFERENCE
An Imprint of IGI Global

Managing Director:	Lindsay Johnston
Senior Editorial Director:	Heather Probst
Acquisitions Editor:	Erika Gallagher
Book Production Manager:	Sean Woznicki
Development Manager:	Joel Gamon
Development Editor:	Myla Harty
Typesetters:	Deanna Jo Zombro
Print Coordinator:	Jamie Snavely
Cover Design:	Nick Newcomer, Greg Snader

Published in the United States of America by
Medical Information Science Reference (an imprint of IGI Global)
701 E. Chocolate Avenue
Hershey PA 17033
Tel: 717-533-8845
Fax: 717-533-8661
E-mail: cust@igi-global.com
Web site: http://www.igi-global.com

Copyright © 2012 by IGI Global. All rights reserved. No part of this publication may be reproduced, stored or distributed in any form or by any means, electronic or mechanical, including photocopying, without written permission from the publisher. Product or company names used in this set are for identification purposes only. Inclusion of the names of the products or companies does not indicate a claim of ownership by IGI Global of the trademark or registered trademark.

Library of Congress Cataloging-in-Publication Data

Systemic approaches in bioinformatics and computational systems biology : recent advances / Paola Lecca, Dan Tulpan, and Kanagasabai Rajaraman, editors.
    p. cm.
  Summary: "This book presents new techniques that have resulted from the application of computer science methods to the organization and interpretation of biological data, covering three subject areas: bioinformatics, computational biology, and computational systems biology"-- Provided by publisher.
  Includes bibliographical references and index.
  ISBN 978-1-61350-435-2 (hardcover) -- ISBN 978-1-61350-436-9 (ebook) -- ISBN 978-1-61350-437-6 (print & perpetual access) 1. Bioinformatics. 2. Systems biology. 3. Computational biology. I. Lecca, Paola, 1973- II. Tulpan, Dan, 1976- III. Rajaraman, Kanagasabai, 1968-
  QH324.2.S947 2012
  572.80285--dc23
                                    2011036916c

This book is published in the IGI Global book series Advances in Bioinformatics and Biomedical Engineering (ABBE) (ISSN: 2327-7033; eISSN: 2327-7041)

British Cataloguing in Publication Data
A Cataloguing in Publication record for this book is available from the British Library.

All work contributed to this book is new, previously-unpublished material. The views expressed in this book are those of the authors, but not necessarily of the publisher.

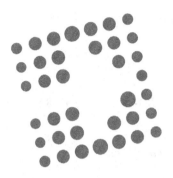

Advances in Bioinformatics and Biomedical Engineering (ABBE) Book Series

Ahmad Taher Azar
Benha University, Egypt

ISSN: 2327-7033
EISSN: 2327-7041

MISSION

The fields of biology and medicine are constantly changing as research evolves and novel engineering applications and methods of data analysis are developed. Continued research in the areas of bioinformatics and biomedical engineering is essential to continuing to advance the available knowledge and tools available to medical and healthcare professionals.

The **Advances in Bioinformatics and Biomedical Engineering (ABBE) Book Series** publishes research on all areas of bioinformatics and bioengineering including the development and testing of new computational methods, the management and analysis of biological data, and the implementation of novel engineering applications in all areas of medicine and biology. Through showcasing the latest in bioinformatics and biomedical engineering research, ABBE aims to be an essential resource for healthcare and medical professionals.

COVERAGE

- Biomechanical Engineering
- Biostatistics
- Chemical Structures
- Computational Biology
- Dental Engineering
- DNA sequencing
- Drug Design
- Genomics
- Rehabilitation Engineering
- Robotics and Medicine

IGI Global is currently accepting manuscripts for publication within this series. To submit a proposal for a volume in this series, please contact our Acquisition Editors at Acquisitions@igi-global.com or visit: http://www.igi-global.com/publish/.

The Advances in Bioinformatics and Biomedical Engineering (ABBE) Book Series (ISSN 2327-7033) is published by IGI Global, 701 E. Chocolate Avenue, Hershey, PA 17033-1240, USA, www.igi-global.com. This series is composed of titles available for purchase individually; each title is edited to be contextually exclusive from any other title within the series. For pricing and ordering information please visit http://www.igi-global.com/book-series/advances-bioinformatics-biomedical-engineering-abbe/73671. Postmaster: Send all address changes to above address. Copyright © 2012 IGI Global. All rights, including translation in other languages reserved by the publisher. No part of this series may be reproduced or used in any form or by any means – graphics, electronic, or mechanical, including photocopying, recording, taping, or information and retrieval systems – without written permission from the publisher, except for non commercial, educational use, including classroom teaching purposes. The views expressed in this series are those of the authors, but not necessarily of IGI Global.

Titles in this Series

For a list of additional titles in this series, please visit: www.igi-global.com

Technological Advancements in Biomedicine for Healthcare Applications
Jinglong Wu (Okayama University, Japan)
Medical Information Science Reference • copyright 2013 • 382pp • H/C (ISBN: 9781466621961) • US $245.00 (our price)

Biomedical Engineering and Cognitive Neuroscience for Healthcare Interdisciplinary Applications
Jinglong Wu (Okayama University, Japan)
Medical Information Science Reference • copyright 2013 • 472pp • H/C (ISBN: 9781466621138) • US $245.00 (our price)

Pharmacoinformatics and Drug Discovery Technologies Theories and Applications
Tagelsir Mohamed Gasmelseid (King Faisal University, Kingdom of Saudi Arabia)
Medical Information Science Reference • copyright 2012 • 442pp • H/C (ISBN: 9781466603097) • US $245.00 (our price)

Machine Learning in Computer-Aided Diagnosis Medical Imaging Intelligence and Analysis
Kenji Suzuki (University of Chicago, USA)
Medical Information Science Reference • copyright 2012 • 524pp • H/C (ISBN: 9781466600591) • US $245.00 (our price)

Systemic Approaches in Bioinformatics and Computational Systems Biology Recent Advances
Paola Lecca (The Microsoft Research – University of Trento, Centre for Computational and Systems Biology, Italy) Dan Tulpan (National Research Council of Canada, Canada) and Kanagasabai Rajaraman (Institute for Infocomm Research, Singapore)
Medical Information Science Reference • copyright 2012 • 471pp • H/C (ISBN: 9781613504352) • US $265.00 (our price)

Intravascular Imaging Current Applications and Research Developments
Vasilios D. Tsakanikas (University of Ioannina, Greece) Lampros K. Michalis (University of Ioannina, Greece) Dimitrios I. Fotiadis (University of Ioannina, Greece) Katerina K. Naka (University of Ioannina, Greece, and Michaelideion Cardiology Center, Greece) and Christos V. Bourantas (University of Ioannina, Greece)
Medical Information Science Reference • copyright 2012 • 478pp • H/C (ISBN: 9781613500958) • US $245.00 (our price)

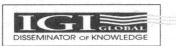

www.igi-global.com

701 E. Chocolate Ave., Hershey, PA 17033
Order online at www.igi-global.com or call 717-533-8845 x100
To place a standing order for titles released in this series, contact: cust@igi-global.com
Mon-Fri 8:00 am - 5:00 pm (est) or fax 24 hours a day 717-533-8661

Editorial Advisory Board

Francesco Amato, *University of Catanzaro, Italy*
Robert Beiko, *Dalhousie University, Canada*
Alessandra Orsoni, *Kingston University, UK*
Monika Heiner, *Brandeburg University, Germany*
Joao Manuel R. S. Tavares, *University of Porto, Portugal*

List of Reviewers

Andrea Pugliese, *University of Trento, Italy*
Guylaine Poisson, *University of Hawaii, USA*
Patricia Evans, *University of New Brunswick, Canada*
Michela Lecca, *Fondazione Bruno Kessler – Center for Information Technology, Italy*
Marina Scarpa, *University of Trento, Italy*

Table of Contents

Section 1

Chapter 1

*Miroslava Cuperlovic-Culf, Institute for Information Technology, National Research Council,
Canada*

Chapter 2

Jose M. Garcia-Manteiga, Protein Transport and Secretion Unit, San Raffaele – DIBIT, Italy

Chapter 3

Dan Tulpan, National Research Council of Canada, Canada
Athos Ghiggi, University of Lugano (USI), Switzerland
Roberto Montemanni, Istituto Dalle Molle di Studi sull'Intelligenza Artificiale (IDSIA), Switzerland

Chapter 4

Boris R. Jankovic, King Abdullah University of Science and Technology, Kingdom of Saudi Arabia
John A. C. Archer, King Abdullah University of Science and Technology, Kingdom of Saudi Arabia
Rajesh Chowdhary, Biomedical Informatics Research Center, USA
Ulf Schaefer, King Abdullah University of Science and Technology, Kingdom of Saudi Arabia
Vladimir B. Bajic, King Abdullah University of Science and Technology, Kingdom of Saudi Arabia

Detailed Table of Contents

Section 1

Chapter 1

Miroslava Cuperlovic-Culf, Institute for Information Technology, National Research Council,
Canada

The chapter shows the benefits and limitations of different unsupervised analysis tools currently utilized in qualitative and quantitative metabolomics data analysis. A detailed literature review outlining different applications of unsupervised methods in metabolomics is reported and examples of an application of the major previously utilized unsupervised analysis methods are described.

Chapter 2

Jose M. Garcia-Manteiga, Protein Transport and Secretion Unit, San Raffaele – DIBIT, Italy

Nuclear magnetic resonance and mass spectrometry are the two techniques usually employed to collect metabolomic data. The chapter focuses on the different data analysis tools that can be applied to such data to with the purpose of extracting information relevant to the modern approaches of modeling in systems biology.

The chapter outlines recent algorithms used in microarray probe design and presents an evaluation of the existing probe sequences used in commercial arrays. The authors suggest methodologies that have the potential to improve on existing design techniques.

Conserved families of motifs of for promoter regulatory structures between Homo sapiens, Mus musculus and Drosophila melanogaster have been revealed. Conservation of promoter structures across these vertebrate and invertebrate genomes suggests the presence of a fundamental promoter architecture and provides the basis for deeper understanding of the necessary components of the transcription regulation machinery.

Chapter 5

The chapter deals with the computational identification of translation initiation sites. A new human translation initiation sites recognition model is presented. This model is able to successfully recognize deeply conserved genomic signals that characterize translation initiation sites.

A survey of the recent methodologies proposed for the structure inference and for the parameter estimation of a system of interacting biological entities is reported in this chapter. Furthermore, the recent studies of the authors on model identification and calibration are presented.

The work addresses the question of how to quantify and characterize the structural and dynamical variability in ecological networks. The authors presents a novel process algebra model of the network dynamics and new methods of network analysis that can feed the network structure with quantitative information. The model is supported by the data on a large, real ecological network -, the Prince William Sound in Alaska.

The chapter introduces two ecological food-webs. The concepts of dominator tree, dominance relations and trophic chain are introduced to deal with static analysis of the ecological network. Then, stochastic dynamic simulations are proposed as an alternative approach to static analyses based on food web topology. The work demonstrates that Rranking species importance using stochastic-based simulations partially contradicts the predictions based on network analyses.

The expressive capabilities of process algebra for specifying models of for biological processes are presented. Process algebras complement conventional more established mathematical approaches to systems biology with new insights that emerge from computer science and software engineering. Process algebras allow to specify parallel and concurrent interactions between biological entities as well as the multi-functionality of biological complexes. The stochastic extension of process algebras can model the stochasticity inherent to many biological processes at the micro- and meso-scale. An illustrative example is described: the phagocytosis, an evolutionarily conserved process by which cells engulf larger particles.

Chapter 10

Parthasarathy Subashini, Avinashilingam Deemed University for Women, Thadagam Post, India
Bernadetta Kwintiana Ane, Universität Stuttgart, Germany
Dieter Roller, Universität Stuttgart, Germany
Marimuthu Krishnaveni, Avinashilingam Deemed University for Women, Thadagam Post, India

In many applications, the fusion of multiple relatively simple classifiers has been proved to be achieve better recognition rates than a single sophisticated classifier. The chapter reviews classifiers and classification methods currently in use in bioinformatics and shows models of fusions and their performances.

Chapter 11

Yue Wang Webster, Eli Lilly and Company
Ernst R Dow, Eli Lilly and Company & Indiana University, USA
Mathew J Palakal, Indiana University, USA & Purdue University, USA

The chapter discusses the opportunities and the challenges of translational research applied to link biological basics research and medical/clinical practice. Translational research is presented as a tool enabling knowledge translation between life science and health care domains. Today, translational research has to face the need to provide a conceptual framework to fully realize the value of the existent tools and technologies currently implementing it. The authors presents Complex System as a proposal of theoretical foundation of for such a framework. They designed HyGen (Hypotheses Generation Framework) a tool implementing this framework. Heuristic and quantitative tests of this tool in the Ccolorectal Ccancer disease area are presented.

Foreword

The last two decades saw the development of many new experimental technologies in genome sequencing, microscopy, high-throughput analytics, etc. These technologies have given rise to a rapid accumulation of data of various forms, nature, and complexity. Coupled with the advances in computing power, this flow of information should enable scientists to model and understand biological systems in novel ways.

Let me highlight three threads of advances that I find particularly exciting:

- **The appearance of many databases containing information on biological networks.** Such networks are useful to understanding the function of genes and proteins in a more holistic way. For example, as physical protein interactions underlie cellular processes, analysis of protein interaction networks has been shown helpful in the prediction of protein function, the discovery of protein complexes, and detection of epistatic interactions. As another example, as each disease generally has an underlying cause which is expected to be reflected in a biological pathway, combined analysis of biological pathways and gene expression profiling data has been used to enhance the reliability of the inference of disease genes.

- **The appearance of whole-genome sequences of many organisms and many strains of the same organisms.** For example, comparative analysis of these sequences from the greatly increased variety of genomes permits a deeper analysis of conserved gene structures and functional motifs, and translates to improvement in gene finding and recognition of various functional sites. As another example, comparative analysis of multiple strains of an organism such as a pathogen, can provide better insights into the virulence of the pathogen, the identification of genes involved in antibiotic resistance, and discovery of mode of action of novel antibiotic drugs.

- **The appearance of large-scale metabolic profiling data, especially lipid profiles.** When we go for a medical checkup today, only a handful of lipids—e.g., the lipoprotein cholesterols and triglycerides—are measured. Yet there are over three thousand types of lipids in our body. Furthermore, the critical role of lipids in cell, tissue and organ physiology is demonstrated by a large number of genetic studies and by many human diseases involving the disruption of lipid metabolic enzymes and pathways. Examples of such diseases include cancer, diabetes, neurodegenerative and infectious disorders. Novel systems level analysis of lipids and their interaction partners, while still in an early stage, is promising for the identification of biomarkers and drug targets.

Driven by such opportunities and challenges, bioinformatics has rapidly expanded in scope and complexity over the last two decades. This book offers the readers a timely, broad, and useful introduction to these exciting developments.

Limsoon Wong
National University of Singapore 30 May 2011

Limsoon Wong *is a provost's chair professor in the School of Computing and a professor in the Yong Loo Lin School of Medicine at the National University of Singapore. Before that, he was the Deputy Executive Director for Research at A*STAR's Institute for Infocomm Research. He is currently working mostly on knowledge discovery technologies and is especially interested in their application to biomedicine. Prior to that, he has done significant research in database query language theory and finite model theory, as well as significant development work in broad-scale data integration systems. Limsoon has written about 150 research papers, a few of which are among the best cited of their respective fields. In recognition for his contributions to these fields, he has received several awards, the most recent being the 2003 FEER Asian Innovation Gold Award for his work on treatment optimization of childhood leukemias and the 2006 Singapore Youth Award Medal of Commendation for his sustained contributions to science and technology. He serves on the editorial boards of Information Systems (Elsevier), Journal of Bioinformatics and Computational Biology (ICP), Bioinformatics (OUP), IEEE/ACM Transactions on Computational Biology and Bioinformatics, Drug Discovery Today (Elsevier), and Journal of Biomedical Semantics (BMC). He is a scientific advisor to Semantic Discovery Systems (UK), Molecular Connections (India), and CellSafe International (Malaysia). He received his BSc(Eng) in 1988 from Imperial College London and his PhD in 1994 from University of Pennsylvania.*

Foreword

Recent developments in biology and bioinformatics have produced a huge amount of data on the static structure of the living matter and the research community is now facing the challenge of providing their appropriate interpretation, integration, and system-level understanding. Deep interdisciplinary skills are required to attain the goal, spanning from biology to computer science and touching upon mathematics, engineering, and physics.

The thorough expertise of the editors of the book, Paola Lecca, Dan Tulpan, and Kanagasabai Rajaraman, clearly shows in the thoughtful selection of contributions in this book.

Paola Lecca, with whom I had the pleasure of collaborating on many occasions over the latest few years, has a rich research record on stochastic biochemical kinetics, biological networks inference, optimal experimental design in biochemistry, and computational cell biology.

Dan Tulpan is an expert on computational biology, microarray probe design, comparative genomics, and data analysis.

Kanagasabai Rajaraman is a prolific and skilled researcher in data mining, semantic technologies, and bio-ontologies.

The three of them carefully choose an outstanding excerpt of topics and of contributions which make this book a unique reference on the most challenging areas at the convergence of biology and computational sciences.

Paola Quaglia
University of Trento, Italy, 23 April 2011

Paola Quaglia, PhD in Computer Science, is Associate Professor at the Faculty of Science, University of Trento, Italy. Her research interests are mainly in the area of the application of formal methods to model and analyze the dynamics of biological behaviours, and to study and validate service-oriented distributed systems. In particular, she has been active in the following areas: application of mobile process calculi to systems biology; specification of biochemical interactions; analysis of service-oriented coordination and interaction protocols; application of typing disciplines to specification languages for distributed systems; semantics for mobile processes; probabilistic and stochastic process calculi. Her major contributions are relative to: investigation and definition of primitives and formal languages for modelling biological systems; specification, analysis, and simulation of complex systems exhibiting stochastic or probabilistic behaviour; comparative analysis of the expressiveness of distinct interaction paradigms.

Preface

Computer science methods along with traditional mathematical approaches support the organization and the interpretation of biological data. This book presents a collection of recent studies on three main areas of convergence of computer science and mathematics with systems biology. The subject areas are: (1) experimental data analysis, (2) knowledge inference, (3) modeling and simulations, and (4) computational sequence design and analysis. Although these areas have different biological application contexts, different aims and make use of different computational tools and techniques, they share the common rationale that is the construction of conceptual models of real biological systems to disentangle their complexity.

Modeling is an attempt to describe an understanding of the elements of a system of interest, their states, and their pair wise interactions. The model should be sufficiently detailed and precise so that it can in principle be used to simulate the behavior of the system on a computer. In the context of molecular cell biology, a model may describe the mechanisms involved in transcription, translation, cell regulation, cellular signaling, DNA damage and repair processes, the cell cycle or apoptosis. At a higher level, modeling may be used to describe the functioning of a tissue, organ, or even an entire organism. At a still higher level, models can be used to describe the behavior and time evolution of populations of individual organisms. At the beginning of a modeling project, the first issue to confront is to decide which features to include in the model and the level of detail the model is intended to capture. So, for example, a model of an entire organism is unlikely to describe the detailed functioning of every individual cell, but a model of a cell is likely to include a variety of very detailed description of key cellular processes. Even then, however, a model of a cell is unlikely to contain details of every single gene and protein. In order to show how it is possible to think about a biological process at different levels of detail, let us consider the photosynthesis process. It can be summarized by a single chemical reaction mixing water with carbon dioxide to get glucose and oxygen. The reaction is catalyzed by the sunlight. This single reaction is a summary of the overall effect of the process. Although the photosynthesis consists of multiple reactions, the above descriptive equation it is not really wrong. It globally represents the process at higher level than the more detailed description biologists often prefer to work with. Whether a single overall equation or a full breakdown into component reactions is necessary depends on whether intermediate reagents are elements of interest to the modeler. In general, we can state that the "art" to build a good model consists in the ability to capture the essential features of the biology without burdening the model with non-essential details. However just because of the omission of the details, every model is to some extent a simplification of the biological process it represents. Nevertheless, models are valuable because they take ideas that might have been expressed verbally or diagrammatically, and make them more explicit, so they can begin to be understood in a quantitative rather than purely qualitative way. The features of a model depend very much on the aims of the modeling. Modeling and simulation appeared on the scientific horizon much earlier than the emergence of molecular and cellular biology. Their genesis is in the physical sciences and engineering. In the physical sciences, besides theoretical and experimental studies, modeling and simulation are considered as the third indispensable approach because not all hypotheses are amenable for confirmation or rejection by experimental observations. In biology, researchers are facing the same or maybe even a worse situation. On one hand experimental studies are unable to produce a sufficient amount of data to support theoretical interpretations, and on the other hand, due to data insufficiency, theoretical research cannot provide substantial guidance and insights for experimentation. Therefore computational modeling takes a more important role in biology by integrating experimental data, facilitating theoretical hypotheses, and addressing "*what if*" questions.

Another important aim of modeling is to shed light on the current state of knowledge regarding a particular system, by attempting to be precise about the elements involved and the interactions between them. Such an approach can be an effective way to highlight gaps in our somewhat limited understanding. Our understanding of the experimental observations of any system can be measured by the extent to which our model simulation mimics the real behavior of that system. Behaviors of computer-executable models are at first compared with experimental values. If at this stage inconsistency is found, it usually means that the assumptions representing our knowledge of the system, are at best incomplete, or that the interpretation of the experimental data is wrong. Models surviving this initial validation stage can then be used to make predictions to be tested by experiments, as well as to explore configurations of the system that are not easy to investigate by *in vitro* or *in vivo* experiments. Creation of predictive models can give opportunities for unprecedented control over the system. In contrast to physics, biology still lacks a clear explicit framework for the fundamental laws on which it is based. Modeling can provide valuable insights into the workings and general principles of organization of biological systems. Although we will always need real experiments to advance our understanding of biological processes, conducting *in silico*, or computer-simulated experiments can also help guide the wet-lab experimental processes by narrowing down the experimental search space.

More than fifty years ago, the structure of DNA was identified, thus paving the way for the molecular biology and genetics. Grounding the biological phenomena on molecular basis made it possible to describe the different aspects of biology, such as heredity, diseases and development, as the result of the coherent interactions between sets of elements that are either functionally different or most often multifunctional. Grounding biological phenomena on a molecular basis made it possible to include biology in a consistent framework of knowledge based on fundamental laws of physics. Since then, the field of molecular biology has emerged and enormous progress has been made in this direction. Molecular biology enables us to understand biological systems as molecular machines. Large numbers of genes and the function of transcriptional products have been identified. DNA sequences have been fully identified for various organisms such as mycoplasma, E.coli, C.elegans, Drosophila melanogaster, and Homo sapiens. Measurements of protein levels and their interactions are also making progress. In parallel with such efforts, new methods have been invented to disrupt the transcription of genes, such as loss of function via knockout of specific genes and RNA interference that is particularly effective for C.elegans, a process that is now applied for other species. Nevertheless, such knowledge is not sufficient to provide us with a complete understanding of biological systems *as systems per se*. Cells, tissues, organs and organisms as well as ecological webs are systems of components whose specific interactions have been defined by evolution. Thus, a system-level understanding should be the prime goal of biology.

System-level understanding is the paradigm of systems biology and requires a set of principles and methodologies that links the behaviors of molecules to system characteristics and function. These principles and methodologies should be developed in the following four areas of investigation.

1. **System structures.** These include the network of gene interactions and biochemical pathways, as well as the mechanisms by which such interactions modulate the physical properties of intracellular and multicellular structures.
2. **System dynamics**, describing the time-evolution of the system components. How a system behaves over time under various conditions can be understood through metabolic analysis, sensitivity analysis, and dynamic analysis methods such as portrait and bifurcation analysis. Specifically, the system behavior analyses aim at addressing the following questions: how does a system respond to changes in the environment? How does it maintain robustness against potential damage, such as DNA damage and mutations? How do specific interaction pathways exhibit the observed functions? It is not a trivial task to understand the behaviors of complex biological networks. Computer simulation and a set of theoretical analyses are essential to provide in-depth understanding of the mechanisms behind the pathways.
3. **Control methods.** The identification of mechanisms that systematically control the state of the cell is necessary for two reasons. First, their understanding can be exploited to modulate them so to minimize malfunctions, and second, they involve potential therapeutic targets for treatments of diseases.
4. **The design methods.** Strategies to modify and construct biological systems with desired properties can be developed on definite design principles and simulations, instead of blind trial-and-error approaches.

Any progress in each of the above areas requires breakthroughs in our understanding not only of molecular biology, but also of measurement technologies and computational sciences. Although advances in accurate, quantitative experimental approaches will doubtlessly continue, insights into the functioning of biological systems will not result from purely intuitive assaults. The reason resides in the intrinsic complexity of biological systems expected to be solved by combinations of experimental and computational simulation approaches. Biologists are getting enthusiastic about mathematical modeling, as modelers are getting excited about biology. The complexity of molecular and cellular biological systems makes it necessary to consider dynamic systems theory for modeling and simulation of intra- and inter-cellular processes. Modeling of complex systems has to be taken as a priority by modelers and computational biologists, if we want to reach the important milestones of the research in computational systems biology. To describe a system as "complex" has become a common way to either motivate new approaches or to describe the difficulties in making progress. Currently, before we can fully explain and understand the functioning and the functions of cells, organs or organisms from the molecular level upwards, the major difficulties are technological and methodological. Sometime the temptation is thinking that the complexity of these systems ensures that there is no way around mathematical and computational modeling in this endeavor.

The contributions presented in this book are going in the opposite direction, directly facing the problem of modeling biological complexity and attest the progress of the fruitful convergence of biology and computational sciences.

Paola Lecca
The Microsoft Research – University of Trento, Centre for Computational and Systems Biology, Italy

Dan Tulpan
National Research Council, Canada

Kanagasabai Rajaraman
Institute for Infocomm Research, Singapore

Acknowledgment

The editors would like to thank the Editorial Advisory Board that supported us in the review process. Francesco Amato of University of Catanzaro (Italy), Robert Beiko of Dalhousie University (Canada), Alessandra Orsoni of Kingston University (UK), Monika Heiner of Brandeburg University (Germany), Joao Manuel R. S. Tavares of University of Porto (Portugal) took part on the Editorial Advisory Board and offered their time and their scientific guidance to make the contents of the book homogenous and current. The editors are also extremely grateful to the reviewers that revised accurately and always in time the chapter proposals and the full manuscripts. In particular the editors would like to thank Andrea Pugliese of University of Trento, Guylaine Poisson of University of Hawaii (USA), Patricia Evans of University of New Brunswick (Canada), Michela Lecca of Fondazione Bruno Kessler – Center for Information Technology (Italy) and Marina Scarpa of University of Trento (Italy). Finally, the editors would like to express their thanks to all the authors that submitted their manuscript and made the realization of this book possible.

Paola Lecca
The Microsoft Research – University of Trento, Centre for Computational and Systems Biology, Italy

Dan Tulpan
National Research Council, Canada

Kanagasabai Rajaraman
Institute for Infocomm Research, Singapore

Section 1

Chapter 1
Unsupervised Data Analysis Methods used in Qualitative and Quantitative Metabolomics and Metabonomics

Miroslava Cuperlovic-Culf
Institute for Information Technology, National Research Council, Canada

ABSTRACT

Metabolomics or metababonomics is one of the major high throughput analysis methods that endeavors holistic measurement of metabolic profiles of biological systems. Data analysis approaches in metabolomics can broadly be divided into qualitative – analysis of spectral data and quantitative – analysis of individual metabolite concentrations. In this work, the author will demonstrate the benefits and limitations of different unsupervised analysis tools currently utilized in qualitative and quantitative metabolomics data analysis. Following a detailed literature review outlining different applications of unsupervised methods in metabolomics, the author shows examples of an application of the major previously utilized unsupervised analysis methods. The testing of these methods was performed using qualitative as well as corresponding quantitative metabolite data derived to represent a large set of 2,000 objects. Spectra of mixtures were obtained from different combinations of experimental NMR measurements of 13 prevalent metabolites at five different groups of concentrations representing different phenotypes. The analysis shows advantages and disadvantages of standard tools when applied specifically to metabolomics.

DOI: 10.4018/978-1-61350-435-2.ch001

Copyright © 2012, IGI Global. Copying or distributing in print or electronic forms without written permission of IGI Global is prohibited.

INTRODUCTION

Over the last decade many new technologies have been developed and utilized in order to understand and describe the complexity of biological systems. High throughput methods involving the parallel measurement of biological molecule concentrations have been applied to many different systems in different environments (Schena, 1995; Fiehn, 2000; Nicholson, 2002). Large amount of data created by these methods have made data analysis a major part of most biological explorations nowadays. In many examples of high throughput methodology a strong emphasis in the first level of statistical analysis is on unsupervised approaches. Unsupervised data analysis is employed for obtaining connections between samples and/or molecular features without biasing the results by the introduction of prior knowledge. Thus, the development of methods and tools for unsupervised data analysis as well as the exploration of the most optimal methods and their most appropriate uses in the analysis of various high throughput, *i.e.* omics, biological data is an active research area.

One of the major, fast developing high throughput analysis methods, attempts a holistic measurement of metabolic profiles, *i.e.* metabolom or metabonom, of biological systems. Metabolomics, initially defined as the global analysis of all metabolites in a sample (Fiehn, 2001; Oliver, 1998) and metabonomics perceived as the analysis of metabolic responses to drugs or diseases (Nicholson, 1999) are nowadays often interchangeable terms broadly referring to the multi-component analysis of metabolites in a biological system (Beckoners, 2007). Metabolomics provides to systems biology a functional readout of changes determined by genetic code, regulation, protein abundance and modifications as well as environmental influences. Metabolic differences in biological fluids, cells and tissues provide the closest link to the various phenotypical responses showing the actual effects of various phenotype changes, drug effects, toxicological responses or disease states. The other functional genomics technologies, such as transcriptomics and proteomics indicate the potential causes for phenotype response. Metabolomics can be viewed as a "re-invention" or extension of the approaches of analytical biochemistry of the 1960s. However, there are some major differences between modern metabolomics and analytical biochemistry of the past. First, is the introduction of highly advanced and reliable instrumentation such as nuclear magnetic resonance (NMR) and mass spectrometers (MS) for parallel, quantitative analysis of complex biological samples. Second, is the introduction of a novel data driven approach aimed at observing all measurable metabolites without any preconceptions or preselection. Third, is the introduction of various data analysis procedures, computational tools and methodologies that are able to quantitatively and accurately analyze large amounts of data. These tools must handle, store, pre-process and analyze complex and often large datasets (Cuperlovic-Culf, 2010). This new approach to metabolic phenotyping has emerged as a powerful new way to augment genomic, transcriptomic and proteomic methods for the capture of molecular information already applied to a range of biological systems (Bictash, 2009). Similarly to other types of omics methodologies large amounts of data produced in metabolomics experiments require application of appropriate and often complex data analysis tools.

Depending on the type of metabolic data available the data analysis approach in metabolomics can broadly be divided into qualitative and quantitative with the major steps and applications of these two approaches outlined in Figure 1. The type of analysis employed defines the necessary pre-processing steps. In qualitative metabolic analysis complete metabolomics spectra or spectral regions are used. In contrast, quantitative metabolomics initially performs compound identification and quantification. Once metabolite concentration information is obtained these data can be used for various applications including the development of systems biology models or biomarker discovery.

Figure 1. Schematic representation of the major steps in qualitative and quantitative metabolomice experiment. Procedures are divided into experimentation - data generation, data pre-processing – preparation of the dataset ready for analysis and data interpretation – analysis and knowledge generation.

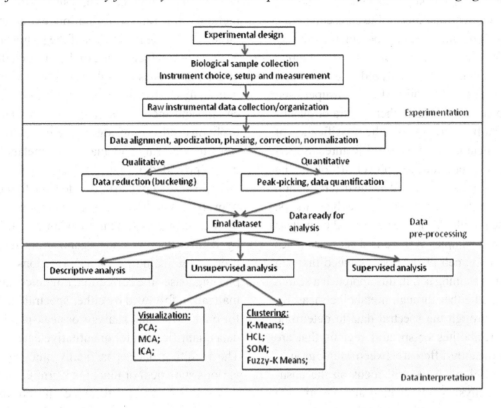

The qualitative approach has a range of clinical applications for direct sample classification. However, the application of spectral data leads to specific problems such as peak drift caused by different experimental conditions and overlapping peaks. In addition, the optimal spectral normalization is still not determined and the application of a suboptimal method can lead to errors in the results. Utilization of spectra also leads to the inclusion of spectral regions that represent background noise in the analysis. This leads to unnecessarily large datasets and can also possibly result in inaccuracies in clustering. Furthermore, overlapping of spectral peaks can lead to erroneous conclusions. Quantitative metabolomics can in principle alleviate some of these issues by determination of concentrations of individual metabolites from spectra. In turn, the availability of metabolite concentrations can lead to many more applications of metabolomics in biomarker discovery, pathway and network analysis, for example. A major concern in quantitative metabolomics is the problem of spectral assignment. Unlike transcriptomics where gene assignment is in principle trivial thanks to highly specific hybridization of genes to specially designed, unique probes, the high throughput analysis of metabolic mixtures, peak assignment and the measurement of abundance for each metabolite requires spectral deconvolution and availability of measurements under the same conditions for all metabolites that can possibly be visible in the measurement. In addition to assignment problems some of the major issues facing the qualitative approach remain in quantitative metabolomics including problems caused by overlapping peaks as well as changes in peak positions of various compounds under different conditions (*i.e.* pH induced changes in ^{1}H NMR spectra). Thus far, the assignment and quantification of metabolites requires comparison with measurements of individual molecules or isotopically labelled standards and thus, unidentified metabolites present a great challenge to quantitative metabolomics analysis.

In both the qualitative and the quantitative approaches data can be analyzed in an unsupervised or supervised fashion. In the unsupervised approach complete data (either spectra or quantified metabolites) are used for the classification of samples, metabolites or spectral features. Supervised methods provide more powerful tools for the sample classification as well as the determination of the major differential features, *i.e.* biomarkers. Supervised methods can be used for the analysis of unknown samples if there is a set of samples with class, *i.e.* cell phenotype, assigned that can be used as a training set. In this approach a search is performed either through metabolite measurements or through the spectral data to determine marker metabolites or spectral regions that are most significantly different between sample groups.

In the following we will focus on the unsupervised analysis of qualitative and quantitative metabolomics data. The goal of the chapter is to describe methods currently used in metabolomics data analysis and show examples of their use in the literature. Finally, we demonstrate for easy comparison, to the best of our knowledge for the first time, with synthetically designed NMR spectra and corresponding quantitative data, the abilities and inabilities of most popular unsupervised methods in metabolomics. Although we will try to cover different methodologies some of the less utilized methods will sadly have to be omitted.

LITERATURE AND METHODOLOGY OVERVIEW

Metabolomics is becoming an increasingly popular tool for functional genomics with new applications regularly appearing. These different applications include widely different types of samples including blood and urine, plant or animal tissues, cells and cell extracts and environmental samples. However, data analysis algorithms and methods for final information extraction are largely the same regardless of the sample origin. Metabolomics faces some of the same challenges as the other types of high-throughput biological data analysis. The use of appropriate data preprocessing and analysis methods is essential in order to obtain useful knowledge. An overview of all the steps in acquiring and analysis of metabolomics data is provided in Figure 1 (based on Goodacre, 2007). These steps can be divided into four groups of processes including experimentation preceded by a careful experimental design and followed by data collection and organization; data preprocessing including data corrections such as phasing, base-line correction, alignment and normalization followed by either spectral bucketing for qualitative data analysis or peak-picking and data quantification for quantitative data analysis. The resulting dataset is finally analyzed using various statistical or machine learning methods.

In the current literature metabolomics, similarly to other omics methods, has as its main objectives:

a. Examination of similarities and difference between samples based on metabolic profiles;

b. Exploration of similarities and difference between metabolites over time or between different phenotypes;

c. Sample classification from metabolic profiles;

d. Determination of major significantly differentially present features.

A majority of metabolomics experiments outlined in Figure 1 do not in general depend on the final goal of the experiment however the final data interpretation *i.e.* analysis, needs to be optimized based on the question of the given metabolomics experiment. The final data interpretation procedures can be divided into descriptive analysis that includes analysis of any correlation between metabolites or samples or general statistical analysis of variances or deviations, for example. A second group of analysis methods include unsupervised analysis approaches that are used for grouping of features (sample, metabolites or spectral points). This group includes the visualization, *i.e.* projection and clustering method. Finally, a third group of methods includes supervised analysis tools that are utilized for sample classification and/or for feature selection for biomarker discovery. The unsupervised methods are most appropriate for accomplishing objectives a. and b. (see above). In general, if sufficient information about the samples is available objectives c. and d. are best accomplished using supervised approaches. In the following literature review we will focus on the use of unsupervised analysis methods in metabolomics aimed at objectives a and b with a separate exploration of application of unsupervised methods for the analysis of samples (objective a) and metabolites (objective b). General brief overview of the major unsupervised methods used in metabolomics is provided in Table 1.

Analysis of Samples

A phenotype is any observable characteristic or trait of an organism such as its morphology, devel-

Table 1. Unsupervised analysis algorithms used in metabolomics

Method	Description	Use
PCA	Principal component analysis PCA makes it possible to extract and display systematic variations in the data while at the same time providing clear and easy-to-interpret graphical representation of data groups. PCA is appropriate only if the biological question is related to the highest variance in the dataset.	Preliminary visualization tool for grouping of samples
HCL	Hierarchical clustering (HCL) is a crisp, hierarchical one or two way clustering method. HCL is rarely used in metabolomics due to its (i) lack of robustness to noise, high dimensionality and outliers; (ii) high expens in terms of computational time and space complexity; (iii) Inability to redo or optimize the results.	Primarily used for clustering of samples when there is no information about the number of clusters and for visualization. In a two way for it can be used for grouping of samples and quantitative metabolic data.
KM	K-Means (KM) clustering, which is a basic crisp, non-hierarchical, one way-method and its adaptation for noisy metabolomics data: bagged K-means. K-means clustering partitions the input data into a user defined number of clusters (K). The solution that K-means clustering reaches can depend on the centroid initialization and this can thus potentially lead to finding only a local rather than a global minimum.	Can be used for clustering samples as well as qualitative and quantitative metabolic data.
SOM	Self organized maps -SOM clustering, which is a crisp, non-hierarchical, one way-method based on neural networks. The SOM method belongs to a class of artificial neural networks which are capable of projecting high-dimensional input data on a two-dimensional map utilizing a single-layered artificial neural network. SOM provides both accurate clustering method as well as powerful visualization tool to a user predefined number of groups and topology. SOM can only reach a local optimum if the initial weights are not chosen properly. In the case of processing a large data, SOM is prone to problems when handling the data abundant in irrelevant and invariant features.	SOM can be used for clustering both samples and metabolites with particularly successful use in clustering based on quantitative metabolic data.
FKM	Fuzzy K-Means (FKM) clustering, which is a fuzzy, non-hierarchical, one way-method. The fuzzy approach allows features to belong to more than one group, cluster. This allows a determination of subtypes for features that belong to major groups and within those groups to subgroups. Fuzzy clustering also allows better assignment of samples that can be divided differently based on different characteristics as is often the case in biological samples. Similarly to crisp KM in F-KM user has to predefine number of clusters and the initial parameters need to be optimized in order to reach the global minimum.	FKM can be used for clustering both samples and metabolites. In the case of qualitative metabolite clustering FKM can provide interesting method for peak grouping leading to assignment.

opment, biochemical or physiological properties, behaviour, and products of behaviour (Mahner, 1997). In order to have an observable difference, *i.e.* different phenotypes, there have to be some metabolic differences in the systems. The only challenge is to find the metabolic differences in general and the ones that lead to the phenotype differences in particular. The goal of metabolomics in this regard is, thus, to measure accurately as many metabolites as possible and to investigate whether the obtained measurements can distinguish between sample types at hand. This type of analysis requires careful consideration of all the steps outlined in Figure 1. In principle, for the analysis of sample differences, including sample clustering and classification it is not essential to quantify individual measured metabolites. The majority of publications dealing with sample analysis presented thus far utilize only qualitative, spectral, metabolic data. The application of quantitative metabolic data does, however, provide some interesting possibilities in terms of interpretation and the analysis of quantitative metabolic data is appearing more often in the literature. In the following both approaches will be presented.

Visualization Methods

Metabolomics, spectral data is generally highly collinear, *i.e.* have highly correlated context-dependent localized structures (Huopaniemi, 2009). At the same time the dimensionality of the data is usually quite large (particularly for the analysis of spectral data) especially in comparison to the number of measurements, *i.e.* samples. In this type of data, visualization of major differences between samples as well as the presence of outliers and erroneous measurements can often be accomplished by projection methods. By far the most commonly used projection, multivariate method in metabolomics is principal component analysis - PCA. PCA makes it possible to extract and display systematic variations in the data (Trygg, 2007) while at the same time

providing clear and easy-to-interpret graphical representation of data groups. In fact the large majority of metabolomics papers to-date include as part of the analysis an application of PCA for sample separation. PCA is a mathematical manipulation of the data matrix where the goal is to represent the variation present in many variables using a small number of "factors". A new space is constructed in which to plot the samples by redefining the axes using factors rather than the originally measured variables. These new axes, *i.e.* principal components (PC), show the true multivatiate nature of the data in a relatively small number of dimensions. With this new presentation visual pattern recognition can be used for identification of data groups (Beebe, 1998). The PC's are calculated such that PC1 explains the maximum amount of variation possible in the dataset in one direction, *i.e.* PC1 direction is the direction that describes the maximum spread of data points.

Mathematically, PCA is defined as a search for matrices of PCA scores, *T,* and loadings, *P,* that decompose data matrix *X* into: $X=TP^{T}+E$. This equation presents data expressed as a linear combination of its basis vectors (*P*). In other words matrix *P* transforms, *i.e.* rotates the original dataset *X* into new dataset *T*. The goal of the procedure is to find P such that the covariance matrix for *T* is diagonalized, *i.e.* all the off-diagonal elements are zero meaning that variables in the matrix *T* do not co-vary. Thus, scores of *T* are orthogonal and the loadings of *P* are orthonormal. The scores *T* and the loadings *P* are together referred to as principal components (PCs). There are several different approaches to solving this problem including the standard approach through calculating the diagnoalized covariance matrix for *T*. A general solution of PCA is provided by the Singular Value Decomposition method (Shlens, 2003). A prominent illustration of basic PCA application include the analysis of human metabolic phenotype diversity and its association with diet and blood pressure (Holmes, 2008) where PCA was used to separate ^{1}H NMR spectra of urine samples for 4,630 subjects involving samples from 17 populations from 4 different countries on three continents. PCA plots showed that geographic differences between two subpopulations in China and Japan and the two western populations from UK and USA are more pronounced than the difference caused by other group differences such as for example, gender. Another example is the use of PCA in the separation of, once again, urine ^{1}H NMR spectra in rats before and after dosing with a drug galactosamine hydochloride (Clayton, 2006). Although in this case PCA once again shows the difference between groups, as expected by the authors, the separation in PCA plots is rather limited and perhaps in this case one of the clustering or supervised analysis methods would have provided more information. PCA was also used for separation between colon carcinomas and normal tissues from MS data leading to almost perfect separation (Denkert, 2008). In this case PCA was used as a method for the initial exploratory analysis of data. In addition the authors have performed Welch's t-test to determine whether principal components PC1 and PC2 are significantly different for cancer and normal tissue measurements. This type of analysis provides an interesting and easy to interpret quantitative addition to the pictorial representation usually utilized for PCA.

PCA can also be utilized as a first step in dimensionality reduction of spectral data. In this case the major variances are determined and combined in PC and then all the other analysis – including unsupervised or supervised analysis is performed on a subset of PC's rather than the spectral data. Assfalg and co-workers (Assfalg, 2008) have presented an application of PCA for data reorganization prior to unsupervised analysis. In this example the ^{1}H NMR spectral buckets were projected into PCA subspace and the samples were clustered using 21 principal components using Hierarchical Clustering (Assfalg, 2008). This analysis has shown clear grouping of sample

obtained from sample individuals at different time points, showing the existence of individual metabolic phenotype.

PCA method is also well positioned for initial investigation of the data in order to examine the variance in the data set without forcing the data into a model for the determination of outliers that potentially need to be removed from further analysis. An example of such exploratory use of PCA prior to supervised classification analysis is given by Giskeødegård et al (Giskeødegård, 2010). In this example, PCA is used to show a general trend in the metabolomic NMR measurements of cancer biopsies from four different subtypes of breast cancers and for the determination of outliers that were removed from further supervised analysis.

Many variations to the PCA method have been proposed for specific applications in metabolomics. For example Multiway Principal Components Analysis (MPCA) has been suggested as a method for multivariate modelling for inter-compartmental analysis of tissues and plasma ^{1}H NMR spectrotypes (Montoliu, 2008). The MPCA analysis allows simultaneous integration of metabolic profiles from diverse biological compartments for each individual subject. PCA analysis was also integrated with wavelet transformation of the data (Xia, 2007). Wavelet decomposition of data leads to denoising and possibly leading to a significant improvement in data separation with PCA. A cause for concern with using this approach is that *a priori* knowledge is utilized for wavelet transformation and thus the WT-PCA is really a semi-supervised method and thus the improvements in data separation observed might be caused by overfitting of data.

The assumption of PCA and projection methods in general is that differences between systems are expressed by a small number of latent variables. Thus, PCA is appropriate only if the biological question is related to the highest variance in the dataset. This assumption does not hold in all the cases and thus other analysis methods should be explored for obtaining additional information. Clustering methods, contrary to the projection methods, consider differences between all the analyzed features. This could cause inaccuracies in datasets where large number of features contain only noise (as is the case in some spectral data) and in those cases projection methods are more appropriate. However, if the data are not overloaded with noise or if the effect of noise can be reduced or removed and/or if differences between samples are caused by large number of variations with possible similarities between multiple groups clustering methods should be used as they can provide better, more accurate, results.

Clustering Methods

Clustering methods aim to assign objects to a smaller number of distinct groups based on their pairwise similarities (Belacel, 2010). Clustering methods are commonly used to search for new associations in biological profile data. However, although in metabolomics literature only a handful of true clustering methods have been applied, they covered a wide variety of types of clustering approaches. The methods previously utilized included both crisp as well as fuzzy clustering; hierarchical as well as partitional clustering; one way and two way clustering (detailed description of clustering methods types is provided in Belacel, 2010). The majority of these applications are general tools however in some cases there were adaptations of methodologies specific for metabolomics analysis. The major clustering tools utilized in metabolomics literature for sample grouping thus far include

- hierarchical clustering (HCL), which is a crisp, hierarchical one or two way clustering method. Examples of its application include a) direct clustering of spectral data (Beckonert, 2003; Damian, 2007; Holmes, 2008; Lu, 2010; Chu, 2006), b) clustering of samples from a subset of major principal

components (Assfalg, 2008) or c) clustering of samples based on statistically selected most significant metabolites (Denkert, 2006);

- K-Means (KM) clustering, which is a basic crisp, non-hierarchical, one way-method and its adaptation for noisy metabolomics data: bagged K-means (Hageman, 2006)
- Self organized maps -SOM clustering, which is a crisp, non-hierarchical, one way-method based on neural networks (Makinen, 2008; Tukiainen, 2008; Suna, 2007),
- Fuzzy K-Means (F-KM) clustering, which is a fuzzy, non-hierarchical, one way-method tested for sample clustering from NMR spectral and MS data (Li, 2009; Cuperlovic-Culf, 2009).

Although hierarchical clustering is by far the most popular method in genomics and transcriptomics applications it is thus far rarely used in metabolomics. Several issues generally problematic in HCL are very significant in HCL applications in metabolomics. The main problems are: (1) lack of robustness to noise, high dimensionality and outliers (Jiang, 2004); (2) HCL is expensive in terms of computational time and space complexity (Xu, 2005). (3) Once the decision is made for merging, it cannot be redone or optimized. To tackle the above problems, several alternative approaches have been proposed (reviewed in Belacel, 2010). In addition, the two-way clustering of samples and features preferred in HCL application in genomics cannot be used on qualitative metabolomics data. Still however, the direct application of HCL on qualitative, spectral metabolomics data can provide interesting information for sample grouping. One of the early examples of an application of HCL is provided by Roessner and co-workers (Roessner, 2001) where HCL and PCA were applied to MS measurements of different plants and the analysis was focused on clustering individual plant systems and determination of relative distances between these clusters in native plants as well as plants following various environmental influences. Other examples of application of HCL include the analysis of toxicity in which case HCL provided a much clearer group of treatments relative to PCA analysis (Beckonert, 2003). HCL analysis in this case provided the groupings of subjects based on all the spectral points rather than only the major variances. In this analysis HCL helped in identifying clear organ-toxicity specific differences and also showed similarities between samples. The HCL results helped explain misclassifications in the k-Nearest Neighbours (kNN) analysis presented in the paper. HCL was also utilized in the analysis of human metabolic phenotype diversity and its association with diet and blood pressure (Holmes, 2008). In this work HCL was a method of choice for clustering of samples directly from normalized NMR spectra and it lead to the clear separation of people from UK and USA relative to subjects from Japan and China. In this case HCL results are in agreement with PCA analysis and thus provide confirmation of the results. In a recent paper contributed by Solberg and co-workers (Solberg, 2010) HCL is combined with K-means for the clustering of MS metabolic profiles of blood plasma for new born piglets following exposure to different oxygen levels. In this case subjects were clustered using HCL and for presentation purposes metabolite data were clustered using K-means grouping. In this analysis ratios of MS measured metabolite values before and after treatment were used for analysis. The heat plots representing the results of this analysis are clear and easy to interpret in terms of both subject and metabolite clustering.

HCL can also be used as a visualization tool for the grouping of metabolites selected using either statistical test (such as t-test) or supervised feature selection. The examples of such application are provided by Denkert and co-workers (Denkert, 2006) where HCL grouping of samples is done based on the measurements of metabolites selected as the most significantly different between two

groups of ovarian carcinomas in that set. Similarly, in the work presented by Lu and co-workers (Lu, 2010) major metabolic features are selected for normal, non-metastatic and metastatic breast cancer cell lines and HCL analysis of these measurements was used to show separation between cell lines. The fact that HCL separates samples in these cases is of course expected and not really relevant, however, HCL analysis provides a nice presentation of results.

HCL analysis can also be utilized for indirect investigation of data produced from other clustering or statistical methods. Assfalg and co-workers (Assfalg, 2008) used HCL for clustering of PC obtained from NMR spectral data. In this case PCA reduces the feature space as well as the influences of noise on the clusters making HCL analysis more robust to noise. At the same time the results obtained from HCL/PCA analysis were easier to interpret in terms of sample groups. HCL has also been utilized in combination with the Clustering Objects of Subsets of Attributes (COSA) method developed by Friedman and Meulman (Friedman, 2004). The COSA method derives a similarity matrix for the features and this matrix can be subsequently used for clustering. Damian and co-workers (Damian, 2007) have shown that HCL grouping of COSA results rather than directly metabolomics data leads to significant improvement in clustering accuracy of the tested dataset.

K-means clustering is a simple clustering method that partitions the input data into a user defined number of clusters (K). The solution that K-means clustering reaches can depend on the centroid initialization and this can thus potentially lead to finding only a local rather than a global minimum. This problem can, however, be alleviated by taking the best solution from multiple random starts. In a typical implementation of the K-means algorithm, the first step is to randomly select K objects, each representing initial cluster centroid. After the initialization step, each object in the data point is assigned to the closest centroid, and a cluster represents a collection of similar points, *i.e.* points assigned to the same centroid. The centroid of each cluster is then recalculated based on the points assigned to the cluster. The assignment and update steps are repeated iteratively until the centroids remain stable. K-means is relatively scalable and efficient when processing large datasets as its time complexity is linear. In addition, K-means can reach a local optimum in a small number of iterations. However, K-means still suffers from several limitations including the requirement to predefine an initial number of clusters K and the dependence of a clustering result to the initial centroid selection. For biological data prior knowledge of the number of clusters is often not available. Thus, in order to detect the optimal number of clusters, an expensive fine-tuning process is necessary. Even more importantly for metabolomics applications, K-means clustering is sensitive to noise and outliers. Finally, K-means often converges at a local optimum thus not necessarily reaching a global optimum. In metabolomics literature K-means clustering is utilized only rarely. An example of K-means clustering of samples from NMR metabolomics spectra with multiple start points is provided by Du et al. (Du, 2005).

A much more popular method for sample clustering in metabolomics is the Self-Organizing Maps (SOM) approach. The SOM method belongs to a class of artificial neural networks (Kohonen, 1982), which are capable of projecting high-dimensional input data on a two-dimensional map utilizing a single-layered artificial neural network. The data objects are located at the input side of the network and the output neurons are organized as a two dimensional grids. Each neuron is associated with a weight known as a reference vector. The weight vectors of neurons are randomly initialized. Each data object acts as a learning example directing the movement of the weight vectors towards the denser areas of the input vector space. Cluster optimization is performed by having neurons compete for data objects. The neuron whose weight vector is closest to the current object becomes the winning unit. Then the weight vector of the best-matching neuron and its set of neighbours move towards the current object. While the training process proceeds, the adjustment of weight vectors is diminished. When the training is complete, the weight vectors trained to fit the distributions of the input dataset and clusters are identified by mapping all data objects to the output neurons. The projection is topology preserving, meaning that input patterns that are located geometrically close to each other in the high-dimensional space will be mapped to close neurons on the resulting feature map. The map is an arrangement of nodes on a grid, where each node represents initially a metabolic pattern with arbitrary records for each metabolite. During an unsupervised training procedure, each metabolic pattern of the input data is connected to a specific node, which shares the highest similarity to it. Afterwards, this specific node adjusts itself to the assigned pattern. Furthermore, it adjusts the patterns of its neighbouring nodes gradually to its own, whereas its influence attenuates with the distance to its neighbours. This process of self-organization is done for several training cycles, resulting in a map that is able to locate any metabolic pattern of the input data with high reliability in its corresponding area on the map. The major advantage of SOM clustering is in cases with large numbers of groups and it has been shown that for the small number of clusters the result of SOM clustering is similar to the result of much simpler K-means clustering (Ultsch, 1999) although the SOM approach is more robust to noise in the data (Jiang, 2004). However, even in these cases map presentation provided by SOM can provide a better visualization of results and approach to connect resulting sample groups with other information available about the samples. Like other conventional clustering algorithms, SOM has its own pitfalls. In order to perform clustering, users have to predefine the initial number of the grids and the topology of the output neurons. The clustering results are closely related to the parameters such as the learning rate and the topology of the neurons. SOM can only reach a local optimum if the initial weights are not chosen properly (Jain, 1999). In the case of processing a large data, SOM is prone to problems when handling the data abundant in irrelevant and invariant features (Jiang, 2004) as those data can dominate majority of clusters. As a result, most of the meaningful patterns might be lost.

Examples of a very interesting application of SOM clustering are provided by the group of Ala-Korpela (Makinen, 2008; Tukiainen, 2008; Suna, 2007) where they have developed a new application of SOM with an ability to relate SOM results with other subject information. It should be kept in mind that additional subject information is only used for visualization and not in the calculations and thus SOM is a true unsupervised analysis method. This method has been used thus far primarily for clustering of binned spectral data with applications in the analysis of the significance of serum metabolic profiles in the development of Alzheimer's disease (Tukiainen, 2008), in the analysis of metabolic profiles in diabetes and their relation to standard clinical measures (Makinen, 2009). SOM analysis is even better positioned for the analysis of quantitative metabolite data as was described in Soininen et al. (Soininen, 2009). Although the majority of applications of SOM in metabolomics are coming from one group, SOM is becoming an increasingly popular method with other groups as well. An example is the use of SOM for sample clustering based on all metabolites measured as well as subset of most differentially present metabolites in the analysis of recombinant *Aspergillus nidulans* (Kouskoumvekaki, 2008).

The majority of clustering analysis in metabolomics was thus far performed using crisp clustering methods. In fact, there were in metabolomics, to the best of our knowledge, only two published applications of only the basic fuzzy K-methods. One by Li and co-workers (Li, 2009) applied to MS data and the other from our group (Cuperlovic-Culf, 2009) applied to NMR

data. The fuzzy approach allows features, in this case samples, to belong to more than one group, cluster. This allows a determination of subtypes for samples that belong to major groups and within those groups to subgroups. Fuzzy clustering also allows better assignment of samples that can be divided differently based on different characteristics as is often the case in biological samples. An example of the application of fuzzy K-means was show by Cuperlovic-Culf and co-workers (Cuperlovic-Culf, 2009) where fuzzy K means analysis of NMR measurements of breast cell lines allowed separation of cancer and normal cell lines as well as subtypes of cancer cell lines. Crisp clustering and PCA on the other hand were able to divide samples in this dataset only by major groups of cancer and normal. Fuzzy clustering provides additional information to, for example PCA analysis, due to the optimization of clusters as well as the fuzziness option. In general, biological samples are not strictly divisible into strongly crisp groups - biological phenotypes are better defined as fuzzy – *i.e.* belonging to one group based on some measure and to another group based on other set of characteristics. Thus fuzzy clustering methods need to be further tested as it warrants a larger place in metabolomics.

Analysis of Metabolites

The clustering of features is a major method of analysis in transcriptomics. In these applications the logic is commonly referred to as "guilt-by-association", *i.e.* genes whose expression measurements co-cluster are likely involved in similar processes. Similar reasoning does not directly apply to metabolomic data due mainly to the fact that metabolite molecules are not necessarily independent – the most closely related metabolites are often related through chemical conversion processes, *i.e.* members of the same metabolic pathway are likely connected through chemical conversion. In addition, obtaining meaningful results from metabolite clustering is difficult due to limited metabolite coverage and large range of concentration changes. Biological systems are composed of thousands of metabolites with current estimates being - yeast 1168 (Herrgard, 2008), plant kingdom 200,000 (Fiehn, 2002), mammals > 6500 (Wishart, 2009) and at the same time current analytical methods can only measure at the most 2,000 metabolites. Further, similarly to the genes, metabolites are involved in multiple processes making it difficult to draw conclusions directly from only clustering in general and crisp clustering in particular.

An additional problem in metabolite clustering is the difficulty in metabolite quantification from the obtained data. If only qualitative spectral data is available, as is often the case, data clustering of metabolite concentrations is not possible. However, there are several published examples of interesting applications of different types of feature correlation analysis in qualitative metabolic data. Furthermore, with an increased availability of quantitative metabolic data there is an increased interest in metabolite clustering either on its own or in combination with other omics data analysis. The unsupervised analysis of metabolites across different samples or in time provides a valuable tool for the analysis of networks and description of biological systems. Quantitative metabolic data contributes valuable information about the actually biological processes and is thus crucial in the description of activated pathways in different phenotypes.

In terms of unsupervised analysis of metabolites the methods can be broadly divided into clustering methods used for metabolite or spectral peaks grouping and network development methods. In clustering methods various tools, for example the ones outlined above, are used to determine groups of features, *i.e.* metabolites that have similar behaviour. In the network development methods various similarity analysis tools are used to determine proximity between pairs of features, *i.e.* metabolites. The pair-wise associations are then utilized to develop networks

of connected features. In the following we will continue to focus on unsupervised, clustering methods. Due to space constraints the exploration of network development methods will not be included in this work.

Metabolite Clustering Methods

In metabolomics applications the correct structural assignment of spectroscopic data is paramount to obtaining molecular level biological information. However, although for an increasing number of metabolites NMR and MS data are becoming available in databases (Wishart, 2009), the direct assignment and quantification of metabolites from the spectra is still difficult and not readily available for the general case. The problems include large signal overlap in complex mixtures particularly in NMR spectra; peak position changes under different pH, solvent and temperature conditions; complexity of spectra in both MS and NMR experiments; multiple derivatization of products and spectrometer drifting in MS, *etc*. A recent highly detailed review dealing with many issues in metabolomics, including current developments in terms of spectral assignment and quantification, has been provided by Dunn and co-workers (Dunn, 2010).

In NMR spectra molecules in general have multiple peaks. This makes NMR analysis highly specific in the case of one molecule. However, in crowded spectra of mixtures it could present problems. At the same time multiple peaks for one compound are correlated across samples and this feature was explored as a property useful for assignment by group of Nicholson with a method for statistical correlation and analysis of peaks - STOCSY (Cloarec, 2005). In STOCSY and related methods correlation coefficients are calculated between all spectral intensities across a set of complex mixture spectra. In this approach a high statistical correlation between intensities at two chemical shift values would imply that the two signals either derive from the same molecule or that there is some external correlation between molecules measured at the two peaks. In this way the STOCSY approach provides a statistical signal separation complementary to physical or multidimensional experiment spectral separation. STOCSY was utilized for structural assignment in many applications and many publications. Thus, in just one issue of Analytical Chemistry (the ACS Journal) STOCSY applications range from deconvolution of overlapping chromatographic peaks in LC-NM (Cloarec, 2007), over delineation of drug metabolism in epidemiological studies (Smith, 2007) to separation or different molecular signatures in diffusion-edited spectroscopy (Holmes, 2007). Although the STOCSY method is a very interested approach for the general case where many related measurements are available for specific cases it is possible to develop faster and more informative metabolite assignment and quantification tools based on regression calculations from standard measurements. An example of this approach was championed by the group of Ala-Korpela for metabolite quantification specifically for serum samples (Soininen, 2009). This method relies on the fact that in NMR measurements of serum there is a limited number of well defined metabolites and lipoproteins and thus their quantification from the spectra can be obtained very accurately and quickly from comparison with standards. MS-based quantification of a large number of metabolites is not trivial either. The commonly used electrospray ionization (ESI) technique is prone to interference and ion suppression. For analysis of a small number of metabolites stable isotope-labelled (SIL) analogues are often used as the internal standards to overcome the matrix and ion suppression effects. However, the number of available SIL standards is very limited. Some efforts are being put into developing a differential isotope labelling (DIL) method which uses a chemical reaction to introduce an isotope tag to the analyte in one sample and another mass-different isotope tag to the same analyte in another, reference, sample, followed

by mixing the two labeled samples for mass spectrometric analysis. This technique requires specific chemistry for different groups of molecules and thus further development of chemistry techniques is needed (Guo, 2009). In MS analysis, metabolite quantification depends critically on the existence of searchable spectral databases as well as on having labelled standards for quantification. The collection of metabolite standards and tools for analysis are being contributed by several groups most notably by group of Fiehn (fiehnlab.ucdavis.edu) as well as together with NMR data at the Human Metabolome Database (Wishart, 2009). In addition, MS experimentation is highly sensitive to experimental procedures and thus requires extensive sample preprocessing and regular application of controls. Recommended practices have recently been outlined by Brown et al. (Brown, 2009 and references therein) Due to issues in both NMR and MS metabolite assignment, quantitative metabolic data is still not generally available in metabolomics with only a handful of examples have been published (see below). Thus, only a few unsupervised analysis methods have been explored including hierarchical clustering (HCL), K-means, and Self-organized maps (SOM) methods.

HCL can be applied as a one- or two-way clustering method. In analysis of qualitative metabolic data one-way clustering is, in the large majority of cases, the only sensible approach. However, quantitative metabolic two-way clustering provides valuable insight in terms of the relation between groups of metabolites and sample types and thus has been preferred in the literature. Two-way HCL has been utilized for the analysis of MS data by Chu et al (Chu, 2006). In this work the authors used GC-MS measurements of urine samples from neonates with and without asphyxia. Quantitative measurements of urinary organic acids were used for hierarchical clustering of samples and metabolites showing clear separation of asphyxiated and normal neonates. The authors used visualization provided by HCL to determine the major groups of metabolites indicative of the conditions under study. Although supervised approaches would be more appropriate for the determination of major features, HCL analysis still lead to a visually clear clustering and indicated a clear separation between sample groups. HCL was also used for arranging the metabolites on the basis of their relative levels across samples in a highly publicized study presented by Sreekumar and co workers (Sreekumar, 2009). Once again, the HCL visual presentation, *i.e.* a heat map, rather than one of many supervised approaches, was used for feature selection. For the analysis of similarities between metabolites, HCL analysis of the results of ANOVA was also explored (Altmaier, 2008). The approach of ANOVA/HCL allowed determination of groups of metabolites that exhibit similar response profiles to disease or drug treatment.

K-Means clustering is highly affected by noise in the data and thus it is rarely used in metabolomics clustering. An attempt has been made by a group headed by Age Smilde to use a resampling technique that can deal with noise and in this way improve the accuracy of K-means clustering (Hageman, 2006). This approach resulted in the Bagged K-Means clustering method that has been shown by the authors to be much less sensitive to noise than the original K-means method. In the original publication, Bagged K-means was used for metabolite clustering from quantitative data. However, this method might be even more useful in the sample clustering from noisy spectral, qualitative data.

SOM clustering has been used by several groups for metabolite analysis. In the majority of cases the authors developed alternative SOM approaches and thus the majority of applications present their own software. An example of utilization as well as the tool is provided by Meinicke et al. (Meinicke, 2008). Meinicke and co-workers presented a 1-dimensional SOM method for metabolite-based clustering and visualization of marker candidates. 1D SOM assigns metabolites to groups. These groups of features are used for the determination of meaningful groups of markers. The 1D SOM provides a visualization of the variation of intensity profiles along the array of prototypes. Another tool developed for SOM analysis in metabolomics, called eSOMet, has been contributed by Haddad and co-workers (Haddad, 2009). eSOMet is an application of emergent SOM (eSOM, Ultsch, 1999). SOM clustering was used for the analysis of time-resolved metabolomics data in the analysis of rice foliage (Sato, 2008). In this example, SOM analysis revealed the synchronous dynamics among metabolic modules and elucidated the underlying biochemical functions. An application of SOM initially developed for gene expression analysis, called Gene Expression Dynamics Inspector (GEDI), was used for metabolites analysis by Patterson and co-workers (Patterson, 2008). GEDI presents a map of features, *i.e.* genes or metabolites, grouped based on their behaviour presented in sample static or longitudinal measurements. GEDI groups metabolites while preserving information about the samples, *i.e.* it is effectively providing a map, or signature, for metabolites in the sample. The work of Patterson *et al.* presented an application of GEDI for the analysis of metabolic changes in cell cultures following exposure to different levels of radiation exposures.

UNSUPERVISED METHODS TESTING AND COMPARISON

The goal in this section is to show the benefits and limitations as well as differences in results obtained from different unsupervised analysis tools currently utilized in metabolomics data analysis. All the methods for unsupervised analysis of either samples or metabolites described above will be tested using spectral, *i.e.* qualitative as well as corresponding quantitative metabolite data. For method testing we have developed a large dataset obtained from different mixtures of experimental NMR measurements of 13 metabolites at five different groups of concentrations. A random component is added to concentrations for each metabolite in order to simulate variations in metabolite concentrations observed in biological samples. Assuming that there is no chemical interaction between molecules in the mixture, the resulting NMR spectrum of a mixture is a direct sum of spectra from the components. The Human Metabolomics DataBase (HMDB, Wishart, 2009) contains information about many individual metabolites including their NMR spectra. We have selected 13 water soluble, *i.e.* hydrophilic metabolites (Table 2 for list and concentrations in five groups of samples). These 13 metabolites were consistently observable in standard 1D ^{1}H NMR in several publications dealing with cell culture metabolomics (Duarte, 2009; Griffin, 2002; Yang, 2007; Gotschalk, 2008; Tiziani, 2009).

Free induction decay (FID) measurements for those compounds obtained at 600MHz at pH 7, dissolved in D_2O at different concentrations were obtained from Human Metabolic Data Bank (HMDB, http://www.hmdb.ca/). All the spectra were processed in the same way, with neither apodization nor spectral filling followed by Fou-

rier transform (using MNova software). Spectra for individual molecules were imported into Matlab. Spectra were scaled in order to represent the concentration of the metabolite in the mixture as well as the number of hydrogen's in the molecules. Scaling was performed for the peak heights rather than peak areas, however in these spectra representing small molecules with very narrow peaks this is a good approximation. Spectra for the 13 compounds after scaling are provided in Figure 2.

In order to simulate different biological situations we have created 2,000 combinations of spectra with 5 different groups of concentrations for 13 compounds with 400 subjects in each group obtained by adding a random value (representing the concentration fluctuations in biological samples) to each concentration of the compound. The final spectra of mixtures were obtained by multiplying concentrations for each compound with each data point in the spectrum. The obtained spectra were combined, *i.e.* summed, leading to 2,000 combination spectra (here referred to as subjects). For each of these subjects we of course had also the exact concentration information for

Table 2. Metabolites used for the creation of the model and their concentrations in five groups of samples

#	Metabolite	Group I conc. (mM)	Group II conc. (mM)	Group III conc. (mM)	Group IV conc. (mM)	Group V conc. (mM)
1	Choline	230	115	172.5	172.5	172.5
2	Glutathione	49	49	49	73.5	98
3	Alanine	50	50	50	75	50
4	Glutamic Acid	50	50	75	50	75
5	Glutamine	50	50	50	50	50
6	Leucine	45	45	45	45	90
7	Valine	37.5	37.5	50	50	50
8	Asparagine	31.5	31.5	42	42	42
9	Isoleucine	26.25	26.25	35	35	35
10	Lactic Acid	37.5	37.5	50	50	50
11	Proline	25.5	21.25	21.25	25.5	25.5
12	Succinic Acid	37.5	37.5	50	50	50
13	Taurine	71.46	142.92	107.19	71.46	142.92

Figure 2. ¹H 1D NMR spectra for 13 metabolites included in the formation of analysed dataset. All spectra are obtained as FID's from HMDB.

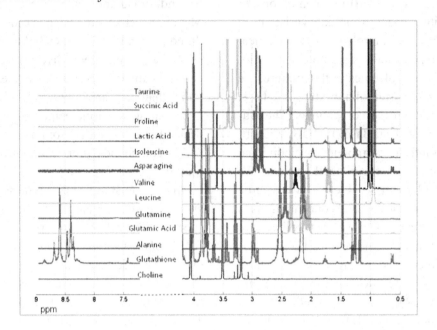

metabolites thus the corresponding quantified metabolic data. The spectra where further binned with different bin sizes and analyzed using different methodologies. Quantified metabolic data were also analyzed using the complete set and also using sets with some metabolic measurements missing.

The metabolite concentrations for 5 groups are provided in Table 2. The concentration changes in 2,000 subjects following the addition of a random concentration alteration value as well as average NMR spectrum for each group are shown in Figure 3.

These qualitative and quantitative data is used for the presentation of results obtained with different unsupervised analysis methods. The analysis is performed on qualitative, spectral data with different bin sizes as well as quantitative metabolomics data with information about all the metabolites as well as some of the metabolites missing in quantification as would likely be the case in the majority of metabolite quantification efforts.

Data Visualization

PCA is an appropriate overview tool used for initial analysis of the outliers, groups and trends in the data. PCA is not however a classification method and thus, although it can provide some information about the sample types it does not lead to separation of clusters of data. In addition, as it is focusing only on the major differences in the data it can lead to loss of information. Results of PCA analysis of samples from our dataset are presented in Figure 4. Figure 4A shows the principal components (PC) 1 to 3 for spectral data with small bins (0.0018ppm); Figure 4B shows PC1, PC2 and PC3 for spectral data with 1000 times larger bins (0.1838ppm); Figure 4C shows the results of PCA for quantitative metabolite data for all 13 observed metabolites and Figure 4D shows PCA for 11 out of 13 metabolites included.

PCA provides a clear separation of Group 5 (Figure 3) in all the datasets tested and separation of Groups 3 and 4, 5 (Figure 3) in the analysis of data arrangement A and C. In addition PCA pro-

Figure 3. Spectra and metabolite concentrations for five groups of samples. Spectra represent average values for 200 samples included in each group. Metabolite concentrations are represented as a heath map for each of 200 samples divided into five groups. Here as well as in all the following figures and text groups are assigned with Roman numerals (I-V).

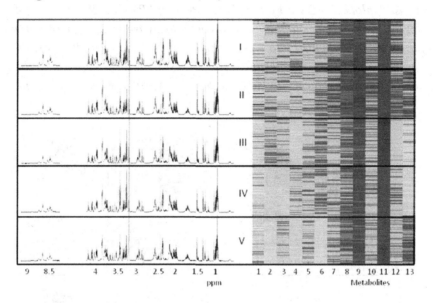

vided similar data separation with the analysis of spectral and quantitative data. However PCA was unable to clearly separate the other groups - 1 and 2 as the differences between these two groups are less prominent then between other groups.

PCA is always recommended as a starting point for analyzing multivariate data and will rapidly provide an overview of the information concealed in the data. However, in many metabolomics papers the PCA method is the only tool applied. Additional information can often be extracted by using more advanced multivariate methods and thus other methods should generally be used in addition to PCA (Trygg, 2007). In a typical PCA analysis, data separation is performed based on the first two or three principal components, *i.e.* major sources of variance in the data. If the variance in the data cannot be adequately included in a few PC's, PCA can result in inaccurate data separation (as can be seen for groups 1 and 2 in the dataset). In addition if there is one dominant source of separation in the data, PCA will show

data division only based on this feature and will ignore other differences in the data.

Data Clustering

The clustering process in general consists of assembling features (samples or entities) in restricted classes so that patterns within one class are less dispersed than between classes. Classes of entities should be homogeneous and, ideally, well separated. In the following we will not present any new tools. Rather our goal is to present differences in results that are obtained from using different contemporary methods. The analysis tools will be applied to both spectral and quantitative data whenever possible.

K-means is a very straightforward, commonly used partitional clustering method. The advantage of K-means clustering is that it quickly assigns data to a predefined number of clusters with the possibility for many different measures of distances between features and different starting and finishing points of optimization. Thus, it was possible

Figure 4. PCA analysis of synthetic metabolomics data. Five groups of samples are labelled in different colours. Data is log scaled prior to analysis. (A) PCA of spectral data with small bin size (0.0018ppm). Boxes are (clockwise) the average spectrum used; plot of PC2 v.s. PC1; PC1 v.s. PC3 and PC2 v.s. PC3; (B) PCA of spectral data with 1000 times larger bin sizes (0.1838ppm). Boxes are (clockwise) the average spectrum used; plot of PC2 v.s. PC1; PC1 v.s. PC3 and PC2 v.s. PC3; (C) PCA of quantitative metabolite data for all 13 observed metabolites. Boxes are (clockwise) values for 13 metabolites included in the analysis for all subjects divided into 5 groups; plot of PC2 v.s. PC1; PC1 v.s. PC3 and PC2 v.s. PC3; (D) PCA for 11 out of 13 metabolites included. Boxes are (clockwise) values for 11 metabolites included in the analysis for all subjects divided into 5 groups; plot of PC2 v.s. PC1; PC1 v.s. PC3 and PC2 v.s. PC3.

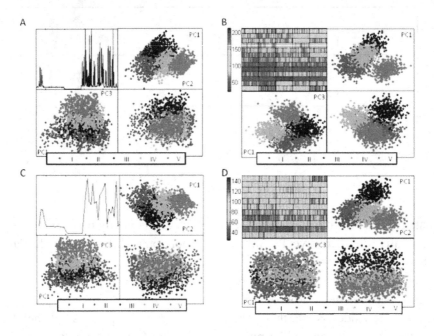

obtain very quickly K-means derived clusters for features from spectral as well as metabolic data (Figure 5). However K-means method is highly sensitive to noise and thus, although it can be used for clustering of very large feature space, as is the case with spectral data, it gives highly suboptimal clustering results (Figure 5A,B). Clustering accuracy is improved for metabolic data with very clear separation of group 2 and 5 as well as good separation of other groups (Figure 5C,D).

Although the K-means method in its basic form does not provide a satisfactory clustering for basic metabolomics data presented here several extensions of this method have been introduced in order to reduce the sensitivity to noise

as well as rigidness of crisp clustering. The *Bagged K-Means* method introduced by a highly prolific Biosystems Data Analysis group at University of Amsterdam intends to deal with noisy metabolomics data through bootstrap aggregation (bagging) resampling. Originally the method was developed for clustering metabolites but the same approach can also be used for sample clustering. The clustering result in the case of bagged K-means shows a heat map of a histogram measuring how often a feature was clustered in each group in different resampling steps. Histograms for the dataset analyzed here with clustering results shown for the complete spectral dataset with small and large bin sizes as well as for the corresponding quan-

Figure 5. Result of K-means clustering of studied dataset. Red lines represent sample cluster belonging, blue represents that the same does not belong to the cluster. Plot is divided by clusters (1-5) and sample groups (I-V). (A) K-Means clustering for spectral data with small bin size (0.0018ppm); (B) K-Means clustering for spectral data with larger bin sizes (0.1838ppm); (C) K-Means clustering for quantitative metabolite data for all 13 observed metabolites; (D) K-Means clustering for 11 out of 13 metabolites included.

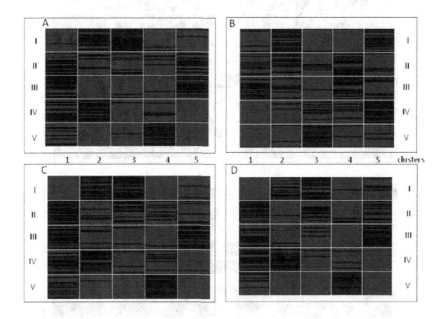

titative metabolic data with all metabolites and with information for 2 metabolites missing.

It is clear from Figure 6 that for quantified data the bagged K-means method provides a better result than standard K-means in all cases. For the complete set of quantitative metabolic data (Figure 6C) bagged K-means methods provided an excellent classification result unlike standard K-means or PCA. For a large spectral data set (small bin sizes) there is clear separation of sample Groups 1 and 5 (defined in Figure 3) but hard to distinguish clusters for other sample groups. The problem in this case could possibly be resolved with a larger number of resampling steps but the dataset size in this case makes this impossible. Removal of information by either increasing the bin size or by the removal of information for two metabolites leads to loss of accuracy in sample separation.

Self-Organizing Maps

Self-Organizing Maps (SOM) application specifically developed for sample clustering in metabolomics (Makinen, 2008) is utilized here as an example of several very interesting and freely available SOM applications. The method of Makinen and co-workers was developed for clustering of samples based on either the quantitative metabolics data or spectral data with large bin sizes, *i.e.* data sets with a relatively small number of features for each sample. Thus, it was not possible to use this method for the analysis of large spectral data. However this approach gave excellent separation of subjects by groups for the other three data presentations. Figure 7 shows the SOM analysis results labelled for 5 groups of samples. The colour of areas in the map represent the percentage of subjects in a group

Figure 6. Heat-map representation of the results of Bagged K-means clustering. (A) Histogram measure for spectral data with small bin size (0.0018ppm); (B) Histogram measure for spectral data with larger bin sizes (0.1838ppm); (C) Histogram measure for quantitative metabolite data for all 13 observed metabolites; (D) Histogram measure for 11 out of 13 metabolites included.

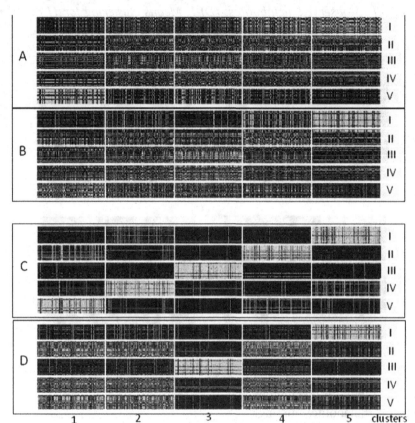

relative to the total number of subjects assigned to the area with dark red colour representing a large percentage (~100%) and the dark blue representing a low percentage (~0%) of subjects from the studied group.

Figure 7 clearly shows that SOM provides excellent clustering results when using quantified metabolic data as well as good sample separation for binned spectral data. Similarly to the other methods when information about metabolites 1 and 13 is removed the information is insufficient to separate groups 1 and 2. However, SOM does separate clearly other groups of subjects even with data for these two metabolites missing. The presentation approach in SOM allows projection of other information on the maps providing "geographical" presentation of various feature properties in relation to characteristics used for data clustering. In this way the clusters of subjects determined from SOM can be explored in combination with other information about the subjects. For the analysis of metabolites the information about pathways or results of analysis from other methodologies can also be overlaid. In terms of crisp clutering tools, *i.e.* when ambiguity in the clustering is not expected SOM provides excellent cluster quality as well as a good presentation tool, particularly for quantitative metabolic data. SOM is not, however, an optimal method for large spectral data and for the investigation of co-

Figure 7. Feature separation determined by SOM analysis. Each map represents positions of samples for one group. (A) Histogram measure for spectral data with larger bin sizes (0.1838ppm); (B) Histogram measure for quantitative metabolite data for all 13 observed metabolites; (C) Histogram measure for 11 out of 13 metabolites included.

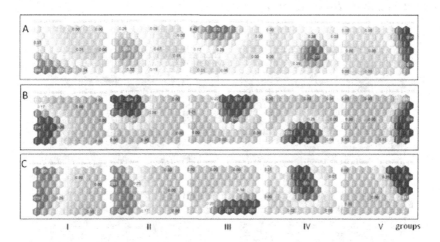

clustering of features. In addition to technical issues, SOM is also prone to problems when handling the data abundant in irrelevant and invariant data (Jiang, 2004). These data can dominate the majority of clusters and thus SOM should ideally be used only for quantitative metabolic data.

Fuzzy Clustering

Fuzzy Clustering provides one-to-many mapping where a single feature belongs to multiple clusters with a certain degree of membership. The memberships can further be used to discover more sophisticated relations between the data and its disclosed clusters (Xu, 2005). The fuzzy approach is more desirable in situations where a majority of features, such as metabolites, participate in different networks and are governed by a variety of regulatory mechanisms or in the case of sample clustering for samples that can be assigned to different groups depending on the observed characteristics. Fuzzy clustering is also robust to the high level of noise often present in omics data.

The result of fuzzy clustering calculation is the matrix of membership degrees that describe the level of similarity between each feature and each cluster centroid. F-KM clustering is the simplest fuzzy clustering methods derived for the K-means approach. With this approach each point can possibly have significant belonging to multiple clusters; to only one cluster and even to no cluster (if all membership values for the point are equal to 1/number of clusters) thus preventing overfitting. The F-KM algorithm used here is freely available as a Matlab routine from Matlab Central.

The result of F-KM analysis of 4 different groups of data including spectral data with the small bin size as well as with the large bin size and the quantitative metabolic data with all the metabolites included and with 2 metabolites missing are shown in Figure 8. F-KM clustering is highly efficient and thus it was possible to cluster subjects even with a large number of features. Furthermore, similarly to standard K-means it is possible to choose different distance matrix calculation methods – in this case we have used Euclidian distances but other measures can be tested for different cases.

Figure 8. Heat map representation of the membership values obtained from F-KM analysis. Plot is divided by clusters (1-5) and sample groups (I-V). (A) Membership values for spectral data with small bin size (0.0018ppm); (B) Membership values for spectral data with larger bin sizes (0.1838ppm); (C) Membership values for quantitative metabolite data for all 13 observed metabolites; (D) Membership values for 11 out of 13 metabolites included.

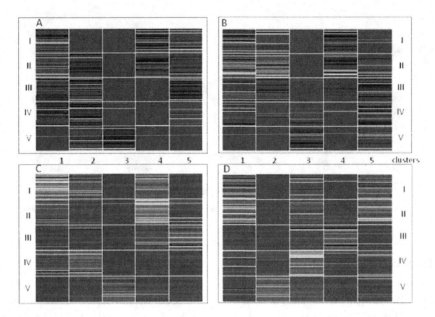

The results of F-KM can be viewed on two levels. On the first level it is important to investigate cluster belonging for subjects based on the top membership value. This result provides information about the most significant cluster assignment. The second level of investigation is the analysis of the other memberships for each subject. This information can lead to discoveries of additional co-clustering partners. It is clear from Figure 8 that F-KM provides an excellent method for subject clustering for either qualitative or quantitative data. F-KM was able to very quickly provide clustering results for subjects from large size spectral data as well as adequate clustering based on large bin size data. F-KM clustering of the quantitative metabolic data for all 13 metabolites provides perfect separation of all 5 groups. Similarly to the other methods removal of metabolites 1 and 13 lead to the loss of separation for groups I and II. The graphical presentation of the results of F-KM is not quite as pleasing as

those presented by SOM. In Figure 8 we show the membership values for each subject and for each cluster. Although this presentation clearly indicates the co-clustering of subjects improvement to the presentation approach of results obtained by F-KM is needed. Still, the F-KM methodology provided as good a sample separation based on the top membership value as SOM and bagged-K-means for quantified metabolite data and better results for complete spectral data. In addition, fuzzification of results can be utilized for further investigation of data properties either for sample or for metabolite classification.

FUTURE RESEARCH DIRECTIONS AND CONCLUSION

Algorithms do not drive metabolomics investigation; however the objectives of these investigations can only be achieved by utilizing an appropriate data treatment and analysis strategy at every step. Unfortunately, a perfect method for unsupervised analysis does not exist. However, many methods have been developed for various applications with new and improved tools regularly presented in the literature. Thus, it is crucial to explore different algorithms for each application rather than relying completely on conclusions drawn from only one methodology. In metabolomics, PCA is still by far the most popular unsupervised method with only a few true clustering tools even tested. The analysis on the synthetic data presented in this work shows that clustering tools can provide additional information to PCA and should thus become regularly exploited part of metabolomics investigations. PCA is fast and informative for the analysis of qualitative, spectral data however the analysis using for example bagged K-means, SOM or fuzzy K-means presented here shows that these methods can lead to better feature clustering with both spectral data and particularly with quantitative metabolic data. Currently, several groups are working of obtaining as large as possible quantitative metabolic datasets. For these types of data unsupervised tools such as SOM, bagged K-means and fuzzy K-means should be preferred as they provide much more information and much more accurate feature grouping then PCA.

The quality of the final result depends on the data characteristics and thus it is not possible to draw conclusions about the best method for a general case. At the same time each of the three methods showing the best results here, *i.e.* SOM, bagged K-means and F-KM provide some unique advantage and some additional information and should be explored in different metabolomics applications. Furthermore, it is very important to understand the limitations of unsupervised methods and to use them only for feature clustering and grouping and to perform the feature selection and classification with more appropriate supervised tools. In the future applications of metabolomics it will be important to take advantage of methods shown here as well as many other methods that have been developed for other applications and not to rely exclusively on one methodology. Only by utilization of the most appropriate unsupervised analysis tools for each application of metabolomics will it be possible to transform metabolomics into truly the "greatest omics of them all" (Ryan, 2006).

ACKNOWLEDGMENT

Author would like to thank Dr.'s A. Smilde, G. Zwanenburg and J. Hageman for providing me with the Matlab scripts for running Bagged K-means method. I would also like to thank Dr. A. Culf for carefully reviewing the manuscript.

REFERENCES

Altmaier, E., Ramsay, S. L., & Graber, A. (2008). Bioinformatics analysis of targeted metabolomics – uncovering old and new tales of diabetic mice under medication. *Endocrinology*, *149*, 3478–3489. doi:10.1210/en.2007-1747

Assfalg, M., Bertini, I., & Colangiuli, D. (2008). Evidence of different metabolic phenotypes in humans. *Proceedings of the National Academy of Sciences of the United States of America*, *105*, 1420–1424. doi:10.1073/pnas.0705685105

Beckoners, O. (2007). Metabolic profiling, metabolomic and metabonomic procedures for NMR spectroscopy of urine, plasma, serum and tissue extracts. *Nature Protocols*, *2*, 2692–2703. doi:10.1038/nprot.2007.376

Beckonert, O., Bollard, M. E., & Ebbels, T. M. D. (2003). NMR-based metabonomic toxicity classification: hierarchical cluster analysis and k-nearest neighbor approaches. *Analytica Chimica Acta*, *490*, 3–15. doi:10.1016/S0003-2670(03)00060-6

Beebe, K., Pell, R. J., & Seasholtz, M. B. (1998). *Chemometrics: A practical guide*. New York: John Wiley & Sons.

Belacel, N., Wang, C., & Cuperlovic-Culf, M. (2010). *"Clustering". Invited book chapter in Statistical Bioinformatics.* New York: John Wiley & Sons.

Bictash, M., Ebbels, T. M., Chan, Q., Loo, R. L., & Yap, I. K. S. (2009). Opening up the "Black Box": Metabolic phenotyping and metabolomie-wide association studies in epidemiology. *Journal of Clinical Epidemiology, 63,* 970–979. doi:10.1016/j.jclinepi.2009.10.001

Brown, M., Dunn, W. B., & Dobson, P. (2009). Mass spectrometry tools and metabolite-specific databases for molecular identification in metabolomics. *Analyst (London), 134,* 1322–1332. doi:10.1039/b901179j

Bylesjo, M., Rantalainen, M., & Cloarec, O. (2006). OPLS discriminant analysis combining the strength of PSL-DA and SIMCA classification. *Journal of Chemometrics, 20,* 341–351. doi:10.1002/cem.1006

Cavill, R., Keun, H. C., & Holmes, E. (2009). Genetic algorithms for simultaneous variable and sample selection in metabolomics. *Bioinformatics (Oxford, England), 25,* 112–118. doi:10.1093/bioinformatics/btn586

Chu, C. Y., Xiao, X., & Zhou, X. G. (2006). Metabolomics and bioinformatic analysis in asphyxiated neonates. *Clinical Biochemistry, 39,* 203–209. doi:10.1016/j.clinbiochem.2006.01.006

Clayton, T. A., Lindon, J. C., & Cloarec, O. (2006). Pharmaco-metabonomic phenotyping and personalized drug treatment. *Nature, 440,* 1073–1077. doi:10.1038/nature04648

Cloarec, O., Campbell, A., & Tseng, L. H. (2007). Virtual chromatographic enhancement in clyoflow LC-NM experiment via statistical total correlation spectroscopy. *Analytical Chemistry, 79,* 5682–5689. doi:10.1021/ac061928y

Cloarec, O., Dumas, M., & Craig, A. (2005). Statistical total correlation spectroscopy: an exploratory approach for latent biomarker identification from metabolic 1H NMR data sets. *Analytical Chemistry, 77,* 1282–1289. doi:10.1021/ac048630x

Cuperlovic-Culf, M., Belacel, N., & Culf, A. (2009). NMR metabolomic analysis of samples using fuzzy K-means clustering. *Magnetic Resonance in Chemistry, 47,* S96–S104. doi:10.1002/mrc.2502

Cuperlovic-Culf, M., Chute, I., & Barnett, D. (2010). Cell culture metabolomics. *Drug Discovery Today, 15,* 610–621. doi:10.1016/j.drudis.2010.06.012

Damian, D., Oresic, M., & Verheij, E. (2007). Applications of a new subspace clustering algorithm (COSA) in medical systems biology. *Metabolomics, 3,* 69–77. doi:10.1007/s11306-006-0045-z

Denkert, C., Budczies, J., & Kind, T. (2006). Mass spectrometry-based metabolic profiling reveals different metabolite patterns in invasive ovarian carcinomas and ovarian borderline tumors. *Cancer Research, 66,* 10795–10804. doi:10.1158/0008-5472.CAN-06-0755

Denkert, C., Budczies, J., & Weichert, W. (2008). Metabolite profiling of human colon carcinoma – deregulation of TCA cycle and amino acid turnover. *Molecular Cancer, 7,* 72–87. doi:10.1186/1476-4598-7-72

Dr, S., Sajda, P., Stoyanova, R., et al. (2005). *Recovery of metabolomics spectral sources using non-negative matrix factorization.* Proc 2005 IEEE.

Duarte, I. F., Marques, J., & Ladeirinha, A. F. (2009). Analytical approaches toward successful human cell metabolome studies by NMR spectroscopy. *Analytical Chemistry, 81,* 5023–5032. doi:10.1021/ac900545q

Dunn, W. B., Broadhurst, D. I., & Atherton, H. J. (2010). Systems levels studies of mammalian metabolomes: the roles of mass spectrometry and nuclear magnetic resonance spectroscopy. *Chemical Society Reviews.* doi:.doi:10.1039/b906712b

Fiehn, O. (2001). Combining genomics, metabolome analysis, and biochemical modelling to understand metabolic networks. *Comparative and Functional Genomics, 2,* 155–168. doi:10.1002/cfg.82

Fiehn, O. (2002). Metabolomics – the link between genotypes and phenotypes. *Plant Molecular Biology, 48,* 155–171. doi:10.1023/A:1013713905833

Fiehn, O., Kopka, J., & Dormann, P. (2000). Metabolite profiling for plant functional genomics. *Nature Biotechnology, 18,* 1157–1161. doi:10.1038/81137

Friedman, J. H., & Meulman, J. J. (2004). Clustering objects on subsets of attributes. *Journal of the Royal Statistical Society. Series B. Methodological, 66,* 1–25. doi:10.1111/j.1467-9868.2004.02059.x

Giskeødegård, G. F., Grinde, M. T., & Sitter, B. (2010). Multivariate modeling and prediction of breast cancer prognostic factors using MR metabolomics. *Journal of Proteome Research, 9,* 972–979. doi:10.1021/pr9008783

Goodacre, R., & Broadhurst, D. (2007). Proposed minumum reporting standards for data analysis in metabolomics. *Metabolomics, 3,* 231–241. doi:10.1007/s11306-007-0081-3

Gottschalk, M.; Ivanova, G.& Collins, D.M. et al. (2008). *Metabolomic studies of human lung carcinoma cell lines using in vitro 1H NMR of whole cells and cellular extracts.* NMR Biomed.

Griffin, J. L., Bollard, M., Nicholson, J. K., & Bhakoo, K. (2002). Spectral profiles of cultured neuronal and glial cells derived from HRMAS 1H NMR spectroscopy. *NMR in Biomedicine, 15,* 375–384. doi:10.1002/nbm.792

Guo, K., & Li, L. (2009). Differential 12C/13C-isitope dansylation labeling and fast liquid chromatography/MS for absolute and relative quantification of the metabolome. *Analytical Chemistry, 81,* 3919–3932. doi:10.1021/ac900166a

Haddad, I., Killer, K., Frimmersdorf, E., et al. (2009). An emergent self-organizing map based analysis pipeline for comparative metabolome studies. In *Silico Biol. 9,* 0014.

Hageman, J.A.; van den Berg, R.A.& Westerhuis, J.A. et al. (2009). *Genetic algorithm based two-mode clustering of metabolomics data.* Metabolomics

Hageman, J. A., van den Berg, R. A., & Westerhuis, J. A. (2006). Bagged K-means clustering of metabolome data. *Clinical Rev Anal Chem, 36,* 211–220. doi:10.1080/10408340600969916

Herrgard, M. J., Swainston, N., & Dobson, P. (2008). A consensus yeast metabolic network reconstruction obtained from a community approach to systems biology. *Nature Biotechnology, 26,* 1155–1160. doi:10.1038/nbt1492

Holmes, E., Loo, R. L., & Cloarec, O. (2007). Detection of urinary drug metabolite (xenometabolome) signatures in molecular epidemiology studies via statistical total correlation (NMR) spectroscopy. *Analytical Chemistry, 79,* 2629–2640. doi:10.1021/ac062305n

Holmes, E., Loo, R. L., & Stamler, J. (2008). Human metabolic phenotype diversity and its association with diet and blood pressure. *Nature, 453,* 396–401. doi:10.1038/nature06882

Huopaniemi, I., Suvitaival, T., & Nikkila, J. (2009). Two-way analysis of high-dimensional collinear data. *Data Mining and Knowledge Discovery, 19,* 261–276. doi:10.1007/s10618-009-0142-5

Jain, A. K., Murty, M. N., & Flynn, P. J. (1999). Data Clustering: A Review. *ACM Computing Surveys, 31*(3), 264–323. doi:10.1145/331499.331504

Jiang, D., Tang, C., & Zhang, A. (2004). Cluster Analysis for Gene Expression Data: A Survey. *IEEE Transactions on Knowledge and Data Engineering, 16*(11), 1370–1386. doi:10.1109/TKDE.2004.68

Kohonen, T. (1982). Self-organized formation of topologically correct feature maps. *Biological Cybernetics, 43*, 59–69. doi:10.1007/BF00337288

Kouskoumvekaki, I., Yang, Z., & Jonsdottir, S. O. (2008). Identification of biomarkers for genotyping Aspergilli using non-linear methods for clustering and classification. *BMC Bioinformatics, 9*, 59. doi:10.1186/1471-2105-9-59

Li, X., Lu, X., & Tian, J. (2009). Application of Fuzzy c-means clustering in data analysis of metabolomics. *Analytical Chemistry, 81*, 4468–4475. doi:10.1021/ac900353t

Lu, X., Bennet, B., & Mu, E. (2010). Metabolomic changes accompanying transformation and acquisition of metastatic potential in a syngeneic mouse mammary tumour model. *The Journal of Biological Chemistry, 285*, 9317–9321. doi:10.1074/jbc.C110.104448

Madsen, R., Lundstedt, T., & Trygg, J. (2010). Chemometrics in metabolomics – A review in human disease diagnosis. *Analytica Chimica Acta, 659*, 23–33. doi:10.1016/j.aca.2009.11.042

Mahner, M., & Kary, M. (1997, May 7). What exactly are genomes, genotypes and phenotypes? And what about phenomes? *Journal of Theoretical Biology, 186*(1), 55–63. doi:10.1006/jtbi.1996.0335

Mäkinen, V. P., Soininen, P., & Forsblom, C. (2008). 1H NMR metabonomics approach to the disease continuum of diabetic complications and premature death. *Molecular Systems Biology, 4*, 167. doi:10.1038/msb4100205

Meinicke, P., Lingner, T., & Kaever, A. (2008). Metabolite-based clustering and visualization of mass spectrometry data using one-dimensional self-organized maps. *Algorithms for Molecular Biology; AMB, 3*, 9. doi:10.1186/1748-7188-3-9

Montoliu, I., Martin, F. J., & Collino, S. (2008). Multivariate modeling strantegy for intercompartmental analysis of tissue and plasma 1H NMR spectrotypes. *Journal of Proteome Research, 8*, 2397–2406. doi:10.1021/pr8010205

Nicholson, J. K. (1999). 'Metabonomics' understanding the metabolic responses of living systems to pathophysiological stimuli via multivariate statistical analysis of biological NMR spectroscopic data. *Xenobiotica, 29*, 1181–1189. doi:10.1080/004982599238047

Nicholson, J. K., Connelly, J., Lindon, J. C., & Holmes, E. (2002). Metabonomics: a platform for studying drug toxicity and gene function. *Nature Reviews. Drug Discovery, 1*, 153–161. doi:10.1038/nrd728

Oliver, S. G., Winson, M. K., & Kell, D. B. (1998). Systematic functional analysis of the yeast genome. *Trends in Biotechnology, 16*, 373–378. doi:10.1016/S0167-7799(98)01214-1

Patterson, A. D., Li, H., & Eichler, G. S. (2008). UPLC-ESI-TOFMS-based metabolomics and gene expression dynamics inspector self-organizing metabolomic maps as tools for understanding the cellular response to ionizing radiation. *Analytical Chemistry, 80*, 665–674. doi:10.1021/ac701807v

Roessner, U., Luedemann, A., Brust, D., Fiehn, O., Linke, T., Willmitzer, L., & Fernie, A. R. (2001). Metabolic profiling allows comprehensive phenotyping of genetically or environmentally modified plant systems. *The Plant Cell, 13*, 11–29.

Ryan, D., & Robards, K. (2006). Metabolomics: the greatest omics of them all? *Analytical Chemistry, 78*, 7954–7958. doi:10.1021/ac0614341

Sato, S., Arita, M., & Soga, T. (2008). Time-resolved metabolomics reveals metabolic modulation in rice foliage. *BMS Syst Biol, 2*, 51. doi:10.1186/1752-0509-2-51

Schena, M., Shalon, D., Davis, R. W., & Brown, P. O. (1995). Quantitative monitoring of gene expression patterns with a complementary DNA microarray. *Science, 270*, 467–470. doi:10.1126/science.270.5235.467

Shlens, J. (2003). *A tutorial on PCA*. Retrieved from http://www.snl.salk.edu/~shlens/pca.pdf

Smith, L. M., Maher, A. D., & Cloarec, O. (2007). Statistical correlation and projection methods for improved information recovery from diffusion-edited NMR spectra of biological samples. *Analytical Chemistry, 79*, 5682–5689. doi:10.1021/ac0703754

Soininen, P., Kangas, A. J., & Wurtz, P. (2009). High throughput serum NMR metabonimics for cost-effective holistic studies on systemic metabolism. *Analyst (London), 134*, 1781–1785. doi:10.1039/b910205a

Solberg, R., Enot, D., & Deigner, H.-P. (2010). Metabolomic Analyses of Plasma Reveals New Insights into Asphyxia and Resuscitation in Pigs. *PLoS ONE, 5*, e9606. doi:10.1371/journal.pone.0009606

Somorjai, R. L., Alexander, M., & Baumgartner, S. (2004). A data-driven, flexible machine learning strategy for the classification of biomedical data. In Dubitzky, W., & Azuaje, F. (Eds.), *Artificial Intelligence Methods and Tools for Systems Biology* (pp. 67–85). Dordrecht: Springer.

Sreekuman, A., Poisson, L. M., & Rajendiran, T. M. (2009). Metabolomic profiles delineate potential role for sarcosine in prostate cancer progression. *Nature, 457*, 910–915. doi:10.1038/nature07762

Suna, T., Salminen, A., & Soininen, P. (2007). 1H NMR metabonomics of plasma lipoprotein subclasses – elucidation of metabolic clustering by SOM. *NMR in Biomedicine, 20*, 658–672. doi:10.1002/nbm.1123

Tiziani, S., Lodi, A., & Khanim, F. L. (2009). Metabolic profiling of drug response in acute myeloid leukemia cell lines. *PLoS ONE, 4*, e4251. doi:10.1371/journal.pone.0004251

Trygg, J., Holmes, E., & Lundstedt, T. (2007). Chemometrics in Metabonomics. *Journal of Proteome Research, 6*, 469–479. doi:10.1021/pr060594q

Tukiainen, T., Tynkkynen, T., & Makinen, V.-P. (2008). A multi-metabolite analysis of serum by 1H NMR spectroscopy: early systemic signs of Alzheimer's disease. *Biochemical and Biophysical Research Communications, 375*, 356–361. doi:10.1016/j.bbrc.2008.08.007

Ultsch, A. (1999). Data mining and knowledge discovery with emergent self-organizing feature maps for multivariate time series. In Oja, E., & Kaski, S. (Eds.), *Kohonen Maps* (pp. 33–45). Elsevier. doi:10.1016/B978-044450270-4/50003-6

Wishart, D. S., Knox, C., & Guo, A. C. (2009). HMDB: a knowledgebase for the human metabolome. *Nucleic Acids Research, 37*(Database issue), D603–D610. doi:10.1093/nar/gkn810

Xia, J., Wu, X., & Yuan, Y. (2007). Integration of wavelet transform with PCA and ANN for metabolomics data-mining. *Metabolmics, 3*, 531–537. doi:10.1007/s11306-007-0090-2

Xu, R., & Wunsch, D. (2005). Survey of Clustering Algorithms. *IEEE Transactions on Neural Networks*, *16*(3), 645–678. doi:10.1109/TNN.2005.845141

Yang, C., Richardson, A. D., Smith, J. W., & Osterman, A. (2007) Comparative metabolomics of breast cancer. *Pacif Symp Biocomp 12*, 181-192.

Zou, W., & Tolstikov, W. (2008). Probing genetic algorithms for feature selection in comprehensive metabolic profiling approach. *Rapid Communications in Mass Spectrometry*, *22*, 1312–1324. doi:10.1002/rcm.3507

Chapter 2
Data Analysis and Interpretation in Metabolomics

Jose M. Garcia-Manteiga
Protein Transport and Secretion Unit, San Raffaele – DIBIT, Italy

ABSTRACT

Metabolomics represents the new 'omics' approach of the functional genomics era. It consists in the identification and quantification of all small molecules, namely metabolites, in a given biological system. While metabolomics refers to the analysis of any possible biological system, metabonomics is specifically applied to disease and physiopathological situations. The data collected within these approaches is highly integrative of the other higher levels and is hence amenable to be explored with a top-down systems biology point of view. The aim of this chapter is to give a global view of the state of the art in metabolomics describing the two analytical techniques usually used to give rise to this kind of data, nuclear magnetic resonance, NMR, and mass spectrometry. In addition, the author will focus on the different data analysis tools that can be applied to such studies to extract information with special interest at the attempts to integrate metabolomics with other 'omics' approaches and its relevance in systems biology modeling.

1. INTRODUCTION

Metabolomics is a relatively new 'omics' strategy aimed at the identification and quantification of potentially all small metabolites in a given biological system. As for genomics, transcriptomics,

and proteomics before, metabolomics represents a picture, a downstream snapshot of the molecular biology dogma flow of information, from genes to proteins and beyond. Small metabolites of almost all kinds, amino acids, lipids, sugars, nucleotides, organic acids, amines etc., define the metabolic composition of a biological system and its changes are governed by chemistry, physiology, biochem-

DOI: 10.4018/978-1-61350-435-2.ch002

Copyright © 2012, IGI Global. Copying or distributing in print or electronic forms without written permission of IGI Global is prohibited.

istry, molecular biology, and genetics in the end. It is therefore one of the most integrative 'omics' approach available today since very small changes in the upstream levels, the transcriptome and the proteome, which could be hardly detectable with the current technologies, could give rise to detectable changes in the levels of metabolites. Hence, metabolomics pursues the highest level of integration within the functional genomics field and is therefore, alone or in combination with other techniques, perfectly suitable to systems biology approaches for their use at different levels such as ecology, physiology, biochemistry, and cell biology studies amongst others.

The metabolomics field puts together a relevant amount of scientific skills, from analytical chemistry, cell biology, physiology, and biochemistry, passing through bioinformatics, statistics, and mathematics. Beginning with good study design and sampling procedures, not only is mandatory to obtain good quality data but to have good expertise in analytical chemistry, such as nuclear magnetic resonance or mass spectrometry skills, which will be required after samples are obtained. Once spectra are acquired, a good statistical and bioinformatics approach will distinguish a success from a failure. Moreover, we must define the goal of our metabolomics study in an early state since there are plenty of bioinformatics and chemometric approaches to apply to the huge amount of data that the analytical high-throughput techniques are currently able to supply with. Each of these approaches is best fitted for different outputs of the study. For example, in clinical metabolomics, PCA (Principal Component Analysis), which will be discussed later in this chapter, is currently the most frequently used tool for extracting metabolic information combined with PLS-DA (Partial Least Square Discriminant Analysis) in a first approach to the data. If big data matrices are available, however, other statistical tools, such as SVM (Support Vector Machines) or genetic algorithms are best suited for the discovery of biomarkers, which is very often the final goal in clinical metabolomics

approaches. One of the goals of this chapter is to bring about a discussion of the state of the art data analysis and interpretation in metabolomics studies, focusing on the attempts to integrate the metabolome information with the proteome and its application at the systems biology level.

In this chapter I will try to give an overall prospective of metabolomics studies, beginning with some definitions and historical approaches to the field as well as its several applications. I will describe the process from the study design and sampling procedures for the different types of approaches covering also the two main analytical techniques, NMR and Mass Spectrometry. I will show their advantages and disadvantages, discussing their technical challenges for the future of the field, such as single-cell metabolomics applications. I will then highlight the most recent aim of combining NMR and MS techniques to get as close to the global metabolomics goal as possible. In the final section I will describe the databases and mining software solutions for data interpretation with special focus on the modeling uses of metabolomics data for systems biology and the integrative approaches with other 'omics' techniques such as proteomics.

1.1 Background: History and Applications

Although the term metabolomics is widely accepted in the research community as a scientific area focused on the analysis and interpretation of metabolite levels in biological samples, the different approaches to such a goal have received different names, giving rise to a vast terminology during the last 20 years, i.e. metabolic profiling, fingerprinting, footprinting etc. I will define a few of the most used approaches in the field but for a good review on their historical hints you can refer to Oldiges (Oldiges et al., 2007). According to Fiehn (Fiehn, 2002), metabolomics technologies are subdivided into *target analysis*, aimed at quantitative analysis of substrate and/or product metabolites of a target protein; *metabolic profiling*, focusing at the analysis of a set of predefined metabolites belonging to a class or a linked group of metabolites and the ideal *metabolomics* approach, striving for a an unbiased overview of whole-cell metabolic patterns. In a reduced approach to metabolomics, metabolic fingerprinting can be used to reduce the analytical effort to those metabolites with biochemical relevance (Fiehn, 2001). In the last years, some other approaches have been added to the list, such as metabolic footprinting, which differs from the approaches mentioned above by analyzing extracellular metabolites instead of intracellular pools. Since true metabolomics is indeed unreachable in practice due to the high complexity of the metabolome, namely the complete set of metabolites of a biological system, the actual unbiased techniques are reduced to metabolic profiling on one hand, and metabolic finger/footprinting on the other. The major difference between those resides in the need for metabolite quantification in metabolic profiling whereas for the finger/footprinting strategies only semi-quantitative data is required. Besides, for the latter, there is no need to actually identify metabolites either, since absolute amounts of identified metabolites and semi-quantitative data of spectral peaks can be analyzed and processed equally, before any further biochemical identification is made.

Despite these last ten years of growing interest, metabolomics is not completely a brand new field. Before the analytical techniques gave the possibility to analyze even thousands of different metabolites per sample in high-throughput manner, the presence and amount of certain specific metabolites of interest in biological samples had been studied for many years, especially in pathological investigations. Classical biochemical blood tests are not other than what is called targeted metabolic profiling, a reduced form of metabolic profiling, where a set of informative, *a priori* chosen, metabolites are detected and quantified. Of course, a more global metabolic approach has

been possible only with the occurrence of highly accurate and high throughput mass spectrometers coupled to high performance chromatography and high field nuclear magnetic resonance.

The historical application of the analysis of the metabolome has been the study of disease, from inborn metabolic errors, through toxicology and nutrigenomics. Nowadays, the modern interest in metabolomics has spread over several other fields. In the clinical field, metabonomics can be used to test cohorts of patients with different diseases and compare their metabolic profiles to "normal" cohorts to find out metabolic markers of disease. In a first approach, it could not be necessary to obtain the whole metabolic profile but just the metabolic fingerprint that distinguishes one group from the others. Initially thought to be useful for pathologies regarding metabolic imbalances, now it starts to be applied to a number of other diseases with success. Also in the field of toxicology, metabolomics is widely applicable and numerous studies are using it to assess in a high-throughput manner the effects of liver and kidney toxins. For a review of metabolomics in the field of toxicology please refer to (Griffin & Bollard, 2004). In fermentative processes and strain development, key studies for biotechnology, the analysis of the metabolome, both intra and extracellular pools, is of great relevance for fundamental investigation of metabolism, regulatory networks, and improvement of production organisms and processes. Finally, targeted and non-targeted analyses contribute to systems biology studies which not only are interested in large global networks organization but also in small subsystems and their links like the biochemical pathways in central metabolism.

1.1.1 Clinical Applications

In the field of cardiovascular diseases, the use of metabolomics on blood and urine samples has facilitated the discrimination between individuals with hypertension and normal blood pressure and finding potential new biomarkers of hypertension. Moreover, it was also demonstrated to be even more effective than the conventional risk factors in establishing the severity of coronary heart disease. In the diabetes and obesity field, serum metabolomics gives the possibility to study large human populations both rapidly and cheaply as well as to interpret the biochemical changes that occur not only in one organ but also in the systemic metabolism (Goldsmith et al., 2010).

Some attempts are being made to use metabolomics as a useful diagnostic tool also in the field of neurology, not only using cerebrospinal fluid analyses but also combining classical MRI (Magnetic Resonance Imaging) tools with MRS (Magnetic Resonance Spectroscopy) to give a more functional picture of the brain metabolism (Ando & Tanaka, 2005; Tsang, Haselden, & Holmes, 2009; X. Zhang et al., 2009).

In the field of organ transplantation, metabolomics has been initially used to enhance early non functional primary grafts diagnosis. This kind of approach has been used with success in liver and kidney transplantations with the particular goal of detecting acute rejection, chronic rejection and knowing about operational tolerance with the minimal invasiveness. However, no information of the etiology of the rejection can be extracted from the different metabolic profiles. Besides, metabolomics tests do not yield enough sensitivity and specificity due to a number of confounding factors, although several attempts to cope with these issues are being currently taken. Despite the difficulties, the challenge of using metabolomics in transplantation for early rejection detection is worth the effort, since the transplantation biopsies, the other reliable method, present a high risk for both the patient and the graft (Sarwal, 2009; Wishart, 2005).

Not surprisingly, metabolomics has revealed an enormous potential in oncologic studies. Since tumors are highly metabolic tissues, the presence of cancer cells can be diagnosed and followed systemically by finding different metabolic patterns in several biofluids, from blood to urine. Metabolic profiling can also be used to get new insights of the cancer cell biology and biochemistry by studying cell lines and tumor tissues. The use of metabolomics in oncology advances in two main fronts: on one hand the search for new biomarkers of disease, disease progression, prognosis or treatment evaluation, and on the other hand the use of fingerprints, the complete metabolic pattern, as hallmarks of the different pathological situations in cancer. A number of studies using cell lines, tissues and biofluids have been published demonstrating the ability of metabolomics to cluster apart samples derived from healthy donors from cancer patients, different grades or stages in the disease or cancer cell lines from their normal counterparts. The studies using patients can go from small pilot studies showing reduced cohorts to large studies where the statistical power and the post-processing analysis pursue the finding of new biomarkers to be used in the clinics. For a recent review on applications of metabolomics in clinical oncology please refer to (Spratlin, Serkova, & Eckhardt, 2009).

1.1.2 Pharmacology, Toxicology and Nutrition

In preclinical drug studies, metabolomics can provide information of the toxic effects of a drug, identifying the site and the timing of action. If we know the metabolic profile associated with a disease, we can use metabolomics to follow pharmacological treatment and its metabolic responses, with special attention to treatment fine tuning and caring of side-effects. An interesting new branch of such studies is called pharmaco-metabolomics, which is aimed at using metabolic profiles to determine *a priori* the response of an individual to xenobiotics with the final goal of improving drug use and getting closer to customized treatment (Griffin & Bollard, 2004; Kaddurah-Daouk, Kristal, & Weinshilboum, 2008).

Several metabolomics studies have demonstrated the effects of diet on metabolism. Not only these results are relevant to other metabolomic studies, where different dietary habits of individuals can be an important source of noise in the data, but also to nutritionists, who can use it to establish individual nutrition phenotypes. In addition, metabolomics of nutrition can give us an overall view of how diet interacts with metabolism and provide a comprehensive definition of nutritional status as well as predicting health and disease outcomes (German, Roberts, Fay, & Watkins, 2002; German, Roberts, & Watkins, 2003; German, Watkins, & Fay, 2005).

1.1.3 Biotechnology

In microbiology, metabolic profiling is used in strain identification and metabolic phenotyping of genetic variants. *Escherichia coli* (E. coli) strains with mutations in genes that are closely related to metabolism can be identified by their metabolic patterns. This feature becomes even more relevant for the identification of biologically and biochemically 'silent' mutations, with no detectable phenotypic parameters in terms of cell growth, proliferation rate, etc. Fast discrimination between strains is also an important issue in industrial biotechnology, where identifying more efficient strains is of great relevance. Besides, with the analysis of extracellular pools, the exometabolome, the classification of strains directly reflects commercially important traits. In the same industrial biotechnological field, metabolomics is helping the discovery of new metabolic pathways producing or degrading chemicals of industrial interest. Then, metabolomics is combined to transcriptomics and genomics to identify and further characterize the pathways. A number of other applications in the field of microbiology and microbial ecology are currently being explored, such as bioremediation and biosurfactants discovery and characterization (Mapelli, Olsson, & Nielsen, 2008; Pope et al., 2007; Pope, MacKenzie, De-

fernez, & Roberts, 2009; Villas-Boas & Bruheim, 2007; Winder et al., 2008).

1.1.4 Systems Biology

In the new top-down approach to biological questions, called systems biology, metabolomics can be used as a data source which could be integrated to data coming from other 'omics' levels aiding to construct metabolic networks and kinetic models. This kind of approach can help the researcher to identify new underlying kinetic biological mechanisms and to generate new hypotheses based on empirical data. How metabolomics data is currently being used to reach this goal will be the focus of the last part of the chapter, within the data analysis and interpretation section.

2. DATA ANALYSIS AND INTERPRETATION

2.1. Study Design

Before any metabolomics study starts, a good study design is mandatory. This preparatory part of the research is of key relevance since it will define the parameters of our study such as the type of samples, numbers, protocols, and analytical techniques to be used. A normal metabolomic study may comprise many classes of samples and several replicates. The number of replicates may vary depending on statistical power calculations that take the natural variance of the metabolite concentrations into account. The typical number of replicates ranges from a minimum of six for low variance samples coming from well controlled laboratory conditions, in vitro cell culture etc., to large cohorts of human samples, usually tissues or biofluids, subjected to high variation. Having a low number of replicates with a high variance can yield poor statistical results leading our study to failure.

The analysis of the different samples must be randomized to avoid bias due to possible instruments drift in sensitivity and resolution of the analysis and all sample identifiers recorded accordingly to follow sample results properly. We must also define the classes of samples to study depending on the type of analysis required. For a typical clinical study, for instance, a healthy group and a patients group is the most common organization, but many modifications can be made to that scheme. Besides, defining the best clinical controls for our study can be critical for the interpretation of results, especially in human metabolomics, since the controls must match the sample group in a vast number of parameters, such as age, dietary habits, gender, etc. Numerous papers have been published regarding the possible confounding variables in human metabolomics studies, and have to be taken into consideration when designing the control groups and the sampling conditions (Bijlsma et al., 2006; Gullberg, Jonsson, Nordstrom, Sjostrom, & Moritz, 2004; van Velzen et al., 2008). For clinical metabolomics studies, some authors consider that the best control for a patient sample should be coming from the same individual prior to the disease state. Of course, whenever possible, this is the optimum control since all possible confounding variables as dietary habits, gender, race, and age would be reduced to a minimum. However, it is rather difficult to have access to these, so called, baseline samples, defining a healthy state for each individual and, hence, this control is nearly absent in clinical metabolomics with human patients. Rather, this kind of analysis, namely crossover design, can be done when dealing with toxicological and pharmacological studies, where the control group may be the same individual before the administration of a given drug or in nutritional studies (van Velzen et al., 2008). Finally, statistical analyses have to be chosen according to the classes in study, and in the case of crossover designs, a multivariate version of a paired t-test should be the right one (van Velzen et al., 2008). The different statistical approaches to analyze metabolomics data will be discussed in the following sections.

If different individuals are chosen as control groups, a good clinical knowledge of the pathology in study is very important for their choice, since very often an age, gender, and race matching of healthy groups are not enough to avoid misinterpretation of results. In fact, when studying a complex disease such as cancer, there may be various clinical variables occurring in patients and not in healthy individuals which could confuse the study and hence give us false positives. For example, different diets of hospitalized patients with particular diets versus normal diets from healthy donors, tissues with high inflammation in cancer patients versus normal tissues, intense drug therapies of patients versus healthy individuals, who are obviously not under the same drug treatment, and so on. Therefore, the choice of the control group has to be dramatically appropriate and perfectly suit the goal of the study, which should be defined *a priori*.

Another key element of the study design is the choice of the type of sample. Samples may come from human or laboratory animal's biofluids, or tissues, or from *in vitro* cell cultures of different origins. Different kinds of samples for analysis can produce different information according to the clinical problem, if this is the application of our study, or in the case of biotechnological applications of metabolomics the type of culture, phase of growth, composition of the medium, etc., have to be completely defined and standardized. In the next section I will focus on sampling and quenching methods and the efforts that have been taken to standardize them.

2.2 Sampling and Quenching Methods

A number of studies have been published so far that address the problem of the sampling conditions in metabolomics (Castrillo, Hayes, Mohammed, Gaskell, & Oliver, 2003; Sellick et al., 2009;

Villas-Boas, Hojer-Pedersen, Akesson, Smedsgaard, & Nielsen, 2005; Winder et al., 2008). The metabolome can be highly modified during the sampling procedure due to enzymatic activities present in the sample, chemical modifications, and temperature. Metabolite sampling and extraction procedures have to be well chosen depending on the desired sub-field of metabolomics while letting us have the most informative picture of the system in study. In an optimum situation, the sampling procedure will freeze the metabolome of a biofluid, tissue, or cell extract until the extraction protocol ideally isolates and extracts from the matrix all metabolites with similar efficiencies. Since this goal has not been reachable so far, we have to choose the type of extraction procedure which fits our approximation to global metabolomics, choosing the one that maximizes efficiency and reproducibility in obtaining the highest number of metabolites while minimally altering the metabolome all over the process. Of course, different sampling and extraction procedures may give different results although coming from the same samples, thus making a standardization process in metabolomics mandatory to compare results from studies using different methodologies. Fiehn and collaborators have proposed a draft of minimal requirements to describe the context of metabolomics studies aimed to help with the task of evaluating, understanding, comparing and repeating metabolomics studies (Sansone et al., 2007). For a complete set of guidelines, please refer to the Metabolomics Standards Initiative web page (http://msi-workgroups.sourceforge.net/).

Following the guidelines of this standardization initiative, one can point out the different relevant points about the sampling procedure. The first important point takes into consideration the time passed between the removal of the sample from its environment to the moment in which metabolic activity will be actually stopped by the chosen quenching procedure. Minimizing this time will help in taking an exact picture of physiologically relevant metabolite concentrations, since

cell cultures tend to change metabolic rates very quickly when removed from their controlled *in vitro* environments. Although *in vivo* tissues have slower metabolic rates, it is recommended to minimize the time passed until the metabolism is quenched in the sample in these studies, too. After the sampling, the quenching step permits to stop metabolism prior to the extraction procedures. This step is mandatory in all metabolomics studies and is usually made via application of low to very low temperatures. When working with tissues or adherent cell cultures, snap freezing in liquid nitrogen is the most useful approach whenever possible. Should liquid nitrogen not be available, during human surgery tissue sampling for instance, -80 C degrees freezing is advisable. Samples can be then stored at -80 C degrees until processed for extraction. There is no available information yet about the effect of long (months to years) storage periods at -80 C degrees on metabolite concentration changes. Another important step of the sampling procedure to be properly considered is the separation technique of the intracellular metabolites from the extracellular medium. This point is of high relevance when working with adherent and suspension cell cultures, since contamination with highly rich culture mediums could mess up the results. For adherent cell cultures, quickly aspirating extracellular medium and adding a cold washing step is the usual approach, whereas the mildest centrifugation is required to separate cells from growth medium avoiding metabolite leakage. Several methodological studies have been published to address this relevant issue concerning microbiological growth for biotechnological applications of metabolic profiling, proposing different filtration technologies and quenching methods which maximize separation while minimizing the time between sampling and quenching (Castrillo et al., 2003; Faijes, Mars, & Smid, 2007; Sellick et al., 2009; Winder et al., 2008). However, few technological advances are available when working at the tissue culture dish or flask level and a cold quick wash and a cold centrifugation step are the only techniques available so far with minimized time between sampling and quenching. Direct quenching using diverse methanol-buffered solutions at -40 C degrees have been proposed and tested for bacterial and yeast cultures but all of them show a rather relevant degree of cell breakage, thus precluding its use for consistent global metabolic profiling. Besides, mammalian cell membranes are even more vulnerable to methanol quenching solutions and hence a cold centrifugation step in suspension mammalian cultures is currently the method of choice for consistent global metabolic profiling. Recently a combined cold glycerol-saline quenching and sampling step, combined to a fast filtration step have been described for the analysis of microbial cells (Smart, Aggio, Van Houtte, & Villas-Boas, 2010) reporting low leakage of metabolites which could be potentially applied to mammalian cell cultures as well.

2.3. Extraction Procedures

Different extraction procedures exist depending on the type of sample analyzed and the analytical platform used. While for the analyses of biofluids such as serum, plasma and urine with NMR no extraction is needed, the processing of tissue samples will usually imply an extraction step consisting in homogenization of the tissue in either acetonitrile, perchloric acid or methanol/chlorophorm (Beckonert et al., 2007). For LC-MS analyses, deproteinization of the sample is mandatory, therefore different extraction protocols have been described for serum, plasma and tissue samples (Michopoulos, Lai, Gika, Theodoridis, & Wilson, 2009; Want et al., 2006; Zelena et al., 2009). Rather, urine samples do not require further extractions since proteins are efficiently filtered by the kidney (Want et al., 2010).

As for cell culture extraction procedures, different protocols have been described and analyzed, especially for microbial cultures analyses. The different protocols include extraction in cold

methanol, hot ethanol or methanol, perchloric acid, chloroform/water, and chloroform/methanol (Faijes et al., 2007; Villas-Boas et al., 2005). For mammalian cell cultures, some adaptations of the methanol/chloroform extraction method described by Viant for tissues, (Viant, 2007) are often used with success. Very briefly, after quenching of cells, pellets are extracted using a mix of methanol/chloroform/water and separated into polar and non-polar fractions. Fractions are then freeze-dried and stored at -80 C. They will be then dissolved in deuterated solvents for NMR analysis. When using LC-MS, acenotrile extractions are preferred over methanol/chloroform methods.

There is not a perfect protocol of sampling, quenching and extraction which could give a complete view of the metabolome whatsoever using either NMR or MS related technologies. The procedures have to be chosen depending on the type of sample and analytical platform to be used which give the best results regarding reproducibility and robustness. If a more complete view of the metabolome is required, a combination of both analytical techniques and extraction procedures must be used.

2.4. Analytical Techniques

The main analytical techniques used in metabolomics studies are based on NMR spectroscopy and Mass Spectrometry (MS). MS usually requires a previous separation step, normally liquid or gas chromatography with the derivatization of the sample. Other more specialized techniques, as Fourier Transform infrared (FTIR) are available, too. Both NMR and MS techniques are good for metabolomics purposes but a list of analytical strengths and weaknesses can be distinguished for both of them. For an extensive review of both techniques applied to metabolomics please refer to (Lenz & Wilson, 2007).

2.4.1 NMR

^{1}H-NMR enables the detection of proton containing metabolites within a given sample. NMR produces also detailed information of the structure of the metabolite, both in pure samples and in mixtures. The general advantage of NMR in metabolomic studies is its ease and simplicity. One dimensional ^{1}H-NMR spectra are collected and acquired after the addition of deuterated buffered solutions to the sample. Modern 1D-^{1}H-NMR spectroscopy is able to analyze with sufficient resolution and sensitivity one sample in no more than 20 minutes (Griffin, 2003; Ludwig et al., 2009; Serkova, Spratlin, & Eckhardt, 2007; Viant, 2003). This feature makes NMR a good high-throughput technique. Furthermore, NMR is not biased to any chemical structure and so it is not selective. One important drawback, however, is the low sensitivity as it has the limit of detection at the low micromolar range. One important feature of NMR in metabolomics, especially for systems biology applications, is its ability to obtain easily absolute quantifications of the compounds identified in a mixture. Although it is also possible using MS, the procedure is often far more difficult and complicated (Chalcraft, Lee, Mills, & Britz-McKibbin, 2009; Weljie, Newton, Mercier, Carlson, & Slupsky, 2006).

Different types of NMR analysis are available when dealing with metabolomics studies. The use of either of them will depend on the type of study. For metabonomic studies aimed at finding biomarkers of disease or merely exploratory experiments, one dimensional ^{1}H-NMR spectra are usually acquired. This kind of spectrum can be obtained in less than 20 minutes per sample and gives global information of the metabolic composition of a mixture. When information is required about metabolic fluxes, ^{13}C-NMR is often used in what is called ^{13}C stable isotope-resolved metabolomics (SIRM) (Fan et al., 2009; Fan et al., 2010). In such an analysis, the medium is enriched in ^{13}C metabolites by use of ^{13}C-glucose or other metabolites and a one dimensional ^{13}C-NMR spectrum is acquired.

Another important drawback of NMR spectrum for metabolomics is that different metabolites give several peaks throughout the spectrum which tend to be highly overlapped in complex mixtures. This overlapping issue makes identification and quantification of poorly represented metabolites very hard. The overlapping issue can be overcome by using two-dimensional correlation spectroscopy. There are different types of 2D NMR experiments, TOCSY (Total Correlation Spectroscopy), STOCSY (Statistical Total Correlation Spectroscopy), HSQC (Heteronuclear Single Quantum Coherence spectroscopy), and J-resolved, all of them permitting the partial solving of the overlapping problem (Xia, Bjorndahl, Tang, & Wishart, 2008). However, almost all of them require longer acquisition times, from one to several hours and make them not suitable for high-throughput metabolomics studies. They are usually used to aid identification of peaks in highly overlapped regions of the spectra by acquiring one representative sample of the study. J resolved NMR spectra is acquirable in shorter times and has been used also in a high-throughput basis. Some recent attempts are made to enhance the speed of acquisition in two-dimension NMR experiments to solve the overlapping of signals (Ludwig et al., 2009).

Since quantification of metabolites is the key point for a systems biology approach of metabolomics, I will discuss further the NMR absolute quantification procedures. In an NMR spectrum, the peak integrals relate directly to the number of protons giving rise to the peak and thus to the concentration of the metabolite in the sample. Absolute concentrations can be obtained when an external standard of known concentration is included in every sample, or an internal standard compound concentration is already known by other independent means. Recently, a synthetic electronic reference signal has been introduced to improve quantification (ERETIC, Electronic

REference To asses In vivo Concentrations) and this method does not require any internal standards (Barantin, Le Pape, & Akoka, 1997).

In high-throughput 1D-^{1}H-NMR experiments, three NMR pulse sequence are most frequently used: 1D-NOESY, which gives normally the best overview of all kind of molecules in either biofluids and extracts, CPMG (Carl Purcell Meiboom Gill) spectra, which uses fast relaxation of protons to filter particularly those signals coming from macromolecules, and diffusion edited to select for macromolecular signals (lipids and lipoproteins, mainly). For absolute quantification of samples NOESY pulses can be used with external standards but CPMG pulses should better be used with the aid of electronic references. This is because DSS and TSP, the most commonly used external standards for both chemical shift reference and concentration can interact with high molecular weight components such as proteins. In samples enriched in proteins or lipoproteins, as serum or plasma, CPMG pulses could be underestimating the amount of standard and hence overestimating the amount of metabolites of unknown concentration. Although CPMG pulses can be used anyway if demonstrated that this effect is similar in all samples of our study, an external standard as ERETIC is advisable for absolute determination of the concentration (Beckonert et al., 2007).

2.4.2 Mass Spectrometry

In mass spectrometry, a separation step using either liquid or gas chromatography often precedes the entry of metabolites in a mass spectrometer. High performance and Ultra High performance liquid chromatography are currently the methods of choice if one MS technique has to be used (UPLC-TOFMS)(Denkert et al., 2006; Want et al., 2010). UPLC-MS techniques can give accurate and reproducible results which overcome the problem of sensitivity, the most important drawback of NMR approaches. On the other hand, MS techniques need a previous preparation of

the samples, as extraction or dilution and in the end the separative chromatography. The choice of the separation technique could depend on the type of sample we have to analyze. For a good analysis of a complete set of lipid metabolites, gas chromatography would be a good global choice; however, if analyzing urine metabolites, liquid chromatography is preferred, since polar solutes have to be separated in a liquid phase. Different columns for liquid chromatography can give different outputs and thus they have to be chosen carefully. Along with classical UPLC and HPLC columns, capillary electrophoresis can be used to separate metabolites prior to the mass spectrometry. Whatever the separation technique is used, metabolites have to be ionized, since Time of Flight MS works with ions. Electro spray ionization (ESI) is the most commonly used technique but there are several different ways of introducing ions into the MS that can be used. Please refer elsewhere for specific reviews on Mass Spectrometry for metabolic profiling (Oldiges et al., 2007) and the different specific applications.

The use of MS techniques provides the highest sensitivity and amount of metabolites detected in the samples. However, one important drawback is that the technique is far from being straightforward; a good expertise in mass spectrometry and chromatography is required with special focus on identification of unknown metabolites. Although modern MS devices yield high resolution in mass to charge measures, the post-processing of such a huge amount of raw data is time consuming and more manual work has to be done. Although MS devices are often accompanied by processing and analysis software packages, usually the time dedicated to interpret raw data is more than the time needed for the samples to be analyzed.

Another important feature of MS metabolite profiling is that of quantification. While semi-quantitative data, or relative concentrations data is often used for metabonomic studies or biomarker discovery and simply peak areas or heights are used in arbitrary units, the use of reference standards for every single compound to absolutely quantify is mandatory. This fact is due to differences in efficiency of ionization and separation of the different metabolites. Besides, the concentrations produced are prone to suffer from sample and matrix effects due to the high complexity of ions being analyzed. Although difficult to pursue, absolute quantification using MS can be achieved if these problems are taken into consideration and several ways of dealing with absolute concentrations have been published so far as external standard calibration and isotope dilution (Oldiges et al., 2007).

2.5. Data Processing and Analysis: Statistical Analysis

2.5.1 Data Pre-Processing

Metabolomic studies usually produce a huge amount of raw data. The quality and type of the processing applied to raw data will have a high impact on the results of our study. The data processing and analysis can be divided into two parts. A first part of pre-processing which will depend basically on which kind of analytical technique we have chosen and the type of samples we have used. The second part of analysis will depend on the kind of result we want to obtain and hence on the type of application we want for our study.

Raw data are obtained as single files for specific samples and their dimensionality will depend on the platform and type of approach used. For one dimensional ¹H-NMR, we will deal with one dimensional spectrum which gives us a single vector of numbers for each sample, corresponding to either integrals or heights of peaks or regions or absolute concentrations of metabolites. For two dimensional NMR or for MS chromatograms we are dealing with spots, two dimensional peaks which correspond to single ions for MS or protons of single metabolites for non overlapped 2D signals in correlation NMR spectroscopy. Before continuing with the pre-processing step, the fea-

ture to be analyzed must be decided. If we need absolute quantification of known metabolites, we will have to first identify those metabolites using databases and specific profiling software and then we will use the concentration matrix of samples and metabolites for the ulterior analysis steps. Rather, if we prefer to proceed with the analysis before the actual identification of metabolites, we will need to apply noise filtering and peak alignment before reducing the amount of data to analyze using data binning or either automatic or manual peak detection. Data binning, the most usually used data reduction technique, consists in dividing either spectra or chromatogram in discrete regions, or buckets, of normally regular widths or areas. Once this is done, we can proceed with the normalization and scaling steps.

Normalization of the samples is mandatory to avoid bias while preserving biological information. For NMR experiments, the total integral of the whole spectrum is usually used to normalize samples with each other, but other sample parameters can be used if needed, as sample dry weight and cell number for tissues or cellular extracts. While normalization deals with undesired or non informative variation amongst samples, scaling deals with variation and relevance information amongst variables. Scaling is thus used to adjust the importance of the variables within data when fitting the model to be constructed. Scaling is often required for NMR experiments since spectra are usually dominated by highly concentrated species giving multiple peak resonances and is hence advisable if similar relevance is to be given to all metabolites, disregarding its relative concentration in the sample. Several methods can be applied depending on the type of statistical model to be constructed (Bijlsma et al., 2006; Viant, 2003). It is usually used the scaling to unit variance, where every variable is divided by its standard deviation in order to give all variables the same chance to contribute to the model. This kind of scaling is often called scale to unit variance or autoscaling if data is previously mean-centered. This kind of scaling is suitable when equal weights are allocated through the baseline noise. Thus, when dealing with very noisy spectra or with variable baselines, it usually distorts results with noise regions and artifacts. Pareto scaling, is used when detrimental effects of autoscaling are caused by different noise and errors within variables. In Pareto scaling, every variable value is divided by the square root of the standard deviation meaning that the variance is not unity but, actually, the standard deviation of each variable. Different other transformations are desirable if one does not assume normality of the data, as log or power transformations (Boccard, Veuthey, & Rudaz, 2010).

2.5.2 Data Analysis

When dealing with metabolomics, especially when our aim is to have a complete biochemical network under study, the huge amount of data can represent a statistical challenge. The choice of the data analysis depends heavily on the desired application of our study and the kind of data we are using to analyze. The first decision to be made is whether to work either with spectral patterns as peak intensities or integrals and bucketing to reduce the amount of data, or actually identify compounds and quantify them. The first kind of approach is often referred to as chemometric analysis or metabolomics, whereas the second type is often called metabolic profiling or global metabolic profiling or quantitative metabolomics (Trygg, Holmes, & Lundstedt, 2007). Chemometrics has the advantage of avoiding bias for the identifiable metabolites since quantitative metabolomics relies upon the previous identification of metabolites. Chemometrics has also the strength of the automation, high-throughput of analysis, data processing and non biased assessment of data; however, it then suffers from high amounts of noise and internal variations that have to be removed by data pre-processing procedures as peak alignment, noise reduction and so on. Besides, for chemometric analysis, it is usually needed a higher amount

of well controlled specimens with a high grade of standardization to minimize intra-group variability, thus sample uniformity and study design, as discussed above, is crucial for these kind of studies. On the other hand, the key advantage of quantitative metabolomics is that such number of replicates is not often necessary since we reduce the statistical noise due to spectral variations when using actual concentrations of already identified metabolites. The main drawback of quantitative metabolomics, though, is the relative lack of automation when dealing with absolute quantifications and the need for identification of metabolites prior to the data analyses, which introduces bias to the study and makes it harder to apply in a high-throughput manner. Nevertheless, global metabolomics platforms exist that can solve the problem by using relative quantification analysis instead of absolute concentrations of a rather big number of identified metabolites. The number of identifiable metabolites is increasing with time, as specific in house databases are being constructed and updated constantly.

Either in a metabolic profiling or quantitative metabolomics or in a chemometric approach to the study, we are going to deal with a great number of variables. The statistical methods to analyze these data are common to both approaches. The difference resides mainly on the kind of data that are being used. In a chemometric approach, the method is applied to spectral features such as integrals or peak intensities, whereas in metabolic profiling the same method is applied to metabolite concentrations. A first global look to data distribution is often required. With that aim, common chemometric tools as PCA (Principal Component Analysis) are generally proposed by metabolomic commercial solutions in built-in statistical packages as exploratory methods which permit a display of a global vision of our data (Hiller et al., 2009; Izquierdo-Garcia et al., 2009; Werth, Halouska, Shortridge, Zhang, & Powers, ; Zhao, Stoyanova, Du, Sajda, & Brown, 2006). However, other statistical tools are needed for identifying relevant variables within the study. For that purpose, univariate hypothesis testing such as Student test, also known as T-test, one way ANOVA or other non-parametric equivalents can be used although their use tends to be limited when dealing with great numbers of correlated variables which could give false positives. Although some procedures exist to address those issues, such as the Bonferroni correction (Boccard et al., 2010), other multivariate analysis and hypothesis testing are needed for metabolomic studies. In the next paragraphs I will give a general overview of the different statistical approaches currently used in metabolomics.

PCA

Principal component analysis is considered as a starting point in almost all metabolomics studies. It gives a global view of the systematic variation of our data and it helps reducing dimensionality of the data by uncovering internal structures. It constructs new variables, namely principal components, using orthogonal transformations. These new variables are created in such a way that the first one, the first principal component, accounts for as much of the variability in the data as possible. Similarly, the second and next components account for the maximum variability in the data with the constraint that they have to be orthogonal (and hence uncorrelated with) to the preceding components (Idborg-Bjorkman, Edlund, Kvalheim, Schuppe-Koistinen, & Jacobsson, 2003). Through the inspection of PCA scores and loading plots, one can learn from the relationship between the distribution of samples and the correlations between the original variables. It is often used to identify outliers and is usually accompanied by other clustering methods and classifications.

Hierarchical Cluster Analysis

Another unsupervised method of clustering data is hierarchical clustering. In principle, HCA makes subgroups of samples that are similar to one another by producing a hierarchical structure. This clustering can be agglomerative (bottom-up) or divisive (top-down), but agglomerative methods are of wider use. The key part of HCA is how it calculates similarity between groups. It is estimated by a set of distances and a linkage function computed with a specific mathematical problem method, such as Euclidean, correlation or Manhattan. The linkage function then adds the criteria chosen to compute the distance. The outcome is graphically represented as a dendogram, a tree of hierarchical branching groups or clusters (Beckonert, Monnerjahn, Bonk, & Leibfritz, 2003).

Supervised Analyses

PLS and PLS-DA. Unlike unsupervised methods, supervised learning considers the samples as belonging to specific groups, or more generally, with respect to an observed feature. It includes regression and classification problems depending on the feature included. This feature can be a numerical value, a class label or an *a priori* grouping. The classification aims to the construction of models based on training sets of samples and the construction of hypotheses based upon them. The model will be itself described by the variables of our data set. The task is then to learn and map samples of unknown description or grouping, based upon an already constructed model. Different statistical techniques or artificial intelligence algorithms have been developed with that purpose (Westerhuis, van Velzen, Hoefsloot, & Smilde, 2010).

Projection to Latent Structures by means of partial least squares (PLS) is a regression method. It is a well-established statistical approach which is specifically well adapted to situations having fewer observations than detected variables, as usually happens in metabolomics. It works in a similar way as PCA, in the sense that it reduces dimensions to a sub-space based on linear combinations of the original variables but it makes use of the additional information contained in the given grouping or class labels, or additional information contained in the additional observed features. For instance, one can use age of patients as an additional observed feature to supervise learning of the model by including *a priori* groupings as young patients, medium age or old, or by including a Y-variable of age to the X variable of metabolite concentrations. The power of PLS-based classification is that it allows us to make predictions by maximizing the covariance between the data and our previous knowledge about it through the class assignment. In this context, Partial Least Squares Discriminant Analysis (PLS-DA) is performed to enhance the partition between groups of observations such that the maximum separation amongst classes is obtained. Orthogonal-PLS-DA is a modern extension to PLS-DA and is usually used in metabolomics with the scope of building diagnostic models. PLS-DA is often used in clinical metabonomics to clearly distinguish patient groups between them or from healthy controls but care has to be taken when using supervised methods in general, since they tend to overfit models and find differences with no statistical meaning or clinical relevance. The best way to avoid this overfitting is to use some cross-validation methods to ensure that PLS-DA clusters are real and robust. If PCA produces good clustering of samples, then PLS-DA and related supervised methods can help and enhance clustering as well as providing a good predictive model to our study. However, when no good clustering is observed with unsupervised methods, PLS-DA and other supervised methods have to be carefully inspected and cross-validated to trust their results (Bijlsma et al., 2006; Xia, Psychogios, Young, & Wishart, 2009).

Machine Learning Tools

Machine learning tools are usually designed for prediction. One of the advantages of these tools is their applicability when the number of variables is much higher than the number of subjects in study, a typical problem in metabolomics. One drawback is that the practical value of the models constructed using them is often unclear. Many of these methods have tunable parameters which give different results depending on the choices made by the model builder. In fact, the model building strategy is very often chosen during the data analysis step. Any data optimization and processing can have a deep impact on the final model and lead to useless models and wrong conclusions. In a recent article Pers and collaborators (Pers, 2009) presented a game of prediction from high-dimensional data to illustrate a proper assessment and validation of the method of machine learning, using as example a study of metabolomics (Pers, Albrechtsen, Holst, Sorensen, & Gerds, 2009). In this game, the metabolomics data is modeled by using three different machine learning tools, random forest, support vector machines and the lasso (least absolute shrinkage and selection operator) algorithm. A conclusion that can be extracted by analyzing this study is that much care has to be taken when using machine learning tools for building statistical models from metabolomics data. In the next paragraphs I describe briefly three of the most used algorithms in metabolomics studies.

Decision Trees

Decision trees are classification algorithms based on logic tests applied to working classes of the training samples characterized by a decision of belonging or not belonging to a class. The decision is made base on a set of attributes that the sample must have to be classified within a given group. Of course, it relies upon the fact that at least one feature is dissimilar amongst groups. The different features can be ranked based upon the ability to discriminate between samples, and the best ones are then selected. The procedure is then repeated recursively and each branch delimit a partition producing sub-trees from the splits. This kind of approach is in essence univariate since it relies upon variation within one single feature, though iteratively, but there are some multivariate alternatives. The random forest approach constitutes another approach to build such multivariate classifiers as it is a collection of decision trees applied in parallel (H. Zhang, Holford, & Bracken, 1996).

Artificial Neural Networks (ANN) and Other Learning Algorithms

Several other classifying algorithms are available. ANN is based on the use of levels of units, called neurons. The neurons are linked together by a network of connections with adjustable weights which give rise to hierarchical structures. ANN works by starting from input units and propagates through the connection with initially random weightings and is adjusted to maximize the correct output. Although highly potent, the interpretation of ANN remains a critical issue (Gallant, Morin, & Peppard, 1998). Other learning methods such as probabilistic algorithms and instance-based algorithms exist and perform rather well in the presence of complex problems (Boccard et al., 2010).

Support Vectors Machines

Support vector machines (SVM) are highly useful algorithms which are being widely applied in metabolomics since they are generally robust to noisy data. It has become a popular technique since it is able to model non linear relationships. They are based upon the selection of a reduced number of critical boundary instances called support vectors (Keerthi & Shevade, 2003; Luts et al., 2010; Mahadevan, Shah, Marrie, & Slupsky, 2008). They rely on the projection of the data in a higher-dimensional space. This transformation is selected to provide separation of the training set classes, and a linear separation in the high-dimensional space can account for a non-linear decision boundary in the original data space. In order to map new points in the high-dimensional space, called the feature space, kernel functions are used, and hence, they

are critical. Several kernel functions can be used with SVMs as linear, polynomial and radial basis. Although SVMs were originally designed to solve binary classifications in machine learning, several algorithms exist to apply them to multiclass cases (Anand & Suganthan, 2009; Guler & Ubeyli, 2007; Land & Verheggen, 2009). In Sreekumar et al. (2009), the authors used SVM to choose the optimal classifiers to include metabolites based on increasing empirical p-values. If combined with cross-validation procedures and visualization of the results, SVM is a good and robust method of obtaining good classifiers in metabolomics. One important drawback of SVM is, however, that the information about the different contribution of variables to the classification is lost. Innovative methods have been recently introduced to overcome this issue (Krooshof, Ustun, Postma, & Buydens, 2010).

2.6. Metabolic Interpretation

2.6.1 Pathway Analysis and Visualization

As a result of our metabolomics study and a good statistical approach, we will obtain a set of metabolites or putative biomarkers, which have to be seen in the context of the entire metabolism. In order to map the metabolites highlighted by the data analysis, good biochemical databases of pathways and reactions are needed along with visualization software to help the scientist to integrate data and extract relevant information (Brown et al., 2009). The metabolic databases are designed to show not only information about the biochemical reactions of a given pathway but also metabolite-gene-protein interactions. This feature is critical when metabolic information is to be integrated with proteomics and transcriptomics high-throughput data. In addition, metabolic databases have to be species specific and could include relevant chemical, clinical or toxicological information regarding concentration of metabolites in biofluids which could give also important information to the clinical scientist. The four main pathway databases are KEGG (Kanehisa et al., 2008), HumanCyc (Karp, Paley, Krieger, & Zhang, 2004), Reactome database (Stein, 2004), and Human Metabolome Database (Wishart et al., 2009)(HMDB), the latter including also metabolomic relevant chemical information such as MS and NMR features for aiding metabolite identification. KEGG database is the biggest of all, it includes extensive pathway, metabolic, chemical information of an extensive number of species. All sub-databases permit queries and the pathway diagrams are entirely hyperlinked with each other. One important drawback is that metabolic pathways are only filtered by species presented as consensus pathways for a given species, making difficult to have information about the concrete reactions taking place in a particular organ or cell type and to distinguish which particular pathway, metabolite or enzyme is specific only for humans or a given species. Despite that, it represents the most valuable and comprehensive view of the entire metabolism.

The Cyc series of databases, which include HumanCyc, BioCyc, EcoCyc and MetaCyc (Caspi & Karp, 2007) are much better manually curated than KEGG and include more information about enzyme kinetics, such as substrate specificity, kinetic properties, regulators, modulators, and links to structure and sequence databases. One particular feature of the Cyc suite of databases is the Omics viewer (Paley & Karp, 2006), which permits the researcher to map metabolomics, proteomics and genomics data onto any organism metabolic network and perform zooms of different resolution concerning the information visualized, ranging from simple reaction diagram to enzyme properties and chemical formulas.

The reactome databases, integrates metabolic reactions with transduction pathways and cell cycle interactions. Like the Omics Viewer of the Cyc database, the Reactome database includes the fantastic tool, *skypainter* (Joshi-Tope et al., 2005), which permits to paste list of genes, proteins or their identifiers and paint the reactome reactions in different ways as to visualize the dynamic changes in the network using the omics data obtained in the study.

2.6.2 Metabolic Modeling

The statistical tools described in the previous section are of particular interest when we are interested in showing metabolic differences between samples, identifying biomarkers or interesting metabolic pathways. However, the vision they give as a model is rather static, a snapshot description of the metabolic space which lacks dynamic information, often of great interest when dealing with metabolism and biochemical networks. To gain more understanding of the dynamics of a system, metabolic modeling is preferred and necessary to try and predict consequences of genetic variations, knock outs, mutations and metabolite or drug interactions. Through metabolic modeling, metabolomics turns into a predictive field with a systems biology approach, which permits the scientist to inspect the system, create a model and generate hypotheses (Wishart, 2007). The main aim of such an approach is to reproduce mathematically a model closely related to our biological system and discover new properties, relationships and hidden patterns. The model can always be tested against empirical data, modified, and completed to include new information coming from experimental data.

Time-Dependent Ordinary Differential Equations

Historically, metabolic modeling or simulation can be done in different ways. All reactions defining our system are written down and solving systems of differential equations in time are used. Some programs exist now that help in constructing models and use differential equations to make simulations: Cell Designer (Funahashi, Jouraku,

Matsuoka, & Kitano, 2007; Kitano, Funahashi, Matsuoka, & Oda, 2005) CellWare (Dhar et al., 2004) COPASI (Hoops et al., 2006) GEPASI (Mendes, 1993), (Alves, Antunes, & Salvador, 2006). The software helps in translating the biochemical and biological knowledge in our system into differential equations describing the kinetics of reactions. Some of them are based upon Michaelis-Menten initial velocity kinetics; some others are only based upon the law of mass action. One relevant feature of all of them is the ability to translate friendly arrow based reaction notation into mathematical notebook interface. The second part of this modeling software is represented by parameter identification algorithms. A good point with modeling software is to have a nice visual and graphical display of the model, which gives a general overview of the system under study which usually helps the scientist to better understand the biochemical network. Some of this software includes also the possibility of storing all information in well annotated databases, which will aid the scientist to share data and make them available for further analysis using different *in silico* tools.

One particular case of biochemical network modeling is the kinetic modeling approach (KM) (Mogilevskaya et al., 2009). The appealing of such approach is the ability to integrate multilevel data into the biochemical network and to include also regulatory loops, feedbacks which for sure will complete and fine tune the *in silico* simulations of our system. When dealing with such an approach, an enormous amount of data has to be obtained, either experimentally, as kinetic parameters not available in the literature, or estimates or kinetic data already published in the literature. One important point of kinetic modeling is the requirement of the catalytic cycle of every enzymatic reaction to be determined. Several ways of determining unknown catalytic cycles will permit us to complete all the kinetic equations. On a third stage of KM, kinetic parameters are evaluated, as K_m, K_i and K_d. Again, if data is not available in the literature, experimentally determined parameters have to be obtained. Finally, software to solve differential equations is used (DBsolve, (Gizzatkulov et al., 2010). The huge amount of kinetical data needed for the kinetic modeling approach is by far its best advantage over other metabolic modeling approaches since temporal dependences in metabolic reactions are highly based upon enzyme catalytic mechanisms and regulatory loops. Besides, kinetic modeling allows mapping high-throughput data onto known networks of organs, tissues and cell systems.

Constraint-Based Models

An alternative to constructing differential equations models is known as constraint-based modeling (Gagneur & Casari, 2005). In such technique, no ordinary differential equations are used but some physicochemical constraints such as mass balance, energy balance and flux limitations to describe the metabolic behavior of the whole system. The advantage of this kind of approach is that of ignoring the rate constants and the time dependence since we are interested in steady-state conditions that satisfy our physicochemical constraints. It is particularly appealing in high complexity systems such as organs or whole organisms since it is almost impossible to know all rates and concentrations of metabolites in time and is therefore involved in large scale metabolomics studies (Wishart, 2010). One particular case of constraint-base modeling that is widely used with these purposes is Flux Balance Analysis (FBA). FBA assumes the knowledge of the stochiometry of all the reactions in the system and a set of constraints which will drive the network to a steady-state (Ruppin, Papin, de Figueiredo, & Schuster, 2010). It normally produces more unknowns than equations, thus yielding an undetermined system. A possible set of solutions is yet found if included information about known fluxes of metabolites or initial and final concentrations become available. Once the solution space is determined, one defines a function to optimize the behavior of the system. This function can be biomass optimization, the levels of the energy compound adenosine triphosphate (ATP) or the production of a given metabolite. The model can be tested and predictions made by altering parameters and observing the results of the perturbations. There are two critical points of FBA to take into consideration to have good models and trustable predictions: the first one is having the proper mass and charge balances within the reactions defining the model, since these balances will guide the equations to be solved and to define the space of solutions. The second point consists in the set of constraints which reduce the space of solutions to be chosen by the optimization function. With a high number of constraints we are reducing the mathematical space of solutions and hence aiding the optimization function to find the right one which will give better *in silico* simulations. Of course, high-throughput metabolomics, and more importantly, fluxomics data, obtained thanks to isotopic labeling experiments, are preferable to inferred or estimated flux ranges and make the model work finer.

3. FUTURE DIRECTIONS

3.1 Combination of NMR and MS

Although there has been a great advance during the last decade in the field, there are still some challenges which are going to be of key relevance for the future development of metabolomics. Metabolomics aims at the identification and absolute quantification of the whole set of metabolites in a biological system. There is still no currently analytical platform which can achieve this goal (Fiehn, 2002). As we have discussed above, NMR is the most unbiased technique, permitting in principle the identification and absolute quantification of metabolites of any chemical types. However, when used alone, the overlap of peaks and the low sensitivity yields no more than 40-60 identifiable

metabolites for cell extracts or tissues. While MS techniques are far more sensitive and the number of compounds analyzed is in the range of thousands, we have to deal with a high number of unidentified peaks. Metabolite identification relies upon good analytical software tools and databases of reference compound that, although growing and improving with time, still are not allowing us to cover the entire metabolome and represent a bias towards identified metabolites. Besides, identification of hits by MS/MS fractionation techniques and spiking of reference compounds require additional extra work and material which makes identification processes expensive and time-consuming, and are often dedicated only to putative biomarkers, already identified by statistical data reduction techniques. It will be therefore necessary to unravel novel analytical techniques that, coupled to the technical improvements in both sensitivity and accuracy of NMR and MS devices, respectively, will aid in the unbiased detection and identification of the highest amount of metabolites as possible. Only following this goal we will really approach to global metabolomics.

In this regard, some attempts have been made to couple both techniques, NMR and MS, to broad the scope of metabolic profiling analyses. In the so called hyphenation studies (Tang, Xiao, & Wang, 2009), parallel samples are run both in LC-MS and NMR devices permitting the analysis of correlated chromatographic peaks extracting structural information from NMR spectra. In this kind of approach we obtain more than just the additive amount of metabolites identified by either of the techniques, we also obtain statistical correlations which can give us further information about the structure of the metabolic space. When it is combined with post column solid phase extraction (SPE), an enrichment in metabolites concentration can be obtained and coupled to cryogenic NMR probes, will improve the NMR sensitivity (Agnolet, Jaroszewski, Verpoorte, & Staerk, 2010). Of course, the need of great amounts of sample material needed for the SPE procedure still precludes the use of this technique in a high-throughput manner but it currently helps the elucidation of the structure of MS unidentified peaks (Godejohann, Tseng, Braumann, Fuchser, & Spraul, 2004).

3.2 Integrative Multi-Omics Analysis

Another important issue in the future of omics studies in general, and hence a perfect complementation of metabolomic studies and modeling network analysis, is going to be the integration of high-throughput data of different levels, such as metabolites, proteins and gene transcripts. In metabolic networks analysis we have to bear in mind that kinetic rates, the rates of transformation of one compound in another, are due to enzymes, which are themselves proteins, whose levels and activities can be themselves measured with proteomics approaches and included in simulations giving rise to an additional level of complexity that can be empirically determined. On the other hand, protein levels are highly regulated also by transcriptional activation of the genes encoding them and hence, transcriptomics data will provide with this additional level of empirically obtainable data. Several types of studies can be made when trying to integrate two or more levels of complexity. For instance, when trying to integrate transcriptomics with proteomics, three types of analyses are usually used. In the first type, one tries to complement one analysis with the other, trying to fill in the gaps that one approach produces with the alternative approaches using the other levels. This is the less integrative, somehow additive kind of approach. A second type is the one that utilizes the different omics levels to cross-validate the other level. When similar results are obtained, for instance, analyzing the transcript of a protein and the protein levels, the result is being validated by both omics techniques. The third kind of analysis is more interesting from a systemic approach point of view, and takes into consideration those cases where the expected correlation between the

transcriptome and the proteome are not present, revealing hidden regulatory information lacking from our previous knowledge of the system. Several studies have tried to integrate proteomics with metabolomics by means of several multivariate unsupervised exploratory tools (W. Zhang, Li, & Nie). Correlation network topology analysis, pattern recognition, PCA and sparsed PLS-regression have been used demonstrating good pattern recognition and improvement in the description of the system when more than one level of complexity is included (Morgenthal, Weckwerth, & Steuer, 2006; Morgenthal, Wienkoop, Wolschin, & Weckwerth, 2007; Weckwerth & Morgenthal, 2005). For example, in fungal and plant biology, it has been demonstrated that transcript and metabolite profiles can be analyzed in parallel and from this pairwise transcript-metabolite correlation analysis functionally relevant genes and metabolites could be identified (Askenazi et al., 2003). In an ideal attempt to cover all possible layers of complexity, DNA microarrays, qPCR for transcriptomics approaches and LC-MS for both proteins and metabolites and flux analysis have been used in a study in *Escherichia coli* (Ishii et al., 2007). This study revealed how robust a metabolic network can be since metabolite and flux levels remained stable even when some enzymatic genes where disrupted causing small changes in mRNA and protein levels. Other studies have been done using the three levels of mRNA, protein and metabolites using thermophillic bacteria in response to thermal adaptation helping to catalogue and correlate the overall molecular changes of the system (Trauger et al., 2008).

But of course, the challenge of integration of omics levels overcomes the mere correlations between data matrices. The lack of correlation between mRNA and protein could be explained not only by post-transcriptional regulation events but also could be due to non proper statistical methodologies to treat different kinds of data as mRNA and protein or metabolites are. Data transformation and normalization are critical points to reach proper correlations between proteins and transcripts, and also handling the non-linearity property of correlations between mRNA amounts and proteins translated from them is a critical issue (Nie, Wu, Culley, Scholten, & Zhang, 2007). Some progresses are being made (Nie, Wu, & Zhang, 2006) and statistical specific approaches as Poisson regression models can be applied to address the issue of lacking information, when dealing with missing proteomics data. Some other studies use co-inertia analysis (CIA) and then gene ontology analysis (GO) coupled to PCA for the visualization of gene expression and protein abundances (Fagan, Culhane, & Higgins, 2007). Recently, another study used stochastic Gradient Boosted Trees approach to uncover possible non-linear relationships between transcriptomics and proteomics data (Torres-Garcia, Zhang, Runger, Johnson, & Meldrum, 2009). In addition to these data-driven methodologies, some studies have taken also into consideration the biological information available using genome-wide models of translation. Mehra et al. (Mehra, Lee, & Hatzimanikatis, 2003) presented a correlation between mRNA and protein levels based on kinetic parameters and concentration of ribosomes. In another study, Mogilevskaya et al. (Mogilevskaya et al., 2009) described an approach to integrate proteomics and mRNA data into metabolic pathways integrating them with enzyme kinetics and kinetic modeling.

Of course, due to the high financial costs of omics studies and the necessity to have in house omics facilities and skills, few multi-omics approaches have been developed so far. Nevertheless, the power of such approaches to better describe models and unravel relevant information is not under discussion. In the future, such integration of multi-omics studies will lead us to a quantified description of the cellular metabolism at a genome scale. Once the foundations of such an analysis, from the statistical and technological point of view, are obtained, the multi-omics integrative approach will prompt us into further hypothesis-

driven research in multiple systems of interest, from microbiology to humans (W. Zhang, Li, & Nie, 2010).

3.3 Single Cell Metabolomics

Almost all omics data obtained in the studies made so far come from populations of cells, from cell cultures or tissues. Cellular heterogeneity arises from stochastic expression of genes, proteins and metabolites and is a fundamental principle of cell biology (Wang & Bodovitz, 2010). In order to study this phenomenon, single cell analysis has been so far beyond our capability for the omics technology. This period is coming to an end with the rapidly changing field of single cell omics. Some emerging technologies such as micronanofluidics, microinterfaces for Mass Spectrometry and next generation DNA sequencing are allowing us in the next future to reach the new frontier in cell omics. This frontier will have the opportunity to transform completely systems biology analysis and finally address the issue of cell heterogeneity.

CONCLUDING REMARKS

Metabolomics is the new omics technique in the functional genomics field. It deals with the quantification and identification of the complete set of metabolites of a biological system. It integrates the other functional genomics levels, the mRNA and the proteins, and hence it represents the best view of the physiology of the cell, which correlates with the central dogma level and represents a highly robust network of biochemical reactions and cross-interactions. The study of the metabolic profile of a given biological state can be addressed in two principal ways. One way is static, a statistical description of the biochemical differences of our samples in study, using different multivariate statistical tools, from data reduction to classification algorithms; the second is the more dynamic way of viewing it of the metabolic and kinetic modeling of the network which can be simulated *in silico* and permits us to inspect and do hypothesis-driven research: the systems biology approach. The first approach drives metabonomic studies, the clinical ones now suffering an exponential growth of interest in the medical community, and although yet in its infancy, representing a promising new field. It is currently contributing not only to the finding of new biomarkers for the clinics, but also unraveling new clinically relevant metabolic pathways which could be used for the discovery of new targeted therapies. The systems biology approach is going to take longer time to achieve applicable results but is the most powerful tool for discovering new patterns in cell biology and biochemistry which will give us the basis, the foundations of the new functional genomics era, which hopefully in the future will integrate at the best level, the genes, the mRNA, the protein and the metabolism in genome-scale studies of cells, tissues, organs and organisms. To deal with this final goal, a great amount of interdisciplinary work has to be done, from mathematics, biostatistics, bioinformatics to analytical chemistry, biochemistry and molecular and cell biology. The challenge of research groups in this field in the future will be to bring together all these skills and to build and participate in big networks of promoting the interdisciplinary research and education of young scientists.

LIST OF ABBREVIATIONS

CPMG: Carr Purcell Meiboom Gill sequence
DSS: 4,4-dimethyl-4-silapentane-1-sulfonic acid
ERETIC: Electronic REference To asses In vivo Concentrations
FBA: Flux Balanced Analysis
FTIR: Fourier Transform Infrarred
HMDB: Human Metabolome Data Base
HSQC: Heteronuclear Single Quantum Coherence spectroscopy

KEGG: Kyoto Encyclopedia of Genes and Genomes
NOESY: Nuclear Overhauser Effect sequence
PCA: Principal Components Analysis
PLS: Partlial Least Square
PLS-DA: Partial Least Square Discriminant Analysis
SIRM: Stable Isotope-Resolved Metabolomics
SPE: Solid Phase Extraction
STOCSY: Statistical Total Correlation Spectroscopy
SVM: Support Vector Machine
TOCSY: Total Correlation Spectroscopy
TSP: Trimethylsilyl propionate
UPLC-TOF-MS: Ultra Performance Liquid Chromatography-Time of Flight-Mass Spectrometry

REFERENCES

Agnolet, S., Jaroszewski, J. W., Verpoorte, R., & Staerk, D. (2010). H NMR-based metabolomics combined with HPLC-PDA-MS-SPE-NMR for investigation of standardized Ginkgo biloba preparations. *Metabolomics*, *6*(2), 292–302. doi:10.1007/s11306-009-0195-x

Alves, R., Antunes, F., & Salvador, A. (2006). Tools for kinetic modeling of biochemical networks. *Nature Biotechnology*, *24*(6), 667–672. doi:10.1038/nbt0606-667

Anand, A., & Suganthan, P. N. (2009). Multiclass cancer classification by support vector machines with class-wise optimized genes and probability estimates. *Journal of Theoretical Biology*, *259*(3), 533–540. doi:10.1016/j.jtbi.2009.04.013

Ando, S., & Tanaka, Y. (2005). Mass spectrometric studies on brain metabolism, using stable isotopes. *Mass Spectrometry Reviews*, *24*(6), 865–886. doi:10.1002/mas.20045

Askenazi, M., Driggers, E. M., Holtzman, D. A., Norman, T. C., Iverson, S., & Zimmer, D. P. (2003). Integrating transcriptional and metabolite profiles to direct the engineering of lovastatin-producing fungal strains. *Nature Biotechnology*, *21*(2), 150–156. doi:10.1038/nbt781

Barantin, L., Le Pape, A., & Akoka, S. (1997). A new method for absolute quantitation of MRS metabolites. *Magnetic Resonance in Medicine*, *38*(2), 179–182. doi:10.1002/mrm.1910380203

Beckonert, O., Keun, H. C., Ebbels, T. M., Bundy, J., Holmes, E., & Lindon, J. C. (2007). Metabolic profiling, metabolomic and metabonomic procedures for NMR spectroscopy of urine, plasma, serum and tissue extracts. *Nature Protocols*, *2*(11), 2692–2703. doi:10.1038/nprot.2007.376

Beckonert, O., Monnerjahn, J., Bonk, U., & Leibfritz, D. (2003). Visualizing metabolic changes in breast-cancer tissue using 1H-NMR spectroscopy and self-organizing maps. *NMR in Biomedicine*, *16*(1), 1–11. doi:10.1002/nbm.797

Bijlsma, S., Bobeldijk, I., Verheij, E. R., Ramaker, R., Kochhar, S., & Macdonald, I. A. (2006). Large-scale human metabolomics studies: a strategy for data (pre-) processing and validation. *Analytical Chemistry*, *78*(2), 567–574. doi:10.1021/ac051495j

Boccard, J., Veuthey, J. L., & Rudaz, S. (2010). Knowledge discovery in metabolomics: an overview of MS data handling. *Journal of Separation Science*, *33*(3), 290–304. doi:10.1002/jssc.200900609

Brown, M., Dunn, W. B., Dobson, P., Patel, Y., Winder, C. L., & Francis-McIntyre, S. (2009). Mass spectrometry tools and metabolite-specific databases for molecular identification in metabolomics. *Analyst (London)*, *134*(7), 1322–1332. doi:10.1039/b901179j

Caspi, R., & Karp, P. D. (2007). Using the MetaCyc pathway database and the BioCyc database collection. *Curr Protoc Bioinformatics, Chapter 1*, Unit1 17.

Castrillo, J. I., Hayes, A., Mohammed, S., Gaskell, S. J., & Oliver, S. G. (2003). An optimized protocol for metabolome analysis in yeast using direct infusion electrospray mass spectrometry. *Phytochemistry*, *62*(6), 929–937. doi:10.1016/S0031-9422(02)00713-6

Chalcraft, K. R., Lee, R., Mills, C., & Britz-McKibbin, P. (2009). Virtual quantification of metabolites by capillary electrophoresis-electrospray ionization-mass spectrometry: predicting ionization efficiency without chemical standards. *Analytical Chemistry*, *81*(7), 2506–2515. doi:10.1021/ac802272u

Denkert, C., Budczies, J., Kind, T., Weichert, W., Tablack, P., & Sehouli, J. (2006). Mass spectrometry-based metabolic profiling reveals different metabolite patterns in invasive ovarian carcinomas and ovarian borderline tumors. *Cancer Research*, *66*(22), 10795–10804. doi:10.1158/0008-5472.CAN-06-0755

Dhar, P., Meng, T. C., Somani, S., Ye, L., Sairam, A., & Chitre, M. (2004). Cellware--a multi-algorithmic software for computational systems biology. *Bioinformatics (Oxford, England)*, *20*(8), 1319–1321. doi:10.1093/bioinformatics/bth067

Fagan, A., Culhane, A. C., & Higgins, D. G. (2007). A multivariate analysis approach to the integration of proteomic and gene expression data. *Proteomics*, *7*(13), 2162–2171. doi:10.1002/pmic.200600898

Faijes, M., Mars, A. E., & Smid, E. J. (2007). Comparison of quenching and extraction methodologies for metabolome analysis of Lactobacillus plantarum. *Microbial Cell Factories*, *6*, 27. doi:10.1186/1475-2859-6-27

Fan, T. W., Lane, A. N., Higashi, R. M., Farag, M. A., Gao, H., & Bousamra, M. (2009). Altered regulation of metabolic pathways in human lung cancer discerned by (13)C stable isotope-resolved metabolomics (SIRM). *Molecular Cancer, 8*, 41. doi:10.1186/1476-4598-8-41

Fan, T. W., Yuan, P., Lane, A. N., Higashi, R. M., Wang, Y., & Hamidi, A. B. (2010). Stable isotope-resolved metabolomic analysis of lithium effects on glial-neuronal metabolism and interactions. *Metabolomics, 6*(2), 165–179. doi:10.1007/s11306-010-0208-9

Fiehn, O. (2001). Combining genomics, metabolome analysis, and biochemical modelling to understand metabolic networks. *Comparative and Functional Genomics, 2*(3), 155–168. doi:10.1002/cfg.82

Fiehn, O. (2002). Metabolomics--the link between genotypes and phenotypes. *Plant Molecular Biology, 48*(1-2), 155–171. doi:10.1023/A:1013713905833

Funahashi, A., Jouraku, A., Matsuoka, Y., & Kitano, H. (2007). Integration of CellDesigner and SABIO-RK. *In Silico Biology, 7*(2Suppl), S81–S90.

Gagneur, J., & Casari, G. (2005). From molecular networks to qualitative cell behavior. *FEBS Letters, 579*(8), 1867–1871. doi:10.1016/j.febslet.2005.02.007

Gallant, P. J., Morin, E. L., & Peppard, L. E. (1998). Feature-based classification of myoelectric signals using artificial neural networks. *Medical & Biological Engineering & Computing, 36*(4), 485–489. doi:10.1007/BF02523219

German, J. B., Roberts, M. A., Fay, L., & Watkins, S. M. (2002). Metabolomics and individual metabolic assessment: the next great challenge for nutrition. *The Journal of Nutrition, 132*(9), 2486–2487.

German, J. B., Roberts, M. A., & Watkins, S. M. (2003). Personal metabolomics as a next generation nutritional assessment. *The Journal of Nutrition, 133*(12), 4260–4266.

German, J. B., Watkins, S. M., & Fay, L. B. (2005). Metabolomics in practice: emerging knowledge to guide future dietetic advice toward individualized health. *Journal of the American Dietetic Association, 105*(9), 1425–1432. doi:10.1016/j.jada.2005.06.006

Gizzatkulov, N. M., Goryanin, I. I., Metelkin, E. A., Mogilevskaya, E. A., Peskov, K. V., & Demin, O. V. (2010). DBSolve Optimum: a software package for kinetic modeling which allows dynamic visualization of simulation results. *BMC Systems Biology, 4*, 109. doi:10.1186/1752-0509-4-109

Godejohann, M., Tseng, L. H., Braumann, U., Fuchser, J., & Spraul, M. (2004). Characterization of a paracetamol metabolite using on-line LC-SPE-NMR-MS and a cryogenic NMR probe. *Journal of Chromatography. A, 1058*(1-2), 191–196.

Goldsmith, P., Fenton, H., Morris-Stiff, G., Ahmad, N., Fisher, J., & Prasad, K. R. (2010). Metabonomics: a useful tool for the future surgeon. *The Journal of Surgical Research, 160*(1), 122–132. doi:10.1016/j.jss.2009.03.003

Griffin, J. L. (2003). Metabonomics: NMR spectroscopy and pattern recognition analysis of body fluids and tissues for characterisation of xenobiotic toxicity and disease diagnosis. *Current Opinion in Chemical Biology, 7*(5), 648–654. doi:10.1016/j.cbpa.2003.08.008

Griffin, J. L., & Bollard, M. E. (2004). Metabonomics: its potential as a tool in toxicology for safety assessment and data integration. *Current Drug Metabolism, 5*(5), 389–398. doi:10.2174/1389200043335432

Guler, I., & Ubeyli, E. D. (2007). Multiclass support vector machines for EEG-signals classification. *IEEE Transactions on Information Technology in Biomedicine, 11*(2), 117–126. doi:10.1109/TITB.2006.879600

Gullberg, J., Jonsson, P., Nordstrom, A., Sjostrom, M., & Moritz, T. (2004). Design of experiments: an efficient strategy to identify factors influencing extraction and derivatization of Arabidopsis thaliana samples in metabolomic studies with gas chromatography/mass spectrometry. *Analytical Biochemistry, 331*(2), 283–295. doi:10.1016/j.ab.2004.04.037

Hiller, K., Hangebrauk, J., Jager, C., Spura, J., Schreiber, K., & Schomburg, D. (2009). MetaboliteDetector: comprehensive analysis tool for targeted and nontargeted GC/MS based metabolome analysis. *Analytical Chemistry, 81*(9), 3429–3439. doi:10.1021/ac802689c

Hoops, S., Sahle, S., Gauges, R., Lee, C., Pahle, J., & Simus, N. (2006). COPASI--a COmplex PAthway SImulator. *Bioinformatics (Oxford, England), 22*(24), 3067–3074. doi:10.1093/bioinformatics/btl485

Idborg-Bjorkman, H., Edlund, P. O., Kvalheim, O. M., Schuppe-Koistinen, I., & Jacobsson, S. P. (2003). Screening of biomarkers in rat urine using LC/electrospray ionization-MS and two-way data analysis. *Analytical Chemistry, 75*(18), 4784–4792. doi:10.1021/ac0341618

Ishii, N., Nakahigashi, K., Baba, T., Robert, M., Soga, T., & Kanai, A. (2007). Multiple high-throughput analyses monitor the response of E. coli to perturbations. *Science, 316*(5824), 593–597. doi:10.1126/science.1132067

Izquierdo-Garcia, J. L., Rodriguez, I., Kyriazis, A., Villa, P., Barreiro, P., & Desco, M. (2009). A novel R-package graphic user interface for the analysis of metabonomic profiles. *BMC Bioinformatics, 10*, 363. doi:10.1186/1471-2105-10-363

Joshi-Tope, G., Gillespie, M., Vastrik, I., D'Eustachio, P., Schmidt, E., & de Bono, B. (2005). Reactome: a knowledgebase of biological pathways. *Nucleic Acids Research, 33*(Database issue), D428–D432. doi:10.1093/nar/gki072

Kaddurah-Daouk, R., Kristal, B. S., & Weinshilboum, R. M. (2008). Metabolomics: a global biochemical approach to drug response and disease. *Annual Review of Pharmacology and Toxicology, 48*, 653–683. doi:10.1146/annurev.pharmtox.48.113006.094715

Kanehisa, M., Araki, M., Goto, S., Hattori, M., Hirakawa, M., & Itoh, M. (2008). KEGG for linking genomes to life and the environment. *Nucleic Acids Research, 36*(Database issue), D480–D484. doi:10.1093/nar/gkm882

Karp, P. D., Paley, S., Krieger, C. J., & Zhang, P. (2004). An evidence ontology for use in pathway/genome databases. *Pacific Symposium on Biocomputing. Pacific Symposium on Biocomputing*, 190–201.

Keerthi, S. S., & Shevade, S. K. (2003). SMO algorithm for least-squares SVM formulations. *Neural Computation, 15*(2), 487–507. doi:10.1162/089976603762553013

Kitano, H., Funahashi, A., Matsuoka, Y., & Oda, K. (2005). Using process diagrams for the graphical representation of biological networks. *Nature Biotechnology, 23*(8), 961–966. doi:10.1038/nbt1111

Krooshof, P. W., Ustun, B., Postma, G. J., & Buydens, L. M. (2010). Visualization and recovery of the (bio)chemical interesting variables in data analysis with support vector machine classification. *Analytical Chemistry, 82*(16), 7000–7007. doi:10.1021/ac101338y

Land, W. H. Jr, & Verheggen, E. A. (2009). Multiclass primal support vector machines for breast density classification. *Int J Comput Biol Drug Des, 2*(1), 21–57. doi:10.1504/IJCBDD.2009.027583

Lenz, E. M., & Wilson, I. D. (2007). Analytical strategies in metabonomics. *Journal of Proteome Research, 6*(2), 443–458. doi:10.1021/pr0605217

Ludwig, C., Ward, D. G., Martin, A., Viant, M. R., Ismail, T., & Johnson, P. J. (2009). Fast targeted multidimensional NMR metabolomics of colorectal cancer. *Magnetic Resonance in Chemistry, 47*(Suppl 1), S68–S73. doi:10.1002/mrc.2519

Luts, J., Ojeda, F., Van de Plas, R., De Moor, B., Van Huffel, S., & Suykens, J. A. (2010). A tutorial on support vector machine-based methods for classification problems in chemometrics. *Analytica Chimica Acta, 665*(2), 129–145. doi:10.1016/j.aca.2010.03.030

Mahadevan, S., Shah, S. L., Marrie, T. J., & Slupsky, C. M. (2008). Analysis of metabolomic data using support vector machines. *Analytical Chemistry, 80*(19), 7562–7570. doi:10.1021/ac800954c

Mapelli, V., Olsson, L., & Nielsen, J. (2008). Metabolic footprinting in microbiology: methods and applications in functional genomics and biotechnology. *Trends in Biotechnology, 26*(9), 490–497. doi:10.1016/j.tibtech.2008.05.008

Mehra, A., Lee, K. H., & Hatzimanikatis, V. (2003). Insights into the relation between mRNA and protein expression patterns: I. Theoretical considerations. *Biotechnology and Bioengineering, 84*(7), 822–833. doi:10.1002/bit.10860

Mendes, P. (1993). GEPASI: a software package for modelling the dynamics, steady states and control of biochemical and other systems. *Computer Applications in the Biosciences, 9*(5), 563–571.

Michopoulos, F., Lai, L., Gika, H., Theodoridis, G., & Wilson, I. (2009). UPLC-MS-based analysis of human plasma for metabonomics using solvent precipitation or solid phase extraction. *Journal of Proteome Research, 8*(4), 2114–2121. doi:10.1021/pr801045q

Mogilevskaya, E., Bagrova, N., Plyusnina, T., Gizzatkulov, N., Metelkin, E., & Goryacheva, E. (2009). Kinetic modeling as a tool to integrate multilevel dynamic experimental data. *Methods in Molecular Biology (Clifton, N.J.), 563*, 197–218. doi:10.1007/978-1-60761-175-2_11

Morgenthal, K., Weckwerth, W., & Steuer, R. (2006). Metabolomic networks in plants: Transitions from pattern recognition to biological interpretation. *Bio Systems, 83*(2-3), 108–117. doi:10.1016/j.biosystems.2005.05.017

Morgenthal, K., Wienkoop, S., Wolschin, F., & Weckwerth, W. (2007). Integrative profiling of metabolites and proteins: improving pattern recognition and biomarker selection for systems level approaches. *Methods in Molecular Biology (Clifton, N.J.), 358*, 57–75. doi:10.1007/978-1-59745-244-1_4

Nie, L., Wu, G., Culley, D. E., Scholten, J. C., & Zhang, W. (2007). Integrative analysis of transcriptomic and proteomic data: challenges, solutions and applications. *Critical Reviews in Biotechnology, 27*(2), 63–75. doi:10.1080/07388550701334212

Nie, L., Wu, G., & Zhang, W. (2006). Correlation of mRNA expression and protein abundance affected by multiple sequence features related to translational efficiency in Desulfovibrio vulgaris: a quantitative analysis. *Genetics, 174*(4), 2229–2243. doi:10.1534/genetics.106.065862

Oldiges, M., Lutz, S., Pflug, S., Schroer, K., Stein, N., & Wiendahl, C. (2007). Metabolomics: current state and evolving methodologies and tools. *Applied Microbiology and Biotechnology, 76*(3), 495–511. doi:10.1007/s00253-007-1029-2

Paley, S. M., & Karp, P. D. (2006). The Pathway Tools cellular overview diagram and Omics Viewer. *Nucleic Acids Research, 34*(13), 3771–3778. doi:10.1093/nar/gkl334

Pers, T. H., Albrechtsen, A., Holst, C., Sorensen, T. I., & Gerds, T. A. (2009). The validation and assessment of machine learning: a game of prediction from high-dimensional data. *PLoS ONE, 4*(8), e6287. doi:10.1371/journal.pone.0006287

Pope, G. A., MacKenzie, D. A., Defernez, M., Aroso, M. A., Fuller, L. J., & Mellon, F. A. (2007). Metabolic footprinting as a tool for discriminating between brewing yeasts. *Yeast (Chichester, England), 24*(8), 667–679. doi:10.1002/yea.1499

Pope, G. A., MacKenzie, D. A., Defernez, M., & Roberts, I. N. (2009). Metabolic footprinting for the study of microbial biodiversity. *Cold Spring Harb Protoc, 2009*(5), pdb prot5222.

Ruppin, E., Papin, J. A., de Figueiredo, L. F., & Schuster, S. (2010). Metabolic reconstruction, constraint-based analysis and game theory to probe genome-scale metabolic networks. *Current Opinion in Biotechnology, 21*(4), 502–510. doi:10.1016/j.copbio.2010.07.002

Sansone, S. A., Fan, T., Goodacre, R., Griffin, J. L., Hardy, N. W., & Kaddurah-Daouk, R. (2007). The metabolomics standards initiative. *Nature Biotechnology, 25*(8), 846–848. doi:10.1038/nbt0807-846b

Sarwal, M. M. (2009). Deconvoluting the 'omics' for organ transplantation. *Current Opinion in Organ Transplantation, 14*(5), 544–551. doi:10.1097/MOT.0b013e32833068fb

Sellick, C. A., Hansen, R., Maqsood, A. R., Dunn, W. B., Stephens, G. M., & Goodacre, R. (2009). Effective quenching processes for physiologically valid metabolite profiling of suspension cultured Mammalian cells. *Analytical Chemistry, 81*(1), 174–183. doi:10.1021/ac8016899

Serkova, N. J., Spratlin, J. L., & Eckhardt, S. G. (2007). NMR-based metabolomics: translational application and treatment of cancer. *Current Opinion in Molecular Therapeutics, 9*(6), 572–585.

Smart, K. F., Aggio, R. B., Van Houtte, J. R., & Villas-Boas, S. G. (2010). Analytical platform for metabolome analysis of microbial cells using methyl chloroformate derivatization followed by gas chromatography-mass spectrometry. *Nature Protocols, 5*(10), 1709–1729. doi:10.1038/nprot.2010.108

Spratlin, J. L., Serkova, N. J., & Eckhardt, S. G. (2009). Clinical applications of metabolomics in oncology: a review. *Clinical Cancer Research, 15*(2), 431–440. doi:10.1158/1078-0432.CCR-08-1059

Stein, L. D. (2004). Using the Reactome database. *Curr Protoc Bioinformatics, Chapter 8*, Unit 8 7.

Tang, H., Xiao, C., & Wang, Y. (2009). Important roles of the hyphenated HPLC-DAD-MS-SPE-NMR technique in metabonomics. *Magnetic Resonance in Chemistry, 47*(Suppl 1), S157–S162. doi:10.1002/mrc.2513

Torres-Garcia, W., Zhang, W., Runger, G. C., Johnson, R. H., & Meldrum, D. R. (2009). Integrative analysis of transcriptomic and proteomic data of Desulfovibrio vulgaris: a non-linear model to predict abundance of undetected proteins. *Bioinformatics (Oxford, England), 25*(15), 1905–1914. doi:10.1093/bioinformatics/btp325

Trauger, S. A., Kalisak, E., Kalisiak, J., Morita, H., Weinberg, M. V., & Menon, A. L. (2008). Correlating the transcriptome, proteome, and metabolome in the environmental adaptation of a hyperthermophile. *Journal of Proteome Research, 7*(3), 1027–1035. doi:10.1021/pr700609j

Trygg, J., Holmes, E., & Lundstedt, T. (2007). Chemometrics in metabonomics. *Journal of Proteome Research, 6*(2), 469–479. doi:10.1021/pr060594q

Tsang, T. M., Haselden, J. N., & Holmes, E. (2009). Metabonomic characterization of the 3-nitropropionic acid rat model of Huntington's disease. *Neurochemical Research*, *34*(7), 1261–1271. doi:10.1007/s11064-008-9904-5

van Velzen, E. J., Westerhuis, J. A., van Duynhoven, J. P., van Dorsten, F. A., Hoefsloot, H. C., & Jacobs, D. M. (2008). Multilevel data analysis of a crossover designed human nutritional intervention study. *Journal of Proteome Research*, *7*(10), 4483–4491. doi:10.1021/pr800145j

Viant, M. R. (2003). Improved methods for the acquisition and interpretation of NMR metabolomic data. *Biochemical and Biophysical Research Communications*, *310*(3), 943–948. doi:10.1016/j.bbrc.2003.09.092

Viant, M. R. (2007). Revealing the metabolome of animal tissues using 1H nuclear magnetic resonance spectroscopy. *Methods in Molecular Biology (Clifton, N.J.)*, *358*, 229–246. doi:10.1007/978-1-59745-244-1_13

Villas-Boas, S. G., & Bruheim, P. (2007). The potential of metabolomics tools in bioremediation studies. *OMICS: A Journal of Integrative Biology*, *11*(3), 305–313. doi:10.1089/omi.2007.0005

Villas-Boas, S. G., Hojer-Pedersen, J., Akesson, M., Smedsgaard, J., & Nielsen, J. (2005). Global metabolite analysis of yeast: evaluation of sample preparation methods. *Yeast (Chichester, England)*, *22*(14), 1155–1169. doi:10.1002/yea.1308

Wang, D., & Bodovitz, S. (2010). Single cell analysis: the new frontier in 'omics'. *Trends in Biotechnology*, *28*(6), 281–290. doi:10.1016/j.tibtech.2010.03.002

Want, E. J., O'Maille, G., Smith, C. A., Brandon, T. R., Uritboonthai, W., & Qin, C. (2006). Solvent-dependent metabolite distribution, clustering, and protein extraction for serum profiling with mass spectrometry. *Analytical Chemistry*, *78*(3), 743–752. doi:10.1021/ac051312t

Want, E. J., Wilson, I. D., Gika, H., Theodoridis, G., Plumb, R. S., & Shockcor, J. (2010). Global metabolic profiling procedures for urine using UPLC-MS. *Nature Protocols*, *5*(6), 1005–1018. doi:10.1038/nprot.2010.50

Weckwerth, W., & Morgenthal, K. (2005). Metabolomics: from pattern recognition to biological interpretation. *Drug Discovery Today*, *10*(22), 1551–1558. doi:10.1016/S1359-6446(05)03609-3

Weljie, A. M., Newton, J., Mercier, P., Carlson, E., & Slupsky, C. M. (2006). Targeted profiling: quantitative analysis of 1H NMR metabolomics data. *Analytical Chemistry*, *78*(13), 4430–4442. doi:10.1021/ac060209g

Werth, M. T., Halouska, S., Shortridge, M. D., Zhang, B., & Powers, R. (n.d.). Analysis of metabolomic PCA data using tree diagrams. *Analytical Biochemistry*, *399*(1), 58–63. doi:10.1016/j.ab.2009.12.022

Westerhuis, J. A., van Velzen, E. J., Hoefsloot, H. C., & Smilde, A. K. (2010). Multivariate paired data analysis: multilevel PLSDA versus OPLSDA. *Metabolomics*, *6*(1), 119–128. doi:10.1007/s11306-009-0185-z

Winder, C. L., Dunn, W. B., Schuler, S., Broadhurst, D., Jarvis, R., & Stephens, G. M. (2008). Global metabolic profiling of Escherichia coli cultures: an evaluation of methods for quenching and extraction of intracellular metabolites. *Analytical Chemistry*, *80*(8), 2939–2948. doi:10.1021/ac7023409

Wishart, D. S. (2005). Metabolomics: the principles and potential applications to transplantation. *American Journal of Transplantation*, *5*(12), 2814–2820. doi:10.1111/j.1600-6143.2005.01119.x

Wishart, D. S. (2007). Current progress in computational metabolomics. *Briefings in Bioinformatics*, *8*(5), 279–293. doi:10.1093/bib/bbm030

Wishart, D. S. (2010). Computational approaches to metabolomics. *Methods in Molecular Biology (Clifton, N.J.)*, *593*, 283–313. doi:10.1007/978-1-60327-194-3_14

Wishart, D. S., Knox, C., Guo, A. C., Eisner, R., Young, N., & Gautam, B. (2009). HMDB: a knowledgebase for the human metabolome. *Nucleic Acids Research*, *37*(Database issue), D603–D610. doi:10.1093/nar/gkn810

Xia, J., Bjorndahl, T. C., Tang, P., & Wishart, D. S. (2008). MetaboMiner--semi-automated identification of metabolites from 2D NMR spectra of complex biofluids. *BMC Bioinformatics*, *9*, 507. doi:10.1186/1471-2105-9-507

Xia, J., Psychogios, N., Young, N., & Wishart, D. S. (2009). MetaboAnalyst: a web server for metabolomic data analysis and interpretation. *Nucleic Acids Res, 37*(Web Server issue), W652-660.

Zelena, E., Dunn, W. B., Broadhurst, D., Francis-McIntyre, S., Carroll, K. M., & Begley, P. (2009). Development of a robust and repeatable UPLC-MS method for the long-term metabolomic study of human serum. *Analytical Chemistry*, *81*(4), 1357–1364. doi:10.1021/ac8019366

Zhang, H., Holford, T., & Bracken, M. B. (1996). A tree-based method of analysis for prospective studies. *Statistics in Medicine*, *15*(1), 37–49. doi:10.1002/(SICI)1097-0258(19960115)15:1<37::AID-SIM144>3.0.CO;2-0

Zhang, W., Li, F., & Nie, L. (2010). Integrating multiple 'omics' analysis for microbial biology: application and methodologies. *Microbiology*, *156*(Pt 2), 287–301. doi:10.1099/mic.0.034793-0

Zhang, W., Li, F., & Nie, L. (n.d.). Integrating multiple 'omics' analysis for microbial biology: application and methodologies. *Microbiology*, *156*(Pt 2), 287–301. doi:10.1099/mic.0.034793-0

Zhang, X., Liu, H., Wu, J., Zhang, X., Liu, M., & Wang, Y. (2009). Metabonomic alterations in hippocampus, temporal and prefrontal cortex with age in rats. *Neurochemistry International*, *54*(8), 481–487. doi:10.1016/j.neuint.2009.02.004

Zhao, Q., Stoyanova, R., Du, S., Sajda, P., & Brown, T. R. (2006). HiRes--a tool for comprehensive assessment and interpretation of metabolomic data. *Bioinformatics (Oxford, England)*, *22*(20), 2562–2564. doi:10.1093/bioinformatics/btl428

Chapter 3
Computational Sequence Design Techniques for DNA Microarray Technologies

Dan Tulpan
National Research Council of Canada, Canada

Athos Ghiggi
University of Lugano (USI), Switzerland

Roberto Montemanni
Istituto Dalle Molle di Studi sull'Intelligenza Artificiale (IDSIA), Switzerland

ABSTRACT

In systems biology and biomedical research, microarray technology is a method of choice that enables the complete quantitative and qualitative ascertainment of gene expression patterns for whole genomes. The selection of high quality oligonucleotide sequences that behave consistently across multiple experiments is a key step in the design, fabrication and experimental performance of DNA microarrays. The aim of this chapter is to outline recent algorithmic developments in microarray probe design, evaluate existing probe sequences used in commercial arrays, and suggest methodologies that have the potential to improve on existing design techniques.

INTRODUCTION

The design of DNA oligos is a key step in the manufacturing process of modern microarrays – biotechnology tools that allow the parallel qualification and quantification of large numbers of genes. Areas that have benefited from the use of microarrays include gene discovery (Andrews

DOI: 10.4018/978-1-61350-435-2.ch003

et al., 2000; Yano, Imai, Shimizu, & Hanashita, 2006), disease diagnosis (Yoo, Choi, Lee, & Yoo, 2009), species identification (Pasquer, Pelludat, Duffy, & Frey, 2010; Teletcheal, Bernillon, Duffraisse, Laudet, & Hänni, 2008) and toxicogenomics (Jang, Nde, Toghrol, & Bentley, 2008; Neumanna and Galvez, 2002).

Microarrays consist of plastic or glass slides, to which a large number of short DNA sequences (probes) are affixed at known positions in a matrix

Copyright © 2012, IGI Global. Copying or distributing in print or electronic forms without written permission of IGI Global is prohibited.

pattern. A probe is a relatively short DNA sequence (20-70 bases) representing the complement of a contiguous sequence of bases from a target that acts as its fingerprint. The purpose of each probe is to uniquely identify and bind a target via a process called hybridization. Nevertheless, in practice probes could bind to more than one target via a process called cross-hybridization.

While microarrays could be used for a variety of applications like transcription factor binding site identification (Hanlon & Lieb, 2004), eukaryotic DNA replication (MacAlpine & Bell, 2005), and array comparative genomics hybridization (Pinkel & Albertson, 2005), their main use remains gene transcript expression profiling (Schena, Shalon, Davis, & Brown, 1995; Ross *et al.*, 2000; Aarhus, Helland, Lund-Johansen, Wester & Knappskog, 2010). However, at present, the fundamental understandings of the bio-chemo-physical mechanisms that power this technology are poorly understood (Pozhitkov, Tautz, & Noble, 2007), thus leading to hybridization signal levels that are still not accurately correlated with exact amounts of target transcripts. While most of the microarray research work carried today focuses on the development of reliable and fault-tolerant statistical techniques that could pre-process large data sets (Holloway, van Laar, Tothill, & Bowtell, 2002; Irizarry *et al.*, 2003; Quackenbush, 2002; Yang *et al.*, 2002; Zhao, Li, & Simon, 2005) and identify significant factors relevant to each particular study (Chu, Ghahramani, Falciani, & Wild, 2005; Harris & Ghaffari, 2008; Leung & Hung, 2010; Peng, Li, & Liu, 2007; Zou, Yang, & Zhu, 2006), more work needs to be done on improving the infrastructural aspects of microarray technology, thus reducing the amount of noise earlier rather than later in an experiment based on microarrays data.

Thus, one of the greatest challenges in DNA microarray design resides in how to select large sets of unique probes that distinguish among specific sequences from complex samples consisting of thousands of closely similar targets. The daunting task of designing such large sets of probes is hampered by the computational costs associated with probe efficacy evaluations. Various design strategies are presented that employ the utilization of intricate probe evaluation criteria. Some of these strategies were inspired from design techniques employed for solving similar problems that arise in coding theory (Bogdanova, Brouwer, Kapralov, & Östergård, 2001; Gaborit & King, 2005; Gamal, Hemachandra, Shperling, & Wei, 1987), bio-molecular computing (Feldkamp, Banzhaf, & Rauhe, 2000; Frutos *et al.*, 1997), molecular tagging (Braich *et al.*, 2003; Brenner & Lerner, 1992) and nano-structure design (Reif, Labean, & Seeman, 2001; Yurke, Turberfield, Mills, Simmel, & Neumann, 2000).

In recent years there has been considerable interest in the application of meta-heuristic algorithms for the design of DNA strands to be used in microarray technologies. Most of the proposed algorithms deal with combinatorial constraints only (Frutos *et al.*, 1997; Marathe, Condon, & Corn, 2001; Kobayashi, Kondo, & Arita, 2003), in order to increase the tractability of the problem from a computational point of view. On the other hand, because of this simplification, the strands obtained do not always have the desired characteristics when used in experimental settings. Therefore, thermodynamic constraints are typically employed to have satisfactory results in practice, notwithstanding they tend to destroy most of the combinatorial structures exploited by the algorithms themselves. A summary of state-of-the-art combinatorial algorithms is presented here. We then describe how two algorithms originally developed for combinatorial constraints can be extended to efficiently deal with thermodynamic constraints.

The first approach is a Stochastic Local Search method originally described in (Tulpan, Hoos, & Condon, 2002; Tulpan & Hoos, 2003; Tulpan, 2006), which works on the search space of infeasible solutions. This means it starts with a given number of random strands, violating many constraints. There is a fitness measure estimating the severity of the total constraints violation of the solution. The algorithm iteratively modifies the strands with the target of improving the fitness. In the end, if all the constraints are fulfilled, a feasible solution has been found; otherwise the minimal set of strings causing violations can be deleted in order to have a feasible solution.

The second approach analyzed is a Seed Building procedure, originally described in (Montemanni & Smith, 2008; Montemanni & Smith, 2009a; Ghiggi, 2010). Differently from the Stochastic Local Search, this method works on the space of feasible solutions: it starts from an empty set of strands and iteratively enlarges it with strands, which are feasible with those already added to the set. From time to time the set is partially destroyed in order to diversify the search.

De-novo experimental results are presented for the two meta-heuristic algorithms discussed. Based on a set of combinatorial and thermodynamic criteria presented in literature, we present a case study including the evaluation of existing probe sets used in Affymetrix microarrays where probe and target sequence information is publicly available. Analyses of such sets provide insights on their strengths and weaknesses and also shed light on potential areas of improvement that can only empower the existing technologies thus increasing their impact in the specific areas of applicability. For example, high throughput similarity searches performed on Affymetrix probe sets of Human Gene arrays and the most recent gene sequence information available in public databases (NCBI, Ensembl) reveal that close to 5-10% of the probes used on some arrays are either not unique or they do not identify the correct target (Wang *et al.*, 2007). Here, we present further evidence, that a careful re-analysis and re-consideration of the microarray probe design techniques for different microarrays should be explored in greater detail.

RELATED WORK

A large number of computational probe design techniques (see Table 1) have been developed over the past 15 years and their impact on the microarray-based experimental results is massive. A number of review papers (Kreil, Russell, & Russell, 2006; Lemoine, Combes, & Le Crom, 2009) collect and describe the particular features of each package, including the set of constraints used for probe design, their versatility, usability and availability.

From a software design perspective, typically, probe design applications can be grouped into two categories: (1) client-server applications; and (2) autonomous software.

Client-Server Software

The client-server category is well represented by a series of software packages like ChipD (Dufour *et al.*, 2010), FastPCR (Kalendar, Lee, & Schulman, 2009), Gene2Oligo (Rouillard, Lee, Truan, Gao, Zhou, *et al.*, 2004), MPrime (Rouchka, Khalyfa, & Cooper, 2005), OligoDB (Mrowka, Schuchhardt, & Gille, 2002), OligoDesign (Tolstrup *et al.*, 2003), OligoWiz (Nielsen, Wernersson, & Knudsen, 2003), Osprey (Gordon & Sensen, 2004), ProbeWiz (Nielsen & Knudsen, 2002) and ROSO (Reymond *et al.*, 2004) that use various algorithmic techniques and constraint combinations. Due to the computational speed and information transfer limitations via web services, many of these applications are optimized for speed, thus the selection of criteria used for probe design tend to be more combinatorial, heuristic and empirical in nature.

One of the latest software, ChipD (Dufour *et al.*, 2010), is a new probe design web server that facilitates the design of oligos for high-density tilling arrays. The software relies on an algorithm that optimizes probe selection by assigning scores based on three criteria, namely specificity, ther-

Table 1. A selection of popular probe design software packages and their availability as of August 2010. The acronyms used in this table have the following meaning: WD = web download, NA = not available (web site), FA = from authors, CS = client-server

Software	Reference	URL	Status
ARB	(Ludwig *et al.*, 2004)	http://www.arb-home.de/	WD
Array Designer 4.25	(Premier Biosoft)	http://www.softpedia.com/get/Science-CAD/Array-Designer.shtml	WD
ArrayOligoSelector	(Bozdech *et al.*, 2003)	http://arrayoligosel.sourceforge.net/	WD
ChipD	(Dufour *et al.*, 2010)	http://chipd.uwbacter.org/	CS
CommOligo v2.0	(Li, Hel, & Zhou, 2005)	http://ieg.ou.edu/software.htm	WD
Featurama/ProbePicker	(ProbePicker)	http://probepicker.sourceforge.net/	NA
GenomePRIDE v1.0	(Haas *et al.*, 2003)	http://pride.molgen.mpg.de/genomepride.html	FA
GoArrays	(Rimour, Hill, Militon, & Peyret, 2005)	http://www.isima.fr/bioinfo/goarrays/	NA
HPD	(Chung *et al.*, 2005)	http://brcapp.kribb.re.kr/HPD/	NA
MPrime	(Rouchka, Khalyfa, & Cooper, 2005)	http://kbrin.a-bldg.louisville.edu/Tools/MPrime/	CS
OliCheck	(Charbonnier *et al.*, 2005)	http://www.genomic.ch/download.php	WD
Olid	(Talla, Tekaia, Brino, & Dujon, 2003)	NA	FA
OligoArray v2	(Rouillard, Zuker, & Gulari, 2003)	http://berry.engin.umich.edu/oligoarray2/	WD
OligoDb	(Mrowka, Schuchhardt, & Gille, 2002)	http://bioinf.charite.de/oligodb/	CS
OligoDesign	(Tolstrup *et al.*, 2003)	http://oligo.lnatools.com/expression/	CS
OligoFaktory	(Schretter & Milinkovitch, 2006)	http://oligofaktory.lanevol.org/index.jsp	FA
OligoPicker	(Wang & Seed, 2003)	http://pga.mgh.harvard.edu/oligopicker/	WD
OligoSpawn	(Zheng *et al.*, 2006)	http://oligospawn.ucr.edu/	NA
OligoWiz	(Nielsen, Wernersson, & Knudsen, 2003)	http://www.cbs.dtu.dk/services/OligoWiz/	WD, CS
Oliz	(Chen & Sharp, 2002)	http://www.utmem.edu/pharmacology/otherlinks/oliz.html	NA
Osprey	(Gordon & Sensen, 2004)	http://osprey.ucalgary.ca/cgi-bin/oligo_array	CS
PICKY	(Chou, Hsia, Mooney, & Schnable, 2004)	http://www.complex.iastate.edu/download/Picky/index.html	WD
PrimeArray	(Raddatz, Dehio, Meyer, & Dehio, 2001)	http://pages.unibas.ch/wtt/Products/PrimeArray/primearray.html	FA
PRIMEGENS v2	(Srivastava, Guo, Shi, & Xu, 2008)	http://compbio.ornl.gov/structure/primegens/	NA

continues on following page

Table 1. Continued

Software	Reference	URL	Status
ProbeMaker	(Stenberg, Nilsson, & Landegren, 2005)	http://probemaker.sourceforge.net/	WD
Probemer	(Emrich, Lowe, & Delcher, 2003)	http://probemer.cs.loyola.edu/	NA
Probe-sel	(Kaderali & Schliep, 2002)	NA	FA
ProbeSelect	(Li & Stormo, 2001)	http://ural.wustl.edu/resources.html	NA
ProbeWiz	(Nielsen & Knudsen, 2002)	http://www.cbs.dtu.dk/services/DNAarray/probewiz.php	CS
ProMide	(Rahmann, 2003)	http://oligos.molgen.mpg.de/	FA
ROSO	(Reymond *et al.*, 2004)	http://pbil.univ-lyon1.fr/roso/	CS, NA
SEPON	(Hornshoj, Stengaard, Panitz, & Bendixen, 2004)	http://www.agrsci.dk/hag/sepon/	NA
Teolenn	(Jourdren *et al.*, 2010)	http://transcriptome.ens.fr/teolenn/	WD
SLSDNADesigner	(Tulpan *et al.*, 2005)	http://www.cs.ubc.ca/labs/beta/Software/DnaCodeDesign/	WD
YODA	(Nordberg, 2005)	http://pathport.vbi.vt.edu/YODA/	NA

modynamic uniformity and uniform coverage of the genome.

OligoDesign (Tolstrup *et al.*, 2003) provides optimal locked nucleic acid (LNA) probes for gene expression profiling. As a first step, the software reduces probe cross-hybridization effects by employing a genome-wide BLAST analysis against a given set of targets. Next, each probe gets assigned a combined fuzzy logic score based on melting temperature, self-annealing and secondary structure for LNA oligos and targets. At the end, the highest ranking probe is reported.

OligoWiz (Nielsen, Wernersson, & Knudsen, 2003) selects probes based on a set of five criteria: specificity, melting temperature, position within transcripts, sequence complexity and base composition. A score is assigned for each criterion per probe and a weighted score is computed. The probes with the best scores are further selected and visualized in a graphical interface.

Osprey (Gordon & Sensen, 2004) designs oligonucleotides for microarrays and DNA sequencing and incorporates a set of algorithmic

and methodological novelties including hardware acceleration, parallel computations, position-specific scoring matrices, which are combined with a series of filters including melting temperature, dimer potential, hairpin potential and secondary (non-specific) binding.

ProbeWiz (Nielsen & Knudsen, 2002) is a probe design client-server application that relies on a two stage approach. In the first stage, the input sequences (FASTA or GenBank accession numbers) are locally aligned with BLAST (Altschul, Gish, Miller, Myers, & Lipman, 1990) against a selected database and the result is filtered using melting temperature, dimer potential, hairpin potential and secondary (non-specific) binding. The second stage optimizes the input obtained in the previous stage by applying a set of filters including probe length, melting temperature, 3' proximity, a probe quality score obtained with PRIMER3 (Rozen & Skaletsky, 2000) and a paralogy score.

ROSO (Reymond *et al.*, 2004) consists of a suite of 5 probe selection steps. First, it filters out all input sequences that are identical and masks also the repeated bases within them. The second step consists of a similarity search using BLAST. Next step consists of eliminating probes that self-hybridize. The fourth step eliminates all probes that have undesired melting temperatures. The last step selects a final set of probes based on four additional criteria: GC content, first and last bases, base repetitions and self-hybridization free energies.

Autonomous Software

The autonomous software category includes a wider variety of programs that allows the user to have more control over the platform where the application is installed and run, while permitting in the same time the usage of larger input files and better control of the configuration parameters.

OliCheck (Charbonnier *et al.*, 2005) is a program designed to test the validity of potential microarray probes by considering the possibility of cross-hybridization with non-target coding sequences. This analysis can be performed within a single genome or between several different strains/organisms.

OligoArray (Rouillard, Herbert, & Zuker, 2002) takes into account the following criteria: specificity, position within transcript, melting temperature, self hybridization and presence of specific subsequences in the probe. The algorithm runs as follows: it selects a probe starting from the end of the first sequence in the input data set and checks it against all the aforementioned criteria. If the probe satisfies all criteria, the algorithm moves to the next input sequence; otherwise it selects a new probe after a 10 base jump towards the 5' end of the input sequence. The process continues until a probe that satisfies all criteria is found. If no such probe is found, the algorithm selects a probe that has a lower probability for cross hybridization. The second version of OligoArray (Rouillard, Zuker, & Gulari, 2003) introduces thermodynamic constraints in the design of oligos.

The ProbeSelect (Li & Stormo, 2001) algorithm is centered on the specificity of sequences and consists of seven steps. First, the program builds a suffix array for the input sequences, to quickly identify the high similarity regions in the input sequences. Then, the algorithm builds a landscape for each input sequence. A landscape represents the frequency in the suffix array of all subsequences in the query input sequence. The third step consists in selecting a list with 10 to 20 candidate probes for each input sequence that minimizes the sum of the frequencies of their subsequences in the suffix array. The fourth step consists in searching for potential cross-hybridizations between each probe and the set of input sequences. Step 5 marks the cross-hybridizations within the input sequences. The next step consists of melting temperature and self-hybridization free energy computations for each remaining probe. The last step consists in selecting the probes, which have the most stable perfect-match free energy and hybridize the least with all the other potential targets.

Some autonomous oligonucleotide design programs are implemented in scripting languages like Perl or Python and are usually much slower than those implemented in C++. OligoPicker (Wang & Seed, 2003) is a Perl program, which also uses a traditional approach. The criteria taken into account are specificity (use of BLAST), melting temperature and position in the transcripts. ProMide (Rahmann, 2003) consists of a set of Perl scripts, with a C program for basic calculations, which uses the longest common substring as a specificity measure for the oligonucleotides. It uses complex data structures such as 'enhanced suffix array' and some statistical properties of sequences. Oliz (Chen & Sharp, 2002) is also implemented in Perl and uses a classical approach relying on BLAST for specificity testing. It however requires additional software to function, like cap3, clustalw, EMBOSS "prima" and a database in the UniGene format. The originality of the method stems from the fact that the oligonucleotides are searched in the 3' untranslated region of the mRNAs, a very specific area where sequences are largely available through expressed sequence tag projects.

The majority of the client-server and autonomous software described above use a pipelined filtering approach for the design of microarray probes, where at an initial stage a local alignment approach is employed for cross-hybridization avoidance and then each ulterior filter evaluates the quality of each probe and ranks them according to well defined scoring criteria.

DNA SEQUENCE DESIGN: PROBLEM DESCRIPTION

A single stranded DNA molecule is a long, unbranched polymer composed of only four types of subunits. These subunits are the deoxyribonucleotides containing the bases adenine (A), cytosine (C), guanine (G) and thymine (T). The nucleotides are linked together by chemical bonds and they are attached to a sugar-phosphate chain like four kinds of beads strung on a necklace (Figure 1). The sugar-phosphate chain is composed by alternating the ribose and phosphate for each nucleotide. This alternating structure gives each base and implicitly the whole strand a direction from the ribose end (denoted by 5') to the phosphate end (denoted by 3'). When the 5'/3' ends are not explicitly labeled, DNA sequences are assumed to be written in 5' to 3' direction.

The nucleotides composing DNA bind to each other in pairs via hydrogen bonds in a process known as hybridization. Each nucleotide pairs up with its unique complement (the Watson-Crick complement), so C pairs up with G and A with T. C and G pair up in a more stable manner than A and T do, which is due to one extra hydrogen bond in the C-G pair. The Watson-Crick complement of a DNA strand is the strand obtained by replacing each C nucleotide with a G and vice versa, and each T nucleotide with an A and vice versa, and also switching the 5' and 3' ends. For example the Watson-Crick complement of 5'-AACTAG-3' is 3'-TTGATC-5'. Non-Watson-Crick base pairings are also possible. For example, G-T pairs occur naturally in biological sequences (Ho *et al.*, 1985; Pfaff *et al.*, 2008).

Formally, these notions are captured in the following definitions:

A DNA strand w is represented by a string over the quaternary alphabet $\{A, C, G, T\}$. String w corresponds to a single-stranded DNA molecule with the left end of the string corresponding to the 5'-end of the DNA strand.

The complement, or Watson-Crick complement, of a DNA strand w is obtained by reversing w and then by replacing each A with a T and vice versa, and replacing each C in the strand by G and vice versa. We denote the Watson-Crick complement of a DNA strand w with $c(w)$ and we will simply use the terms *complementary strand*, or *complement* in this work. For simplicity, we simply use c_i instead of $c(w_i)$.

Throughout the remainder of the chapter we use symbols $w_1, w_2, ..., w_k$ to denote unique strands and $c_1, c_2, ..., c_k$ to denote the corresponding complements. Thus, strand w_i and complement c_i form

Figure 1. Idealized structure of a pair of hybridized DNA sequences

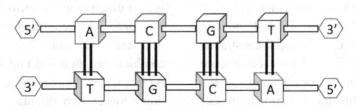

a perfect match (duplex), whereas strand w_i and complement c_j, and complements c_i and c_j, with $j \neq i$, form mismatches. We will call *probes* the strands attached to the surface of microarrays, while *targets* are the corresponding complements floating in the solution. We adopt this terminology because it is widely used in the literature on DNA microarrays.

Finally, we formalize the optimization version of the DNA Strand Design Problem.

The DNA Strand Design (DSD) Problem is defined as follows: with respect to a fixed set C of constraints (which are part of the input and will be detailed in the remainder of the section), given a strand length n, find the largest possible set S with DNA strands of length n, satisfying all the constraints in C.

The constraints used in the design of DNA strands can be grouped into two classes: *combinatorial* and *thermodynamic* constraints. The grouping is based on the measures that estimate the quality of one or more DNA strands upon which the constraint is applied. Combinatorial constraints mostly rely on verifying the presence or absence of certain nucleotides in a strand, and counting of matches and/or mismatches for pairs of DNA strands, whereas thermodynamic constraints take into account the biochemical properties that govern DNA hybridization.

Combinatorial Constraints

Combinatorial constraints are widely used to design large sets of non-interacting DNA strands. The necessity of designing sets of strands that avoid cross-hybridization can be superficially modeled by enforcing a high number of mismatches between all possible pairs of strands and between pairs of strands and the complements of others. The stability and uniformity of DNA strands can be also modeled with combinatorial constraints by either controlling the presence or absence of undesired subsequences or counting specific bases within the same strand. Various types of combinatorial constraints can be considered. In the following paragraphs we will formalize those of interest for our study.

C1: Direct Mismatches: The number of mismatches in a perfect alignment of two strands (also referred to as *Hamming distance*) must be above a given threshold d. Here, a perfect alignment is a pairing of bases from the two strands, where the ith base of the first strand is paired with the ith base of the second strand, and a *mismatch* is a pairing of two distinct bases. For example, G paired with A, C, or T is a mismatch whereas G paired with G is a match. For example, the strands w=5'-AACAA-3' and w^l=5'-AAGAA-3' have one mismatch at position $i = 3$, where $i = 1, 2, \ldots, 5$.

C2: Complement Mismatches: The number of mismatches in a perfect alignment of a strand and a complement must be above a given threshold d. For example, the complement of strand w=5'-AACAA-3', which is c=5'-TTGTT-3' and strand w^l=5'-TTATT-3' have one mismatch at position $i = 3$, where $i = 1, 2, \ldots, 5$. This constraint is also referred to as the *reverse-complement constraint*.

C3: GC Content: The number of G's and/or C's in a strand must be in a given range. For example, all strands presented in (Braich *et al.*, 2003) have 4, 5 or 6 C's. One such strand is w=5'-TTACACCAATCTCTT-3', which contains five Cs.

Constraint C3 can be used to attain desired hybridization. Roughly, the stability of a strand-complement pair increases as the content of G's and C's within strands increases. Constraint C3 is also used to ensure uniform melting temperatures across desired strand-complement pairings. Constraints C1 and C2 can be used in various combinations to avoid undesired hybridization. As it is widely known, the strength of hybridization between two strands (or between bases of the same strand) depends roughly on the number of nucleotide bonds formed (longer perfectly paired regions are more stable than shorter ones; this is modeled by C1 and C2), and on the types of nucleotides involved in bonding.

It can be observed that checking if a combinatorial constraint is satisfied can be done with computational complexity $O(n)$. This makes these constraints extremely tractable from a computational point of view.

Thermodynamic Constraints

While combinatorial constraints provide a good starting point for designing sets of strands for various biotechnological applications, their lack of accuracy is well known. More accurate measures of hybridization are required to efficiently predict the interaction between DNA strands. A higher level of accuracy can be achieved by understanding the thermodynamic laws that govern the interaction between bases of DNA strands. Thermodynamic constraints have been defined and used to design high quality sets of DNA strands.

Before presenting the thermodynamic constraints necessary to obtain such sets, it is necessary to provide a brief introduction to the underlining thermodynamic principles that govern DNA strand interactions.

With the primary goal of predicting secondary structure and DNA / RNA stability from the base sequence, over the past 20 years a number of melting temperature and diffraction based studies have been conducted to estimate the relationship between thermodynamic stability and DNA base sequences, in terms of nearest-neighbor base pair interactions.

The nearest-neighbor (NN) model for nucleic acids was pioneered in the 1960s by (Crothers & Zimm, 1964) and by (Devoe & Tinoco, 1962). Subsequently, several papers and theoretical reports on DNA and RNA nearest-neighbour thermodynamics have been published. In 1986, Breslauer *et al.* reported a first set of nearest-

neighbor sequence-dependent stability parameters for DNA obtained from evaluation of melting curves of short DNA oligomers (Brelauer, Frank, Blöcher, & Marky, 1986). Following that study, further research in the field lead to the development of more complex and accurate sets of DNA and RNA parameters (Gotoh & Tagashira, 1981; Vologodskii, Amirikyan, Lyubchenko, & Frank-Kamenetskii, 1984; Delcourt & Blake, 1991; Doktycz, Goldstein, Paner, Gallo, & Benight, 1992; SantaLucia, Allawi, & Seneviratne, 1996; Sugimoto, Nakano, Yoneyama, & Honda, 1996; SantaLucia, 1998; Tulpan, Andronescu, & Leger, 2010).

Free energies are always lower or equal with zero for any pair of DNA strands. The lower the free energy is for a DNA duplex, the more stable the duplex is.

In this chapter, we use the PairFold program implemented by Mirela Andronescu to compute free energies for DNA duplexes (Andronescu, 2003; Andronescu, 2008). The PairFold program predicts the secondary structure of a pair of DNA molecules based on free energy minimization. The secondary structure for a pair of strands (w, w^l) is a set of base pairs, with each base of w and w^l occurring in at most one pair. PairFold returns four secondary structures, for the pairs (w, w^l), (w^l, w), (w, w), and (w^l, w^l), and their corresponding minimum free energies. The algorithm uses dynamic programming and runs in time bounded by the cube of the lengths of the input strands. A detailed view of the computational model used in this work, which takes into consideration complex interactions between DNA sequences, can be found in (Andronescu, Zhang & Condon, 2005).

Thermodynamic constraints rely on the thermodynamic nearest-neighbor model presented above. We use the DNA parameters of SantaLucia Jr. (SantaLucia, 1998) (a set of unpublished parameters have been previously obtained via private communication with John SantaLucia) and PairFold to calculate minimum free energies of duplexes. We use the parameters and Equation

(3) of (SantaLucia & Hicks, 2004) to calculate melting temperatures, assuming a 1M salt concentration and 1e−07 M concentration of both strands and complements (for a total concentration of 2×1e-07 M). The melting temperature is only calculated for perfectly matched duplexes. Throughout, we use the following notation: T denotes the temperature of the reaction, $R = 1.98717$ kcal/(mol $\cdot$ K) is the gas constant, ΔG_0 (x, y) is the minimum free energy of the duplex xy at standard conditions (room temperature of 24 °C and absolute pressure of 1 atm), and TM_i denotes the melting temperature of strand w_i.

In this chapter we will consider the following thermodynamic constraints:

T1: Complement Mismatch Free Energy: The free energy of a strand and the complement of a distinct strand must be in a given range. For example, the complement mismatch free energy range of the strands in the set S= {TTTAAA, AAAAAA} is [—1.04, —0.33] kcal/mol.

T2: Complement-Complement Mismatch Free Energy: The free energy of a complement-complement duplex must be in a given range. For example, the complement-complement mismatch free energy range of the strands in the set S={AATTCC, GGCCAA, TTCCGG} is [—1.86, —0.81] kcal/mol.

Constraints T1 and T2 are used to restrict undesired hybridization, which can occur between a strand and the complement of a different strand (T1), or between two distinct complements (T2). In the context of microarrays, constraint T2 is the most important one. Constraint T1 is also marginally important although usually not applied against all the possible strand complements.

With respect to combinatorial constraints, checking thermodynamic constraints is more demanding from a computational point of view, since checking a constraint takes up to $O(n^3)$ (free energy has to be computed each time).

STATE OF THE ART OF HEURISTIC ALGORITHMS

There has been considerable interest recently in the application of meta-heuristic algorithms to the DSD problem. Most of the works appeared so far in the literature consider a simplified version of the problem, where only some combinatorial constraints are considered, while the more realistic constraints coming from the thermodynamic interactions among strands are neglected. The choice of not considering these latter constraints come from the consideration that they tend to break the combinatorial structure of the problem, on which most of the methods developed so far were actually based. When only combinatorial constraints are considered, bounds for the size of DNA codes can be obtained by generalizing classic results coming from algebraic coding theory, template-map strategies, genetic algorithms and lexicographic searches (Chee & Ling, 2008; Deaton *et al.*, 1996; Deaton, Murphy, Garzon, Franceschetti, & Stevens, 1999; Faulhammer, Cukras, Lipton, & Landweber, 2000; Frutos *et al.*, 1997; Gaborit & King, 2005; King, 2003; Li, Lee, Condon, & Corn, 2002; Smith, Aboluion, Montemanni, & Perkins; Zhang & Shin, 1998). In (Tulpan *et al.*, 2002) and (Tulpan *et al.*, 2003) a Stochastic Local Search method, able to handle large problems has been developed. In (Montemanni *et al.*, 2008) four new local search algorithms were developed and combined into a variable neighborhood search framework, following ideas originally developed in (Montemanni *et al.*, 2009a) for constant weight binary codes. Further results are presented in (Montemanni & Smith, 2009b), (Montemanni, Smith, & Koul) and (Koul, 2010), where a new simulated annealing procedure and an evolutionary algorithm are discussed.

Other interesting algorithms worth to be mentioned are (the list is not comprehensive): a method based on ant colony optimization discussed in (Ibrahim, Kurniawan, Khalid, Sudin, & Khalid, 2009) and (Kurniawan, Khalid, Ibrahim, Khalid,

& Middendorf, 2008); a global search approach presented in (Kai, Z., Linqiang & Jin, 2007); a randomized algorithm proposed in (Kao, Sanghi, & Schweller, 2009); a particle swarm optimization method discussed in (Khalid, Ibrahim, Kurniawan, Khalid, & Enggelbrecht, 2009).

Only a few algorithms have been presented to handle thermodynamic constraints. These methods are pure meta-heuristic approaches, and connections with coding theory are weaker, since the combinatorial structures of the instances tend to be destroyed by these constraints. They also face intrinsic computational difficulties due to the necessity of calculating free energies (a time consuming task) many times during the execution. The stochastic local search algorithm discussed in (Tulpan *et al.*, 2002) and (Tulpan *et al.*, 2003) is extended to handle thermodynamic constraints in (Tulpan *et al.*, 2005) and (Tulpan, 2006), where results are presented. In (Ghiggi, 2010) one of the local searches originally presented in (Montemanni *et al.*, 2008) - Seed Building - is modified to handle these constraints. These last two algorithms will be detailed and experimentally compared on some test instances in the next sections.

Stochastic Local Search

Stochastic local search (SLS) algorithms strongly use randomized decisions while searching for solutions to a given problem. They play an increasingly important role for solving hard combinatorial problems from various domains of Artificial Intelligence and Operations Research, such as satisfiability, constraint satisfaction, planning, scheduling, and other application areas (Hoos & Stützle, 2004). Over the past years there has been considerable success in developing SLS algorithms as well as randomized systematic search methods for solving these problems, and to date, stochastic local search algorithms are amongst the best known techniques for solving problems from many domains. In particular, SLS

methods are indicated for complex problems, for which a model cannot be directly used to devise solutions. The DSD problem with thermodynamic constraints lies in this category.

The stochastic local search algorithm introduced by Tulpan *et al.* in 2002 (Tulpan, Hoos, & Condon, 2002) performs a randomized iterative improvement search in the space of DNA strand sets. All strand sets constructed during the search process have exactly the target number of strands. It is ensured that all strands in the given candidate set always have the prescribed GC content. The proposed SLS algorithm starts with a target number of strands k and attempts to minimize the number of pairs that violate the given constraint(s). After all the constraint violations have been eliminated, or a given maximum computation time has elapsed, the algorithm stops. In the latter case a post-processing phase has to be run in order to eliminate the smallest possible number of strands, leading to the largest possible residual feasible set of strands. A pseudo-code for the overall algorithm is shown in Exhibit 1.

The initial set of k strands is determined by a simple randomized procedure that generates any DNA strand of length n fulfilling GC content constraints with equal probability. Note that the initial strand set may contain multiple copies of the same strand.

A loop is then entered. At each *step* of the search process, first, a pair of strands violating one of the constraints (either combinatorial or thermodynamics) is selected uniformly at random. Then, for each of these strands, all possible single-base modifications complying with the required GC content are considered. As an example of single-base modifications, consider the strand ACGT of length 4. A new strand TCGT can be obtained by replacing letter A from the first strand with letter T. With a given probability θ, one of these modifications is accepted uniformly at random, regardless of the number of constraint violations that will result from it. In the remaining case (with probability $1 - \theta$), each modification is assigned

Exhibit 1. StochasticLocalSearch()

```
Input: number of strings (k), string length (n), set of combinatorial con-
straints (C)
Output: set S of m strings that satisfy constraints C
For i:= 1 to maxTries do
     S:= initial set of strings
     S':= S
     For j:= 1 to maxSteps do
          If (S satisfies all constraints) then return S
     Randomly select strings w1, w2 ∈ S that violate at least one of the con-
straints
     M1:= all strings obtained from w1 by substituting one base
     M2:= all strings obtained from w2 by substituting one base
     With probability θ do
          Select string  w' from M1 ∪ M2 at random
     Otherwise
          Select string  w' from M1 ∪ M2 such that the number of conflicts is
maximally decreased
     If (w' ∈ M1) then
          Replace w1 by w' ∈ S
     Otherwise
          Replace w2 by w' ∈ S
     If (S has no more constraint violations than S') then
          S':= S
Return S'
```

a score, defined as the net decrease in the number of constraint violations caused by it, and a modification with maximal score is accepted. If there are multiple such modifications, one of them is chosen uniformly at random. Note that using this scheme, in each step of the algorithm, exactly one base in one strand is modified.

The parameter θ, also called the noise parameter, controls the greediness of the search process; for high values of θ, constraint violations are not resolved efficiently, while for low values of θ, the search has more difficulties to escape from local optima of the underlying search space. Throughout the run of the algorithm, the best candidate solution encountered so far, i.e., the DNA strand set with the fewest number of constraint violations, is memorized. Since the algorithm evolves a set of infeasible strings trying to reduce a measure of infeasibility, we say that it works in the infeasible search space. If the algorithm terminates without finding a valid set of size k, a valid subset can always be obtained by applying the following post-optimization phase. The algorithm builds a graph and then solves a maximum clique problem, where the maximum clique corresponds to the largest possible set of mutually feasible strands. The method is detailed in the remainder of this section.

Maximum Clique Post-Optimization

A maximum-clique post-optimization algorithm was introduced by Ghiggi in 2010 (Ghiggi, 2010). The first stage of the algorithm consists of con-

Figure 2. Example of maximum clique problem. The largest maximum clique has size 4 and is the subgraph consisting of vertices 2, 4, 5 and 6.

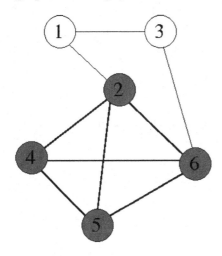

structing a graph $G = \{V, E\}$ as follows. The set V corresponds to the strands retrieved (k in this case). An edge $\{i, j\} \in E$ exists if no constraint violation exists between the strands associated with nodes i and j. An example of such a graph can be found in Figure 2.

After having built the graph as described above, the problem of retrieving the largest possible set of strands mutually fulfilling combinatorial and thermodynamic constraints is equivalent to solving a maximum clique problem on the graph G. In graph theory a maximum clique of a graph G is defined as the largest complete subgraph of G, where complete means that an edge must exist between each pair of vertices of the subgraph (Pardalos & Xue, 1994). In this case, finding a complete subgraph means to look for a subset of strands mutually fulfilling all the constraints, thus we look for the largest possible subset.

The advantage of the problem transformation described above is that very efficient algorithms exist to solve the maximum clique problem. The implementation used in this work adopts the algorithm *cliquer* (Östergård, 2002).

Seed Building

Algorithms that examine all possible strands in a given order, and incrementally accept strands that are feasible with respect to already accepted ones, can often produce fairly good codes when only combinatorial constraints are considered (Gaborit & King, 2005; King, 2003; Montemanni *et al.*, 2009a; Montemanni, Smith, & Koul). For this reason the *Seed Building* (SB) method is based on these orderings, combined with the concept of *seed strands* (Brouwer, Shearer, Sloane, & Smith, 1990). These seed strands are an initial set of strands with the required GC-content and feasible with respect to each other, to which strands are added in the given ordering if they satisfy the necessary criteria. In our implementation we generate strands in a random order. Preliminary experiments suggested that, in contrast to binary codes (Montemanni *et al.*, 2009a), a random order is preferable for DNA codes (Montemanni, Smith, & Koul). In this section we describe how a Seed Building strategy can be modified to deal with thermodynamic constraints, too (Ghiggi, 2010).

Seeds can be selected at random, but experiments on binary codes and on DNA code design problems with combinatorial constraints only, clearly show that there is a better way to proceed: in the seed building algorithm a set of seeds is initially empty, and one random seed (feasible with respect to the previous seeds, and fulfilling the GC-content constraint) is added at a time. If this seed leads to good results, it is kept, and a new random seed is designated for testing, thus increasing the size of the seed set. The same rationale is used to decide whether to keep subsequent seeds or not. In the same way, if after a given number of iterations the quality of the solutions provided by a set of seeds is judged to be not good enough, the most recent seed is eliminated from the set, which results therefore in a reduction in the size of the seed set. In this way the set of seeds is expanded or contracted depending on the quality of the solu-

Exhibit 2. SeedBuilding()

```
Input: maximum time (TimeSB), maximum number of iterations with the same set
of seeds (ItrSeed), set of combinatorial constraints (C)
Output: set S of strings that satisfy constraints CSeeds:= Ø
S:= Ø
ItrCnt:= 0
While (Computation time < TimeSB) do
    ItrCnt:= ItrCnt + 1
Cstring:= random string with proper GC content, compatible with SeedsWordSol:=
Seeds ∪ {Cstring}
    Complete WorkSol by adding feasible strings examined in a random order
    If (|WorkSol| > |S|)
ItrCnt:= 0
S:= WorkSolSeeds:= Seeds ∪ {CString} // Added in the last position
If (ItrCnt == ItrSeed)
    AclSeed:= average code size in the last ItrCnt iterations
    AclAll:= average code size from the beginning
    If (AclSeed >AclAll)
        CString:= random string with proper GC content compatible with Seeds-
Seeds:= Seeds ∪ {CString} // Added in the last position
    Else
        If (|Seeds| > 0)
            CString:= String in the last position of SeedsSeeds:= Seeds \
{CString}
    ItrCnt:= 0
Return S
```

tions provided by the set itself. What happens in practice is that the size of the seed set oscillates through a range of small values. A pseudo-code for the algorithm is shown in Exhibit 2.

The Seed Building algorithm works in an iterative fashion on an adaptive set of seed strands contained in the set *SeedSet*, which is initially empty. At each iteration, a new strand *CString*, compatible with those in *Seeds*, is generated and the partial solution *WorkSol*, initialized with the elements of *Seeds* and *CString*, is expanded by adding feasible strands, examined in a random order. If a new best solution is found, the set *Seeds* is immediately expanded. Every *ItrSeed* iterations, the average size of the codes generated with the set *Seeds* is checked to determine whether *Seeds*

is a promising set (in which case it should be augmented) or not (in which case it is reduced by deleting the most recently added seed). The procedure stops after a fixed computation time of *Time_{SB}* seconds has elapsed.

Preliminary tests clearly suggested (Ghiggi, 2010) that applying the general Seed Building paradigm when dealing with thermodynamic constraints is computationally intractable with current technology: too many time-consuming free energy evaluations would be necessary, leading to a method able to perform just a few iterations in an affordable computation time. This suggested that SB is probably less indicated than SLS to deal with thermodynamic constraints. However, it is possible to implement a workaround able to make SB applicable to problems with thermodynamic constraints. In order to explore the solution space in a satisfactory way, we need to minimize the number of free energy evaluations necessary to understand whether the various constraints are violated or not. In our implementation, we compute only one special case of thermodynamic constraint T2 at each iteration, while we postpone the evaluation of the remaining one into a post-optimization phase. This permits to reduce the number of free energy computations, focusing on those that show to be crucial in shaping up the solutions. The resulting algorithm can be therefore sketched as follows:

1. **Processing phase:** Classic Seed Building algorithm where combinatorial constraints are considered together with a special case of the T2 constraint. Here each string is only checked against itself, but not against the strands already in the solution. The hope is that this particular T2 constraint is sufficient to filter out most of the unfeasible strands, and to shape up the solution in an efficient way.

2. **Post Processing phase:** Starting from the solution obtained in the previous point, a graph is built analogously to what was done before for the Stochastic Local Search approach. At this point we know that all combinatorial constraints and self-T2 are fulfilled, so we need to take care only of the residual T2 thermodynamic constraints. Notice that the number of free energy evaluations is of the order of $O(s^2)$, where s is the number of strands produced at phase 1. This number is intuitively small if the filter provided in phase 1 is efficient. Again analogously to what was done before, it is sufficient now to run a maximum clique algorithm to retrieve the largest possible clique in the graph, which corresponds to a feasible solution for the original problem.

Even when the two phase approach is adopted, we can say that the SB algorithm works in the feasible search space, in the sense that it only produces feasible solutions (according to the constraints considered in phase 1), that are incrementally increased during the computation. This is the main difference with respect to the Stochastic Local Search method described above.

It is important to emphasize that the decomposition described above is not based on any theoretical results guarantying optimality: it is a heuristic criterion that might lead to suboptimal solutions. Everything basically depends on the filter provided by phase 1. Experimental results discussed in the next section clearly suggest that the decomposition approach is effective in practice.

COMPUTATIONAL EXPERIMENTS

In this section we compare the results obtained by the two meta-heuristic methods described in the previous sections.

Experiments Set Up

The comparison between the two algorithms is based on the number of feasible strands retrieved at the end of the computation. Since SLS requires the target number of strands k as input, we provide SLS with $k = \text{res(SB)}$; $k = \text{res(SB)}*1.1$ and $k = \text{res(SB)}*1.2$, where res(SB) is the number of feasible strands retrieved by seed building. In this way we check whether SLS is able to replicate, or improve the results of SB. Notice that the final result returned by SLS is less than or equal to k by definition, since infeasible strands are deleted in the post-optimization phase, as described in the previous section. In order to run experiments, we also have to define feasible free energy values for the thermodynamic constraints T1 and T2. We used the values calculated empirically and reported in (Ghiggi, 2010), which are reported in Figure 3. Notice that the same thresholds have been used

Figure 3. Feasible free energy ranges for constraints T1 and T2

n	4	5	6	7	8	9	10	11	12	13	14	15	16	17	18	19	20
Minimum	-4.50	-5.80	-7.20	-8.70	-8.60	-9.60	-12.60	-10.80	-12.30	-12.60	-13.37	-14.60	-13.90	-15.50	-16.40	-16.40	-19.90
Maximum	0.00	-0.10	-0.60	-1.04	-1.50	-2.00	-2.60	-3.00	-3.50	-4.0	-4.50	-5.00	-5.50	-6.00	-6.50	-6.90	-7.50

for all the thermodynamic constraints considered. The parameter settings used for the algorithms are those reported in (Ghiggi, 2010), where we refer the interested reader for the details.

The other parameter settings used for the algorithms are those reported in (Ghiggi, 2010): for the SLS algorithm probability $\theta = 0.2$, *MaxTries* $= 10$ and *MaxSteps* $= 50000$; *ItrSeed* $= 5$ and *TimeSB* $= 600$ seconds for the SB algorithm.

RESULTS

Theoretical Results

In Figure 4 the results obtained by the different algorithms while considering constraints C1, C2, C3 and T2 are reported. For different values of n (measuring the length of the strands) and of d (the threshold for the distance involved in combinatorial constraints C1 and C2) the results of the Stochastic Local Search algorithm, on the left of each cell, and those of the Seed Building method, on the right, are reported. Notice that for the Stochastic Local Search algorithm the best results among the different values of k considered are reported, with a superscript indicating the configuration that generated the result of each cell. Notice that some of the entries are missing (-) since the corresponding test was not run.

From Figure 4 it emerges that SLS is better in the quasi-diagonal part of the table (i.e. right below the diagonal corresponding to $n=d$), while SB has to be preferred otherwise. The result can be explained by observing that SLS searches in the infeasible search space, making it possible to modify strands, while SB incrementally accepts

strands at each iteration (feasible search space). This makes difficult to find optimal solutions for those settings where only a few combinations of strands are optimal.

As previously observed, in the context of microarrays, the thermodynamic constraint of major interest is T2, nevertheless constraint T1 plays a role, too. For this reason we run some tests of the algorithms we propose also on the combination of constraints C1, C2, C3, T2 and T1. Results are reported in Table 2, where some combinations of n and d values are considered. Notice that for the Stochastic Local Search algorithm the best results among the different values of k considered (the same used for Figure 4) are reported, this time without indicating the configuration that generated the result of each entry.

A comparison of Figure 4 and Table 2 suggests that the introduction of constraint T1 substantially decreases the dimension of the feasible sets of strands. Future research will investigate the reasons for this phenomenon.

Case Study: Computational Evaluation of Affymetrix Probe Sequences

Over the past 15 years Affymetrix microarrays constituted one of the most widely used experimental platforms for gene expression studies. Each array consists of a solid wafer (quartz substrate) to which large numbers of 25mer probes are attached. Gene expression levels are measured by hybridizing mRNA extracted from cells or tissues of interest to the probes on the array. For each expressed transcript Affymetrix assigns one or more probe sets, each consisting of 11-20 series of probe pairs.

Figure 4. Computational results obtained for constraints C1, C2, C3 and T2

n\d	3	4	5	6	7	8	9	10
4	4 ,-	2 ,-	-	-	-	-	-	-
5	9 ,-	2 ,-	1 ,-	-	-	-	-	-
6	21 ,-	9 ,-	3 ,-	2 ,-	-	-	-	-
7	$54 ,40^{0\%}$	$18 ,16^{0\%}$	$5 ,4^{0\%}$	1 ,-	$1 ,2^{0\%}$	-	-	-
8	181 ,-	$53 ,29^{0\%}$	$13 ,8^{0\%}$	$6 ,4^{0\%}$	$1 ,2^{0\%}$	$2 ,3^{0\%}$	-	-
9	$378 ,222^{0\%}$	$126 ,78^{0\%}$	$33 ,23^{0\%}$	$11 ,8^{0\%}$	$4 ,3^{0\%}$	$2 ,3^{0\%}$	$1 ,2^{0\%}$	-
10	1871 ,-	$420 ,179^{0\%}$	$100 ,49^{0\%}$	$34 ,20^{0\%}$	$12 ,8^{0\%}$	$5 ,3^{0\%}$	$1 ,2^{0\%}$	$1 ,2^{0\%}$
11	2247 ,-	$816 ,10^{0\%}$	$238 ,116^{0\%}$	$63 ,25^{0\%}$	$21 ,12^{0\%}$	$7 ,5^{0\%}$	$3 ,3^{0\%}$	$1 ,2^{0\%}$
12	1617 ,-	1054 ,-	$196 ,58^{0\%}$	$46 ,18^{0\%}$	$47 ,17^{0\%}$	$15 ,4^{0\%}$	$7 ,6^{0\%}$	$3 ,2^{0\%}$
13	915 ,-	$771 ,6^{0\%}$	$266 ,74^{0\%}$	$102 ,32^{0\%}$	$20 ,11^{0\%}$	$7 ,5^{0\%}$	$5 ,5^{0\%}$	$3 ,2^{0\%}$
14	1743 ,-	1196 ,-	918 ,-	$235 ,56^{0\%}$	$48 ,17^{0\%}$	$77 ,22^{0\%}$	$27 ,7^{0\%}$	$4 ,4^{0\%}$
15	$1298 ,4^{0\%}$	$803 ,5^{0\%}$	$669 ,101^{0\%}$	$441 ,82^{0\%}$	$111 ,21^{0\%}$	$23 ,7^{0\%}$	$47 ,11^{0\%}$	$22 ,8^{0\%}$
16	1428 ,-	1543 ,-	966 ,-	$639 ,11^{0\%}$	$498 ,61^{0\%}$	$60 ,9^{0\%}$	$21 ,8^{0\%}$	$50 ,8^{0\%}$
17	$5350 ,2^{0\%}$	$1452 ,17^{0\%}$	$1114 ,4^{0\%}$	$460 ,15^{0\%}$	$311 ,39^{0\%}$	$128 ,21^{0\%}$	$264 ,43^{0\%}$	$76 ,9^{0\%}$
18	1296 ,-	1387 ,-	959 ,-	564 ,-	1265 ,-	445 ,-	$103 ,14^{0\%}$	$36 ,6^{0\%}$
19	$1312 ,3^{0\%}$	$1453 ,10^{0\%}$	$529 ,3^{0\%}$	$339 ,3^{0\%}$	$236 ,9^{0\%}$	$123 ,8^{0\%}$	$61 ,6^{0\%}$	$486 ,38^{0\%}$
20	1120 ,-	1220 ,-	700 ,-	424 ,-	329 ,-	1433 ,-	516 ,-	$219 ,14^{0\%}$

n\d	11	12	13	14	15	16	17	18	19	20
4	-	-	-	-	-	-	-	-	-	-
5	-	-	-	-	-	-	-	-	-	-
6	-	-	-	-	-	-	-	-	-	-
7	-	-	-	-	-	-	-	-	-	-
8	-	-	-	-	-	-	-	-	-	-
9	-	-	-	-	-	-	-	-	-	-
10	-	-	-	-	-	-	-	-	-	-
11	$1 ,2^{0\%}$	-	-	-	-	-	-	-	-	-
12	$2 ,3^{0\%}$	$2 ,3^{0\%}$	-	-	-	-	-	-	-	-
13	$1 ,2^{0\%}$	$1 ,1^{0\%}$	$1 ,2^{0\%}$	-	-	-	-	-	-	-
14	$2 ,1^{0\%}$	$2 ,2^{0\%}$	$1 ,2^{0\%}$	$2 ,3^{0\%}$	-	-	-	-	-	-
15	$3 ,2^{0\%}$	$2 ,2^{0\%}$	$1 ,2^{0\%}$	$2 ,3^{0\%}$	$1 ,2^{0\%}$	-	-	-	-	-
16	$20 ,6^{0\%}$	$9 ,4^{0\%}$	$4 ,2^{0\%}$	$1 ,2^{0\%}$	$1 ,2^{0\%}$	$1 ,2^{0\%}$	-	-	-	-
17	$36 ,7^{0\%}$	$12 ,4^{0\%}$	$7 ,2^{0\%}$	$1 ,1^{0\%}$	$1 ,2^{0\%}$	$2 ,2^{0\%}$	$1 ,2^{0\%}$	-	-	-
18	$77 ,11^{0\%}$	$32 ,5^{0\%}$	$14 ,3^{0\%}$	$7 ,2^{0\%}$	4 ,-	$1 ,2^{0\%}$	$1 ,1^{0\%}$	$1 ,2^{0\%}$	-	-
19	$109 ,10^{0\%}$	$57 ,7^{0\%}$	$5 ,5^{0\%}$	$12 ,3^{0\%}$	$5 ,2^{0\%}$	$1 ,2^{0\%}$	$1 ,2^{0\%}$	$2 ,2^{0\%}$	$1 ,1^{0\%}$	-
20	$374 ,21^{0\%}$	$125 ,6^{0\%}$	$52 ,6^{0\%}$	$19 ,3^{0\%}$	$11 ,3^{0\%}$	$5 ,1^{0\%}$	$3 ,2^{0\%}$	$2 ,1^{0\%}$	$2 ,2^{0\%}$	$2 ,1^{0\%}$

Each pair consists of one perfect match probe and one mismatch probe. The perfect match probe corresponds to the complementary sequence of the gene of interest, while the imperfect match probe has the middle nucleotide at position 13 replaced by its Watson-Crick complement.

The array design process employed by Affymetrix technology for Gene Arrays typically includes a series of successive steps, as follows:

- Large numbers of sequences and annotations are collected from publicly available databases including NCBI RefSeq, GenBank and dbEST.
- The sequences are aligned to genome assemblies for each organism and their quality and orientation is evaluated based on consensus splice sites, known polyadenylation sites and confirmed coding sequences.
- Probe selection is typically done from the 600-base region at the 3' end of a consensus sequence

Here we consider the case study where industrially produced microarray probes are evaluated *in-silico* based on 74 out of a total of 86 publicly available probe and target sequence data sets made available by Affymetrix Corporation, Santa Clara, CA. The remaining 12 out of 86 array data was incomplete, meaning that either probe or target sequences (but not both) were available

Table 2. Computational results obtained for constraints C1, C2, C3, T2 and T1

n	d	SB	SLS
12	6	27	13
12	7	9	8
12	8	3	5
12	9	2	2
13	8	5	6
13	9	2	2
13	10	2	2
14	7	34	10
14	8	12	6
14	9	6	5
14	10	2	2
14	11	2	2
15	9	4	3
15	10	2	1
15	11	1	1
16	9	8	3
16	10	5	2
16	11	2	2
17	9	2	1
18	10	9	3
19	11	12	3
19	12	3	2
20	13	2	2
20	14	2	2

on the NetAffx web site. The species covered by Affymetrix microarray technology span a wide taxonomic range including the realms of plants, amphibians, bacteria, birds, fungi, insects, mammals (mouse and human included) and worms. The total number of complete (probe, target) sequence sets made available by Affymetrix for their arrays are 18,460,805 and respectively, 1,492,049. While Affymetrix technology makes use of perfect match and mismatch probe sequences, this study will only analyze the perfect match probes.

Affymetrix Probe and Target Sequence Characteristics

As one of the biggest producers of microarrays in the world, Affymetrix uses a technology employing multiple synthesized oligonucleotide probes, each one being 25 nucleotides long, to identify and discriminate among large numbers of targets. The data analyzed in this chapter shows that the Affymetrix array with the highest number of distinct probe sequences is the Wheat array (674,353 probes), while the array that tests the highest number of targets is the Poplar array (61,413 targets). The lowest number of probe sequences can be found in the RT-U34 rat array (20,464 probes). The lowest number of targets corresponds to the same rat RT-U34 array (1,031 targets).

The following indicators were used for the evaluation of the probe design quality of the Affymetrix arrays:

- Number of duplicate probe and target sequences,
- Probe sequence homology with NCBI RefSeq and Affymetrix target sequences,
- Thermodynamic evaluation of probe sequences: melting temperatures, perfect match minimum free energies, GC-content.

Each one of these indicators can be used to gauge the quality of the probe sequences or the overall quality of a microarray.

Sequence Duplication

The presence of identical probe sequences on a microarray will affect the specificity of those probes and will diminish the signal strength since the same target, if present, could potentially bind to all locations where the given probe is present. A close analysis of the Affymetrix probe sequences (see Table 3) reveals that only those designed for the *P. aeruginosa* array bear no duplications, the remaining 73 arrays containing up to 9.47% (11,696

/ 123,524) probe duplication for the *S.aureus* array. A similar analysis of the Affymetrix targets shows one potential cause of the probe duplication problem, namely that only 7 out of 74 arrays have no duplicated targets. The remaining 67 arrays show up to 1.55% (16 / 1031) target sequence duplication for the rat array RT-U34.

While the use of multiple probes allows Affymetrix technology to better and widely assess the expression levels of numerous target genes, we believe the presence of identical probe sequences as components of various probe sets will negatively influence the final outcomes of the microarray experiments, since the expression signals will have shared components that will act as confounders in the final results analysis.

Sequence Homology between Probes and Non-Targets

In Affymetrix arrays, all probes within a probe set should ideally estimate the expression level of the same target, since their sequences are specifically designed to uniquely identify it. Nevertheless, high levels of variation for probe intensities, which are consistent across multiple array experiments that use the same platform, have been reported in the literature (Li & Wong, 1998; Cambon, Khalyfa, Cooper, & Thompson, 2007). It was hypothesized that among the multiple causes of variability of probes within a probe set, the most prominent one is their unintended affinity to bind non-targets (cross-hybridization). A number of very specific studies that focused on Affymetrix arrays designed for various species like *Rattus Norvegicus* (Cambon, Khalyfa, Cooper, & Thompson, 2007), *Homo Sapiens* (Barnes, Freudenberg, Thompson, Aronow & Pavlidis, 2005; Harbig, Sprinkle, & Enkemann, 2005; Kapur, Jiang, Xing, & Wong, 2008) and *Mus Musculus* (Yee, Wlaschin, Chuah, Nissom, & Hu, 2008), were carried out to test this hypothesis. Here we report our findings based on a mass homology search of all Affymetrix array-specific complemented probe sequences against

their intended Affymetrix targets and NCBI RefSeq coding sequences.

When complements of Affymetrix probe sequences are matched against Affymetrix targets in a homology exact match search using BLAST (*word size* = 25, *e-value* = 1e-04), in average 88.09% of the probes match exactly one target, while 10.52% match more than one target and 1.39% do not have a match. The only array that shows an unusually high percentage of probes without a match (90.92%) corresponds to the Rat230 Affymetrix array. The same array proves also to be the only one with 0% single matches. The array with the lowest percentage of mismatched probes (0%) is the *P.aeruginosa* array, while the array with the highest percentage of probes with multiple matches (89.03%) is the *E.coli* array.

When RefSeq sequences are used as targets in a homology search we notice a drop of the average percentage of probes that match exactly one target (36.75%) as opposed to when Affymetrix targets are considered. The average percentage of probes that do not match any RefSeq target is much higher (46.78%) than in the previous scenario, possibly suggesting that consensus sequences used by Affymetrix at the time when the array probes were designed were different than the ones available today. The average percentage of probes that match more than one target is only 6% higher (16.47%) than in the previous case. We notice again that the highest percentage of probes that do not match any targets corresponds to the same Rat230 array (94.76%), while the array with the lowest percentage (7.64%) is the HG-Focus array. The array with the highest percentage (71.07%) of probes that match exactly one target is the RN-U34 rat array, while the one with the lowest percentage (0.04%) is again the Rat230 array. The array with the highest percentage of probes (35.89%) with multiple hits is the HC-G110 human array, while the one with lowest percentage (1.48%) is the Citrus array.

The impact of probes that either do not identify the corresponding target or identify more than one

Table 3. Duplicate probe and target sequences in Affymetrix arrays

Array	Num probes	Num Dup Probes	%	Num targets	Num Dup Targets	%
ATH1-121501	251,078	212	0.08	22,814	0	0.00
AtGenome1	131,822	894	0.68	8,297	15	0.18
Barley1	251,437	2,575	1.02	22,840	60	0.26
Bovine	265,627	690	0.26	24,128	4	0.02
Bsubtilis	100,584	51	0.05	5,039	9	0.18
C_elegans	249,165	2,987	1.20	22,625	2	0.01
Canine_2	473,162	3,345	0.71	43,035	56	0.13
Canine	263,234	1,254	0.48	23,913	13	0.05
Chicken	424,097	1,879	0.44	38,535	26	0.07
Citrus	341,730	5,269	1.54	30,372	123	0.40
Cotton	265,516	1,719	0.65	24,132	30	0.12
DrosGenome1	195,994	112	0.06	14,010	1	0.01
Drosophila_2	265,400	481	0.18	18,955	15	0.08
E_coli_2	112,488	108	0.10	10,208	2	0.02
E_coli_Antisense	141,629	547	0.39	7,140	9	0.13
E_coli	141,629	547	0.39	7,312	9	0.12
HC-G110	30,313	19	0.06	1,887	15	0.79
HG-Focus	98,149	339	0.35	8,793	0	0.00
HG-U133A_2	247,899	6,062	2.45	22,283	0	0.00
HG-U133A	247,965	6,067	2.45	22,283	0	0.00
HG-U133B	249,502	977	0.39	22,645	0	0.00
HG-U133_Plus_2	604,258	9,726	1.61	54,675	47	0.09
HG-U95A	201,807	1,717	0.85	12,454	15	0.12
HG-U95Av2	201,800	1,727	0.86	12,453	15	0.12
HG-U95B	201,862	2,671	1.32	12,620	24	0.19
HG-U95C	201,867	1,376	0.68	12,646	16	0.13
HG-U95D	201,858	584	0.29	12,644	16	0.13
HG-U95E	201,863	851	0.42	12,639	17	0.13
HT-HG-U133A	247,719	6,058	2.45	22,268	0	0.00
HT-HG-U133B	249,453	972	0.39	22,665	25	0.11
Hu35KsubA	140,010	59	0.04	8,934	16	0.18
Hu35KsubB	139,996	16	0.01	8,924	15	0.17
Hu35KsubC	140,008	107	0.08	8,928	15	0.17
Hu35KsubD	139,985	254	0.18	8,928	16	0.18
HuGeneFL	131,541	200	0.15	6,633	20	0.30
MG-U74A	201,964	1,121	0.56	12,654	16	0.13
MG-U74Av2	197,993	956	0.48	12,488	16	0.13
MG-U74B	201,960	446	0.22	12,636	15	0.12
MG-U74Bv2	197,131	160	0.08	12,477	15	0.12

continues on following page

Table 3. Continued

Array	Num probes	Num Dup Probes	%	Num targets	Num Dup Targets	%
MG-U74C	201,963	1,664	0.82	12,728	15	0.12
MG-U74Cv2	182,797	309	0.17	11,934	15	0.13
MOE430A	249,958	4,471	1.79	22,690	18	0.08
MOE430B	248,704	1,505	0.61	22,575	21	0.09
Maize	265,682	4,830	1.82	17,734	44	0.25
Medicago	673,880	8,878	1.32	61,278	167	0.27
Mouse430A_2	249,958	4,471	1.79	22,690	18	0.08
Mouse430_2	496,468	5,978	1.20	45,101	39	0.09
Mu11KsubA	131,280	75	0.06	6,584	15	0.23
Mu11KsubB	119,580	989	0.83	6,002	53	0.88
P_aeruginosa	77,674	0	0.00	5,900	0	0.00
Plasmodium_Anopheles	250,758	4,017	1.60	22,769	149	0.65
Poplar	674,330	11,539	1.71	61,413	280	0.46
Porcine	265,635	519	0.20	24,123	2	0.01
RAE230A	175,477	502	0.29	15,923	5	0.03
RAE230B	168,984	479	0.28	15,333	4	0.03
RG-U34A	140,317	260	0.19	8,799	21	0.24
RG-U34B	140,312	19	0.01	8,791	15	0.17
RG-U34C	140,284	32	0.02	8,789	15	0.17
RN-U34	21,305	5	0.02	1,322	15	1.13
RT-U34	20,464	57	0.28	1,031	16	**1.55**
Rat230_2	342,410	968	0.28	31,099	9	0.03
Rhesus	668,485	3,801	0.57	52,865	65	0.12
Rice	631,066	17,890	2.83	57,381	352	0.61
S_aureus	123,524	11,696	**9.47**	7,775	67	0.86
Soybean	671,762	5,343	0.80	61,170	102	0.17
Sugar_Cane	92,384	1,425	1.54	8,387	23	0.27
Tomato	112,528	198	0.18	10,209	2	0.02
U133_X3P	673,904	**42,190**	6.26	61,359	**903**	1.47
Vitis_Vinifera	264,387	2,795	1.06	16,602	74	0.45
Xenopus_laevis	249,678	4,143	1.66	15,611	55	0.35
YG-S98	138,412	3,872	2.80	9,335	114	1.22
Yeast_2	120,855	423	0.35	10,928	6	0.05
Zebrafish	249,752	2,282	0.91	15,617	27	0.17
Wheat	674,353	30,278	4.49	61,290	614	1.00
AVG	249,470.34	3,284.30	0.98	20,162.82	54.70	0.25
MAX	67,4353	42,190	9.47	61,413	903	1.55
MIN	20,464	0	0.00	1,031	0	0.00

target shall not be neglected since they will create confounding effects during the data interpretation stage. Even if Affymetrix uses probeset identifiers that flag those probes associated with multiple transcripts ("_s_at", "_x_at" suffixes, Table 4), our results and previous gene mappings (Okoniewski & Miller, 2006) show that many probesets associated with multiple genomic loci are not correctly identified. The probes that identify multiple targets have a common component in expression signals, and thus they can lead to an increased number of incorrect positive correlations between expressed genes (Okoniewski & Miller, 2006; Orlov *et al.*, 2006). The probes that do not identify a correct target will not contribute to the hybridization signal, thus producing lower than expected intensities or allowing cross-hybridization to dominate the overall intensity value.

Thermodynamic Evaluation of Probe Sequences

The thermodynamic evaluation of Affymetrix microarray probe sequences was performed using the Thermodynamic Nearest Neighbour Model, with parameters developed by SantaLucia and Hicks (2004) and Lu, Turner, and Mathews (2006). The calculation of minimum free energies and melting temperatures is based on the MultiRNAFold v1.9 software package (Andronescu, Zhang & Condon, 2005) publicly available at http://www.rnasoft.ca/.

The quality of probe samples is estimated using the following criteria:

- The perfect match melting temperature min-max interval (PM-MT). The narrower the interval is, the better the probes are.
- The perfect match minimum free energy min-max interval (PM-MFE). Similar as above.
- The free energy gap between perfect matches and imperfect matches ($\delta*$). The measure was introduced in (Tulpan *et al.*, 2005) and can be used to gauge the qual-

ity of a set of probes at the design stage. Here, the measure could be used only as a post-processing mechanism to weed out the problematic probes, since the numbers of probes for each array are prohibitively large. The calculation of $\delta*$ is computationally intensive, since the number of imperfect match free energies is proportional to the square of the number of probes, thus only an approximation of this measure could be considered in this study based on a random sampling approach.

One of the most common probe selection criteria used nowadays in probe design software is the choice of melting temperature (Tm) characteristics, such that the interval of Tm values (PM-MT) for all probe sequences is narrow enough to ensure a uniform behaviour for all sequences. Table 5 lists all PM-MT intervals for all 74 Affymetrix arrays studied here. The largest PM-MT value (35.08 °C) corresponds to the HG-U95D human array, while the smallest value (20.7 °C) corresponds to the RAE230A rat array.

Similarly, the perfect match minimum free energy interval (PM-MFE) measures the uniformity of the thermodynamic behaviour for all probes on an array and in general, correlates well with the PM-MT measure. Thus, the largest PM-MFE value (21.54 kcal/mol) corresponds to the same HG-U95D array, while the smallest value (12.75 kcal/mol) was obtained for the MOE430A mouse array.

While the exact melting temperature values, as well as perfect match minimum free energies (and GC-content), are strongly correlated with the nucleotide distribution of each set of targets (e.g. GC-rich targets will have higher melting temperature probes), a tradeoff must be considered between selecting probes for all or some of the targets and increasing or decreasing the melting temperature or the minimum free energy intervals.

Nevertheless, the PM-MT and PM-MFE measures quantify and qualify probe sequences taken

Table 4. Probe and target sequences publicly made available by Affymetrix. The table contains only arrays for which both, probe and target sequences are accessible on the Affymetrix website.

Array	# probes	# targets	# s_at	% _s_at	# x_at	% _x_at
ATH1-121501	251,078	22,746	10,415	4.15	1,408	0.56
AtGenome1	131,822	8,297	22,826	17.32	0	0.00
Barley1	251,437	22,840	39,709	15.79	11,790	4.69
Bovine	265,627	24,128	2,859	1.08	1,012	0.38
Bsubtilis	100,584	5,039	320	0.32	0	0.00
C_elegans	249,165	22,625	60,561	24.31	13,530	5.43
Canine	263,234	23,913	23,858	9.06	5,968	2.27
Canine_2	473,162	43,035	**148,336**	31.35	10,764	2.27
Chicken	424,097	38,535	90,893	21.43	5,071	1.20
Citrus	341,730	30,372	78,759	23.05	17,563	5.14
Cotton	265,516	24,132	102,209	38.49	17,212	6.48
DrosGenome1	195,994	14,010	2,464	1.26	0	0.00
Drosophila_2	265,400	18,955	27,823	10.48	1,204	0.45
E_coli	141,629	7,312	0	0.00	0	0.00
E_coli_2	112,488	10,208	79,267	**70.47**	1,142	1.02
E_coli_Antisense	141,629	7,140	1,025	0.72	0	0.00
HC-G110	30,313	1,887	6,912	22.80	0	0.00
HG-Focus	98,149	8,793	36,301	36.99	4,257	4.34
HG-U133A	247,965	22,283	87,894	35.45	26,719	10.78
HG-U133A_2	247,899	22,283	87,883	35.45	26,708	10.77
HG-U133B	249,502	22,645	27,606	11.06	15,906	6.38
HG-U133_Plus_2	604,258	54,675	124,377	20.58	46,277	7.66
HG-U95A	201,807	12,454	17,984	8.91	0	0.00
HG-U95Av2	201,800	12,453	17,936	8.89	0	0.00
HG-U95B	201,862	12,620	6,480	3.21	0	0.00
HG-U95C	201,867	12,646	7,230	3.58	0	0.00
HG-U95D	201,858	12,644	3,232	1.60	0	0.00
HG-U95E	201,863	12,639	4,992	2.47	0	0.00
HT-HG-U133A	247,719	22,268	87,883	35.48	26,708	10.78
HT-HG-U133B	249,453	22,639	27,595	11.06	15,895	6.37
Hu35KsubA	140,010	8,934	15,915	11.37	0	0.00
Hu35KsubB	139,996	8,924	9,298	6.64	0	0.00
Hu35KsubC	140,008	8,928	15,609	11.15	0	0.00
Hu35KsubD	139,985	8,928	20,852	14.90	0	0.00
HuGeneFL	131,541	6,633	19,950	15.17	0	0.00
MG-U74A	201,964	12,654	5,952	2.95	0	0.00
MG-U74Av2	197,993	12,488	5,936	3.00	0	0.00
MG-U74B	201,960	12,636	1,216	0.60	0	0.00

continues on following page

Table 4. Continued

Array	# probes	# targets	# s_at	% _s_at	# x_at	% _x_at
MG-U74Bv2	197,131	12,477	1,296	0.66	0	0.00
MG-U74C	201,963	12,728	2,464	1.22	0	0.00
MG-U74Cv2	182,797	11,934	1,952	1.07	0	0.00
MOE430A	249,958	22,690	16,189	6.48	16,629	6.65
MOE430B	248,704	22,575	6,919	2.78	10,235	4.12
Maize	265,682	17,734	5,146	1.94	9,535	3.59
Medicago	673,880	61,278	56,729	8.42	20,417	3.03
Mouse430A_2	249,958	22,690	16,189	6.48	16,629	6.65
Mouse430_2	496,468	45,101	22,998	4.63	26,842	5.41
Mu11KsubA	131,280	6,584	71,940	54.80	0	0.00
Mu11KsubB	119,580	6,002	72,260	60.43	0	0.00
P_aeruginosa	77,674	5,900	694	0.89	0	0.00
Plasmodium_Anopheles	250,758	22,769	20,036	7.99	6,476	2.58
Poplar	674,330	**61,413**	99,092	14.69	27,665	4.10
Porcine	265,635	24,123	2,725	1.03	704	0.27
RAE230A	175,477	15,923	1,639	0.93	1,177	0.67
RAE230B	168,984	15,333	1,254	0.74	1,507	0.89
RG-U34A	140,317	8,799	23,488	16.74	0	0.00
RG-U34B	140,312	8,791	4,192	2.99	0	0.00
RG-U34C	140,284	8,789	3,968	2.83	0	0.00
RN-U34	21,305	1,322	6,416	30.11	0	0.00
RT-U34	**20,464**	**1,031**	4,980	24.34	0	0.00
Rat230_2	342,410	31,099	2,860	0.84	2,684	0.78
Rhesus	668,485	52,865	44,589	6.67	9,054	1.35
Rice	631,066	57,381	31,262	4.95	**78,746**	12.48
S_aureus	123,524	7,775	4,491	3.64	57,707	**46.72**
Soybean	671,762	61,170	57,498	8.56	9,373	1.40
Sugar_Cane	92,384	8,387	7,283	7.88	2,739	2.96
Tomato	112,528	10,209	1,441	1.28	154	0.14
U133_X3P	673,904	61,359	73,650	10.93	77,568	11.51
Vitis_Vinifera	264,387	16,602	22,261	8.42	4,327	1.64
Xenopus_laevis	249,678	15,611	6,049	2.42	8,864	3.55
YG-S98	138,412	9,335	7,600	5.49	0	0.00
Yeast_2	120,855	10,928	2,084	1.72	473	0.39
Zebrafish	249,752	15,617	2,929	1.17	5,008	2.01
Wheat	**674,353**	61,290	29,119	4.32	74,492	11.05
AVG	249,470.34	20,161.55	27,919.45	12.07	9,704.58	2.99
Max	674,353	61,413	148,336	70.47	78,746	46.72
Min	20,464	1,031	0	0	0	0

Table 5. Thermodynamic evaluation of random sets of 1000 probes for 74 Affymetrix arrays

Array	PM-MT	PM-MFE	$\delta*$	Array	PM-MT	PM-MFE	$\delta*$
ATH1-121501	23.25	14.19	3.03	MG-U74B	26.86	16.91	-12.12
AtGenome1	23.17	13.75	2.51	MG-U74Bv2	25.17	15.24	-2.73
Barley1	25.00	15.60	2.31	MG-U74C	27.49	16.44	-8.17
Bovine	24.18	13.67	-7.29	MG-U74Cv2	34.65	20.88	-9.03
Bsubtilis	26.75	16.67	-8.80	MOE430A	21.76	**12.75**	-4.22
C_elegans	26.23	15.39	2.86	MOE430B	22.99	14.39	-2.18
Canine	24.70	15.17	4.13	Maize	24.71	14.45	-2.74
Canine_2	27.21	17.62	-3.40	Medicago	23.42	13.97	-5.99
Chicken	29.36	18.11	3.72	Mouse430A_2	23.70	14.36	-6.10
Citrus	26.45	15.73	-6.82	Mouse430_2	26.07	15.92	4.55
Cotton	22.39	13.97	-7.43	Mu11KsubA	27.46	17.25	0.40
DrosGenome1	23.59	14.56	-4.46	Mu11KsubB	27.45	17.15	-8.29
Drosophila_2	24.35	15.28	0.19	P_aeruginosa	22.37	13.85	1.14
E_coli	31.30	19.83	-9.80	Plasmodium_Anopheles	27.24	16.11	0.63
E_coli_2	25.69	16.01	-8.84	Poplar	25.15	16.25	**5.42**
E_coli_Antisense	30.73	18.86	-9.26	Porcine	23.66	14.36	4.99
HC-G110	28.37	17.34	-12.30	RAE230A	**21.70**	13.91	3.06
HG-Focus	28.15	18.44	-1.71	RAE230B	25.24	15.23	3.44
HG-U133A	29.89	17.13	**-12.59**	RG-U34A	26.92	16.61	-7.98
HG-U133A_2	25.16	15.61	-3.67	RG-U34B	29.81	19.39	-5.42
HG-U133B	23.97	15.87	-0.26	RG-U34C	25.77	16.58	-2.25
HG-U133_Plus_2	26.04	16.11	2.67	RN-U34	28.04	17.12	-10.85
HG-U95A	28.04	16.80	-8.42	RT-U34	28.85	17.66	-12.40
HG-U95Av2	28.46	16.72	2.46	Rat230_2	22.80	13.96	-2.98
HG-U95B	26.95	15.93	-10.91	Rhesus	27.18	15.80	-0.02
HG-U95C	27.21	16.55	-4.07	Rice	22.95	14.59	3.01
HG-U95D	**35.08**	**21.54**	-11.69	S_aureus	27.25	16.36	-12.17
HG-U95E	32.48	20.06	-5.78	Soybean	25.62	15.88	2.53
HT-HG-U133A	26.63	15.74	2.88	Sugar_Cane	28.90	16.69	-3.39
HT-HG-U133B	28.60	17.75	1.32	Tomato	23.38	13.68	3.27
Hu35KsubA	28.27	16.26	-6.74	U133_X3P	27.88	17.29	-4.48
Hu35KsubB	26.25	15.41	-4.36	Vitis_Vinifera	22.97	13.89	-7.47
Hu35KsubC	28.61	17.60	-7.63	Xenopus_laevis	26.16	15.54	2.83
Hu35KsubD	29.79	18.78	-11.41	YG-S98	28.46	18.06	-6.17
HuGeneFL	28.20	17.26	-5.83	Yeast_2	22.67	13.89	5.37
MG-U74A	28.29	17.66	-9.45	Zebrafish	25.97	15.86	-2.03
MG-U74Av2	28.86	17.14	-5.65	Wheat	25.24	16.21	-5.30

individually ignoring the potential interaction among sequences, while the δ^* measure allows us to estimate the degree of interaction among pairs of probes and complements and among complements. More, the δ^* measure is not as sensitive to the nucleotide content of the probe and target sequences, as PM-MT and PM-MFE are. From a practical perspective, δ^* plays a very important role because the thermodynamic constraints T1 and T2 allow one to directly design a collection of probe sequences for which δ^* is above a certain threshold, thus limiting cross-hybridization. Negative δ^* values signify that some hybridizations among probe-complement or complement-complement sequences are energetically stronger than perfect match hybridizations, thus the potential of having large quantities of noise caused by cross hybridization in the microarray signals is high since the free energies of DNA duplex hybridization and signal intensities can be directly correlated via the Langmuir model (Halperin, Buhot, & Zhulina, 2006).

By taking random samples containing 1,000 probe sequences for each of the 74 Affymetrix arrays, we obtained under-estimates of δ^* values. Note that exact estimates will imply the exhaustive calculation of all probe-complement and complement-complement hybridization, a process that is very computationally expensive ($O(N^2)$, where N is the total number of probes on an array and is usually above 10,000). Our random sampling approach shows that the largest δ^* value (5.42 kcal/mol) corresponds to the Poplar array, while the smallest value (-12.59 kcal/mol) corresponds to the Human HG-U133A array. The average δ^* for all 74 arrays is -3.57 kcal/mol. We also note that only 4 out of 20 (20%) Human arrays have positive δ^* values, which represents the same percentage as for Mouse arrays (2 out of 10). The highest percentage of positive δ^* values is observed in plant arrays, i.e. 50% (7 out of 14). Also, when δ^* average is considered, plant arrays ($avg(\delta^*)$ = -1.22 kcal/mol) outperform Human ($avg(\delta^*)$ = -5.13 kcal/mol), Mouse ($avg(\delta^*)$ = -5.25

kcal/mol) and other mammalian arrays ($avg(\delta^*)$ = -2.84 kcal/mol). This suggests, that in average, plant arrays may exhibit less cross-hybridization among probes and undesired targets as opposed to Human, mouse and other mammalian arrays, nevertheless we may arrive at a definite conclusion only after an exhaustive rather than a random sample approach is considered.

In the majority of probe design programs, the only control mechanism for cross-hybridization avoidance relies on using local alignment algorithms like BLAST and BLAT (Kent, 2002). Such algorithms, while providing a significant computational speed up, suffer from major drawbacks, like the lack of guarantees with respect to the optimality of the results and more importantly their inability to identify sequence matches shorter than the initial string size (Flikka, Yadetie, Laegreid, & Jonassen, 2004). Thus it is highly recommended to combine traditional probe design criteria with more advanced approaches (e.g. integration of the δ^* measure) that allow better quality control for probes, while still ensuring the computational feasibility of the whole design process.

CONCLUSION AND FUTURE RESEARCH DIRECTIONS

While over the past decade significant advancements in understanding hybridization on microarrays was reported, the adaptation of efficient probe design techniques for generating high quality arrays is still an area that requires special attention. This chapter summarizes existing probe design techniques available in the literature and introduces the general DNA sequence design problem together with combinatorial and thermodynamic constraints relevant for microarrays. The chapter presents promising algorithmic solutions based on stochastic local search approaches that are capable of taking the microarray probe design at the next level, where both, high probe quality and computational efficiency are combined.

The case study considered in this work evaluates existing collections of publicly available probes specific to 74 Affymetrix arrays. While Affymetrix technology provides the necessary means for experimentalists to simultaneously explore impressive numbers of genes (tens of thousands), the analysis of the existing probe and target sequences suggests that probe design can be further improved. Probe and target sequence redundancy can be easily detected and minimized using widely-used local alignment algorithms and overall probe quality can be improved by further restricting (where possible) the intervals of thermodynamic characteristics (e.g. perfect match melting temperatures and minimum free energies). A major improvement in probe quality can be achieved if constraints based on pairwise sequence hybridization are used during the probe design process, either during or after the processing phase, as suggested by the two metaheuristic algorithms presented in this chapter. We also acknowledge that a tradeoff between using a higher number of probes per target (Affymetrix currently uses 11-20 probes per target) or lower numbers of higher quality probes (other technologies use only one long probe per target) must be established.

We conclude, that while an emerging trend in computational work over the past decade focuses on signal interpretation (dealing with errors and inaccuracies) rather than probe sequence design (producing data with less errors and inaccuracies), the next major milestone that will allow microarrays to play a far more important role in health, pharmacology, and systems biology studies, lies in the latter trend, rather than the former.

REFERENCES

Aarhus, M., Helland, C. A., Lund-Johansen, M., Wester, K., & Knappskog, P. M. (2010). Microarray-based gene expression profiling and DNA copy number variation analysis of temporal fossa arachnoid cysts. *Cerebrospinal Fluid Research*, 7(6).

Altschul, S. F., Gish, W., Miller, W., Myers, E. W., & Lipman, D. J. (1990). Basic local alignment search tool. *Journal of Molecular Biology*, 215(3), 403–410.

Andrews, J., Bouffard, G. G., Cheadle, C., Lü, J., Becker, K. G., & Oliver, B. (2000). Gene discovery using computational and microarray analysis of transcription in the Drosophila melanogaster testis. *Genome Research*, 10(12), 2030–2043. doi:10.1101/gr.10.12.2030

Andronescu, M. (2003). Algorithms for predicting the secondary structure of pairs and combinatorial sets of nucleic acid strands. *Master thesis*, University of British Columbia, BC, Canada.

Andronescu, M. S. (2008). Computational approaches for RNA energy parameter estimation. *PhD thesis*, University of British Columbia, BC, Canada.

Andronescu, M., Zhang, Z. C., & Condon, A. (2005). Secondary structure prediction of interacting RNA molecules. *Journal of Molecular Biology*, 345(5), 987–1001. doi:10.1016/j.jmb.2004.10.082

Barnes, M., Freudenberg, J., Thompson, S., Aronow, B., & Pavlidis, P. (2005). Experimental comparison and cross-validation of the Affymetrix and Illumina gene expression analysis platforms. *Nucleic Acids Research*, 33(18), 5914–5923. doi:10.1093/nar/gki890

Bogdanova, G. T., Brouwer, A. E., Kapralov, S. N., & Östergård, P. R. J. (2001). Error-correcting codes over an alphabet of four elements. *Designs, Codes and Cryptography*, 23(3), 333–342. doi:10.1023/A:1011275112159

Bozdech, Z., Zhu, J., Joachimiak, M. P., Cohen, F. E., Pulliam, B., & DeRisi, J. L. (2003). Expression profiling of the schizont and trophozoite stages of Plasmodium falciparum with a long-oligonucleotide microarray. *Genome Biology*, 4, R9. doi:10.1186/gb-2003-4-2-r9

Braich, R., Johnson, C., Rothermund, P., Hwang, D., Chelyapov, N., & Leman, L. (2001). Solution of a satisfiability problem on a gel-based DNA computer. *Lecture Notes in Computer Science, 2054*, 27–42. doi:10.1007/3-540-44992-2_3

Brelauer, K. J., Frank, R., Blöcher, H., & Marky, L. A. (1986). Predicting DNA duplex stability from the base sequence. *Proceedings of the National Academy of Sciences of the United States of America, 83*(11), 3746–3750. doi:10.1073/pnas.83.11.3746

Brenner, S., & Lerner, R. A. (1992). Encoded combinatorial chemistry. *Proceedings of the National Academy of Sciences of the United States of America, 89*(12), 5381–5383. doi:10.1073/pnas.89.12.5381

Brouwer, A. E., Shearer, J. B., Sloane, N. J. A., & Smith, W. D. (1990). A new table of constant weight codes. *IEEE Transactions on Information Theory, 36*, 1334–1380. doi:10.1109/18.59932

Cambon, A. C., Khalyfa, A., Cooper, N. G., & Thompson, C. M. (2007). Analysis of probe level patterns in Affymetrix microarray data. *BMC Bioinformatics, 8*(146).

Charbonnier, Y., Gettler, B., Francois, P., Bento, M., Renzoni, A., & Vaudaux, P. (2005). A generic approach for the design of whole-genome oligoarrays, validated for genomotyping, deletion mapping and gene expression analysis on Staphylococcus aureus. *BMC Genomics, 6*(1), 95. doi:10.1186/1471-2164-6-95

Chee, Y. M., & Ling, S. (2008). Improved lower bounds for constant GC-content DNA codes. *IEEE Transactions on Information Theory, 54*(1), 391–394. doi:10.1109/TIT.2007.911167

Chen, H., & Sharp, B. M. (2002). Oliz, a suite of Perl scripts that assist in the design of microarrays using 50mer oligonucleotides from the 3' untranslated region. *BMC Bioinformatics, 3*(27).

Chou, H. H., Hsia, A. P., Mooney, D. L., & Schnable, P. S. (2004). Picky: oligo microarray design for large genomes. *Bioinformatics (Oxford, England), 20*, 2893–2902. doi:10.1093/bioinformatics/bth347

Chung, W. H., Rhee, S.-K., Wan, X. F., Bae, J.-W., Quan, Z.-X., & Park, Y.-H. (2005). Design of long oligonucleotide probes for functional gene detection in a microbial community. *Bioinformatics (Oxford, England), 21*, 4092–4100. doi:10.1093/bioinformatics/bti673

Chu, W., Ghahramani, Z., Falciani, F., & Wild, D. L. (2005). Biomarker discovery in microarray gene expression data with Gaussian processes. *Bioinformatics (Oxford, England), 21*(16), 3385–3393. doi:10.1093/bioinformatics/bti526

Crothers, D., & Zimm, B. (1964). Theory of the melting transition of synthetic polynucleotides: Evaluation of the stacking free energy. *Journal of Molecular Biology, 116*, 1–9. doi:10.1016/S0022-2836(64)80086-3

Deaton, R., Garzon, M., Murphy, R., Rose, J., Franceschetti, D., & Stevens, S. (1996). Genetic search of reliable encodings for DNA- based computation. *Proceedings of the First Annual Conference on Genetic Programming*, 9–15.

Deaton, R., Murphy, R., Garzon, M., Franceschetti, D., & Stevens, S. (1999). Good encodings for DNA-based solutions to combinatorial problems. *DIMACS Series in Discrete Mathematics and Theoretical Computer Science, 44*, 247–258.

Delcourt, S., & Blake, R. (1991). Stacking energies in DNA. *The Journal of Biological Chemistry, 266*(23), 15160–15169.

Devoe, H., & Tinoco, L. (1962). The stability of helical polynucleotides: base contributions. *Journal of Molecular Biology, 4*, 500–517. doi:10.1016/S0022-2836(62)80105-3

Doktycz, M. J., Goldstein, R. F., Paner, T. M., Gallo, F. J., & Benight, A. S. (1992). Studies of DNA dumbbells. I. Melting curves of 17 DNA dumbbells with different duplex stem sequences linked by T4 endloops: evaluation of the nearest neighbor stacking interactions in DNA. *Biopolymers, 32*(7), 849–864. doi:10.1002/bip.360320712

Dufour, Y. S., Wesenberg, G. E., Tritt, A. J., Glasner, J. D., Perna, N. T., Mitchell, J. C., & Donohue, T. J. (2010). chipD: a web tool to design oligonucleotide probes for high-density tiling arrays. *Nucleic Acids Research, 38* Suppl(), W321-5.

Emrich, S. J., Lowe, M., & Delcher, A. L. (2003). PROBEmer: A web-based software tool for selecting optimal DNA oligos. *Nucleic Acids Research, 31*(13), 3746–3750. doi:10.1093/nar/gkg569

Faulhammer, D., Cukras, A., Lipton, R., & Landweber, R. (2000). Molecular computation: RNA solutions to chess problems. *Proceedings of the National Academy of Sciences of the United States of America, 97*, 1385–1389. doi:10.1073/pnas.97.4.1385

Feldkamp, U., Banzhaf, W., & Rauhe, H. (2000). A DNA sequence compiler. *In Proceedings of the 6th DIMACS Workshop on DNA Based Computers*, 253.

Flikka, K., Yadetie, F., Laegreid, A., & Jonassen, I. (2004). XHM: a system for detection of potential cross hybridizations in DNA microarrays. *BMC Bioinformatics, 27*(5), 117. doi:10.1186/1471-2105-5-117

Frutos, A. G., Liu, Q., Thiel, A. J., Sanner, A. M. W., Condon, A. E., Smith, L. M., & Corn, R. M. (1997). Demonstration of a word design strategy for DNA computing on surfaces. *Nucleic Acids Research, 25*, 4748–4757. doi:10.1093/nar/25.23.4748

Gaborit, P., & King, O. D. (2005). Linear construction for DNA codes. *Theoretical Computer Science, 334*, 99–113. doi:10.1016/j.tcs.2004.11.004

Gamal, A. A. E., Hemachandra, L. A., Shperling, I., & Wei, V. K. (1987). Using simulated annealing to design good codes. *IEEE Transactions on Information Theory, 33*(1), 116–123. doi:10.1109/TIT.1987.1057277

Ghiggi, A. (2010). *DNA strands design with thermodynamic constraints.* Master thesis, Università della Svizzera Italiana.

Gordon, P. M. K., & Sensen, C. W. (2004). Osprey: a comprehensive tool employing novel methods for the design of oligonucleotides for DNA sequencing and microarrays. *Nucleic Acids Research, 32*(17), e133. doi:10.1093/nar/gnh127

Gotoh, O., & Tagashira, Y. (1981). Stabilities of nearest-neighbor doublets in double helical DNA determined by fitting calculated melting profiles to observed profiles. *Biopolymers, 20*, 1033–1042. doi:10.1002/bip.1981.360200513

Haas, S. A., Hild, M., Wright, A. P. H., Hain, T., Talibi, D., & Vingron, M. (2003). Genome-scale design of PCR primers and long oligomers for DNA microarrays. *Nucleic Acids Research, 31*(19), 5576–5581. doi:10.1093/nar/gkg752

Halperin, A., Buhot, A., & Zhulina, E. B. (2006). On the hybridization isotherms of DNA microarrays: the Langmuir model and its extensions. *Journal of Physics Condensed Matter, 18*, S463. doi:10.1088/0953-8984/18/18/S01

Hanlon, S. E., & Lieb, J. D. (2004). Progress and challenges in profiling the dynamics of chromatin and transcription factor binding with DNA microarrays. *Current Opinion in Genetics & Development, 14*, 697–705. doi:10.1016/j.gde.2004.09.008

Harbig, J., Sprinkle, R., & Enkemann, S. A. (2005). A sequence-based identification of the genes detected by probesets on the Affymetrix U133 plus 2.0 array. *Nucleic Acids Research, 33*(3), e31. doi:10.1093/nar/gni027

Harris, C., & Ghaffari, N. (2008). Biomarker discovery across annotated and unannotated microarray datasets using semi-supervised learning. *BMC Genomics, 9*(Suppl 2), S7. doi:10.1186/1471-2164-9-S2-S7

Ho, P. S., Frederick, C. A., Quigley, G. J., van der Marel, G. A., van Boom, J. H., Wang, A. H., & Rich, A. (1985). G.T wobble base-pairing in Z-DNA at 1.0 A atomic resolution: the crystal structure of d(CGCGTG). *The EMBO Journal, 4*(13A), 3617–3623.

Holloway, A. J., van Laar, R. K., Tothill, R. W., & Bowtell, D. (2002). Options available-from start to finish-for obtaining data from DNA microarrays II. *Nature Genetics, 32*(suppl. 2), 481–489. doi:10.1038/ng1030

Hoos, H., & Stützle, T. (2004). *Stochastic Local Search: Foundations and Applications*. San Francisco: Morgan Kaufmann.

Hornshoj, H., Stengaard, H., Panitz, F., & Bendixen, C. (2004). SEPON, a Selection and Evaluation Pipeline for OligoNucleotides based on ESTs with a non-target Tm algorithm for reducing cross-hybridization in microarray gene expression experiments. *Bioinformatics (Oxford, England), 20*, 428–429. doi:10.1093/bioinformatics/btg434

Ibrahim, Z., Kurniawan, T. B., Khalid, N. K., Sudin, S., & Khalid, M. (2009). Implementation of an ant colony system for DNA sequence optimization. *Artificial Life and Robotics, 14*, 293–296. doi:10.1007/s10015-009-0683-0

Irizarry, R. A., Hobbs, B., Collin, F., Beazer-Barclay, Y. D., Antonellis, K. J., Scherf, U., & Speed, T. P. (2003). Exploration, normalization, and summaries of high density oligonucleotide array probe level data. *Biostatistics (Oxford, England), 4*(2), 249–264. doi:10.1093/biostatistics/4.2.249

Jang, H. J., Nde, C., Toghrol, F., & Bentley, W. E. (2008). Microarray analysis of toxicogenomic effects of ortho-phenylphenol in Staphylococcus aureus. *BMC Genomics, 9*, 411. doi:10.1186/1471-2164-9-411

Jourdren, L., Duclos, A., Brion, C., Portnoy, T., Mathis, H., Margeot, A., & Le Crom, S. (2010). Teolenn: an efficient and customizable workflow to design high-quality probes for microarray experiments. *Nucleic Acids Research, 38*(10), e117. doi:10.1093/nar/gkq110

Kaderali, L., & Schliep, A. (2002). Selecting signature oligonucleotides to identify organisms using DNA arrays. *Bioinformatics (Oxford, England), 18*(10), 1340–1349. doi:10.1093/bioinformatics/18.10.1340

Kai, Z., Linqiang, P., & Jin, X. (2007). A global heuristically search algorithm for DNA encoding. *Progress in Natural Science, 17*(6). doi:10.1080/10002007088537469

Kalendar, R., Lee, D., & Schulman, A. H. (2009). FastPCR Software for PCR Primer and Probe Design and Repeat Search. *Genes. Genomes and Genomics, 3*(1), 1–14.

Kao, M.-Y., Sanghi, M., & Schweller, R. (2009). Randomized fast design of short DNA words. *ACS Transactions on Algorithms, 5*(4), 43.

Kapur, K., Jiang, H., Xing, Y., & Wong, W. H. (2008). Cross-hybridization modeling on Affymetrix exon arrays. *Bioinformatics (Oxford, England), 24*(24), 2887–2893. doi:10.1093/bioinformatics/btn571

Kent, W. J. (2002). BLAT--the BLAST-like alignment tool. *Genome Research, 12*(4), 656–664.

Khalid, N. K., Ibrahim, Z., Kurniawan, T. B., Khalid, M., & Enggelbrecht, A. P. (2009). Implementation of binary particle swarm optimization for DNA sequence design. *Lecture Notes in Computer Science, 5518*, 450–457. doi:10.1007/978-3-642-02481-8_64

King, O. D. (2003). Bounds for DNA codes with constant GC-content. *Electronic Journal of Combinatorics, 10*, R33.

Kobayashi, S., Kondo, T., & Arita, M. (2003). On Template Method for DNA Sequence Design. *Lecture Notes in Computer Science, 2568*, 205–214. doi:10.1007/3-540-36440-4_18

Koul, N. (2010). *Metaheuristics for DNA codes design.* Master thesis. Università della Svizzera Italiana, Switzerland.

Kreil, D. P., Russell, R. R., & Russell, S. (2006). Microarray oligonucleotide probes. *Methods in Enzymology, 410*, 73–98. doi:10.1016/S0076-6879(06)10004-X

Kurniawan, T. B., Khalid, N. K., Ibrahim, Z., Khalid, M., & Middendorf, M. (2008). An ant colony system for DNA sequence design based on thermodynamics. *Proceedings of the Fourth IASTED International Conference on Advances in Computer Science and Technology*, 144-149.

Lemoine, S., Combes, F., & Le Crom, S. (2009). An evaluation of custom microarray applications: the oligonucleotide design challenge. *Nucleic Acids Research, 37*(6), 1726–1739. doi:10.1093/nar/gkp053

Leung, Y., & Hung, Y. (2010). A multiple-filter-multiple-wrapper approach to gene selection and microarray data classification. *IEEE/ACM Transactions on Computational Biology and Bioinformatics, 7*(1), 108–117. doi:10.1109/TCBB.2008.46

Li, C., & Wong, W. H. (2001). Model-based analysis of oligonucleotide arrays: expression index computation and outlier detection. *Proceedings of the National Academy of Sciences of the United States of America, 98*(1), 31–36. doi:10.1073/pnas.011404098

Li, F., & Stormo, G. D. (2001). Selection of optimal DNA oligos for gene expression arrays. *Bioinformatics (Oxford, England), 17*, 1067–1076. doi:10.1093/bioinformatics/17.11.1067

Li, M., Lee, H. J., Condon, A. E., & Corn, R. M. (2002). DNA word design strategy for creating sets of non-interacting oligonucleotides for DNA microarrays. *Langmuir, 18*, 805–812. doi:10.1021/la0112209

Li, X., Hel, Z., & Zhou, J. (2005). Selection of optimal oligonucleotide probes for microarrays using multiple criteria, global alignment and parameter estimation. *Nucleic Acids Research, 33*(19), 6114–6123. doi:10.1093/nar/gki914

Lu, Z. J., Turner, D. H., & Mathews, D. H. (2006). A set of nearest neighbor parameters for predicting the enthalpy change of RNA secondary structure formation. *Nucleic Acids Research, 34*, 4912–4924. doi:10.1093/nar/gkl472

Ludwig, W., Strunk, O., Westram, R., Richter, L., & Meier, H., Yadhukumar, *et al.* (2004). ARB: a software environment for sequence data. *Nucleic Acids Research, 32*(4), 1363–1371. doi:10.1093/nar/gkh293

MacAlpine, D. M., & Bell, S. P. (2005). A genomic view of eukaryotic DNA replication. *Chromosome Research, 13*, 309–326. doi:10.1007/s10577-005-1508-1

Marathe, A., Condon, A. E., & Corn, R. M. (2001). On combinatorial DNA word design. *Journal of Computational Biology, 8*(3), 201–219. doi:10.1089/10665270152530818

Montemanni, R., & Smith, D. H. (2008). Construction of constant GC-content DNA codes via a Variable Neighbourhood Search algorithm. *Journal of Mathematical Modelling and Algorithms, 7*, 311–326. doi:10.1007/s10852-008-9087-8

Montemanni, R., & Smith, D. H. (2009). Heuristic algorithms for constructing binary constant weight codes. *IEEE Transactions on Information Theory, 55*(10), 4651–4656. doi:10.1109/TIT.2009.2027491

Montemanni, R., & Smith, D. H. (2009). Metaheuristics for the construction of constant GC-content DNA codes. *Proceedings of the VIII Metaheuristic International Conference (MIC)*.

Montemanni, R., Smith, D.H., & Koul, N. Three metaheuristics for the construction of constant GC-content DNA codes. *Springer volume on metaheuristic algorithms*, S. Voβ and M. Caserta eds., to appear.

Mrowka, R., Schuchhardt, J., & Gille, C. (2002). Oligodb--interactive design of oligo DNA for transcription profiling of human genes. *Bioinformatics (Oxford, England), 18*(12), 1686–1687. doi:10.1093/bioinformatics/18.12.1686

Neumanna, N. F., & Galvez, F. (2002). DNA microarrays and toxicogenomics: applications for ecotoxicology? *Biotechnology Advances, 20*(5-6), 391–419. doi:10.1016/S0734-9750(02)00025-3

Nielsen, H. B., & Knudsen, S. (2002). Avoiding cross hybridization by choosing nonredundant targets on cDNA arrays. *Bioinformatics (Oxford, England), 18*, 321–322. doi:10.1093/bioinformatics/18.2.321

Nielsen, H. B., Wernersson, R., & Knudsen, S. (2003). Design of oligonucleotides for microarrays and perspectives for design of multi-transcriptome arrays. *Nucleic Acids Research, 31*(13), 3491–3496. doi:10.1093/nar/gkg622

Nordberg, E. K. (2005). YODA: selecting signature oligonucleotides. *Bioinformatics (Oxford, England), 21*, 1365–1370. doi:10.1093/bioinformatics/bti182

Okoniewski, M. J., & Miller, C. J. (2006). Hybridization interactions between probesets in short oligo microarrays lead to spurious correlations. *BMC Bioinformatics, 7*, 276. doi:10.1186/1471-2105-7-276

Orlov, Y. L., Zhou, J. T., Lipovich, L., Yong, H. C., Li, Y., Shahab, A., & Kuznetsov, V. A. (2006). A comprehensive quality assessment of the Affymetrix U133A&B probesets by an integrative genomic and clinical data analysis approach. *Proceedings of the Fifth International Conference on Bioinformatics of Genome Regulation and Structure*, Novosibirsk, Inst. of Cytology & Genetics, 1, 126-129.

Östergård, P. R. J. (2002). A fast algorithm for the maximum clique problem. *Discrete Applied Mathematics, 120*, 197–207. doi:10.1016/S0166-218X(01)00290-6

Pardalos, P. M., & Xue, J. (1994). The maximum clique problem. *Journal of Global Optimization, 4*, 301–328. doi:10.1007/BF01098364

Pasquer, F., Pelludat, C., Duffy, B., & Frey, J. E. (2010). Broad spectrum microarray for fingerprint-based bacterial species identification. *BMC Biotechnology, 10*, 13. doi:10.1186/1472-6750-10-13

Peng, Y., Li, W., & Liu, Y. (2007). A hybrid approach for biomarker discovery from microarray gene expression data for cancer classification. *Cancer Informatics, 2*, 301–311.

Pfaff, D. A., Clarke, K. M., Parr, T. A., Cole, J. M., Geierstanger, B. H., Tahmassebi, D. C., & Dwyer, T. J. (2008). Solution structure of a DNA duplex containing a guanine-difluorotoluene pair: a wobble pair without hydrogen bonding? *Journal of the American Chemical Society, 130*(14), 4869–4878. doi:10.1021/ja7103608

Pinkel, D., & Albertson, D. G. (2005). Comparative genomic hybridization. *Annual Review of Genomics and Human Genetics, 6*, 331–354. doi:10.1146/annurev.genom.6.080604.162140

Pozhitkov, A. E., Tautz, D., & Noble, P. A. (2007). Oligonucleotide microarrays: widely applied--poorly understood. *Briefings in Functional Genomics & Proteomics, 6*(2), 141–148. doi:10.1093/bfgp/elm014

Premier Biosoft. Array Designer v4.25. (1994-2011). Retrieved from http://www.premierbiosoft.com/dnamicroarray/index.html, (Retrieved September 20, 2010).

ProbePicker. (n.d.). Retrieved from http://sourceforge.net/projects/probepicker/, (Retrieved September 2010).

Quackenbush, J. (2002). Microarray data normalization and transformation. *Nature Genetics, 32,* 496–501. doi:10.1038/ng1032

Raddatz, G., Dehio, M., Meyer, T. F., & Dehio, C. (2001). PrimeArray: genome-scale primer design for DNA-microarray construction. *Bioinformatics (Oxford, England), 17,* 98–99. doi:10.1093/bioinformatics/17.1.98

Rahmann, S. (2003). Fast large scale oligonucleotide selection using the longest common actor approach. *Journal of Bioinformatics and Computational Biology, 1*(2), 343–361. doi:10.1142/S0219720003000125

Reif, J. H., Labean, T. H., & Seeman, N. C. (2001). Challenges and applications for self-assembled DNA nanostructures. *Lecture Notes in Computer Science, 2054,* 173. doi:10.1007/3-540-44992-2_12

Reymond, N., Charles, H., Duret, L., Calevro, F., Beslon, G., & Fayard, J.-M. (2004). ROSO: Optimizing Oligonucleotide Probes for Microarrays. *Bioinformatics (Oxford, England), 20,* 271–273. doi:10.1093/bioinformatics/btg401

Rimour, S., Hill, D., Militon, C., & Peyret, P. (2005). GoArrays: highly dynamic and efficient microarray probe design. *Bioinformatics (Oxford, England), 21*(7), 1094–1103. doi:10.1093/bioinformatics/bti112

Ross, D. T., Scherf, U., Eisen, M. B., Perou, C. M., Rees, C., & Spellman, P. (2000). Systematic variation in gene expression patterns in human cancer cell lines. *Nature Genetics, 24,* 227–235. doi:10.1038/73432

Rouillard, J.-M., Herbert, C. J., & Zuker, M. (2002)... *Bioinformatics (Oxford, England), 18*(3), 486–487. doi:10.1093/bioinformatics/18.3.486

Rouillard, J.-M., Zuker, M., & Gulari, E. (2003). OligoArray 2.0: design of oligonucleotide probes for DNA microarrays using a thermodynamic approach. *Nucleic Acids Research, 31,* 3057–3062. doi:10.1093/nar/gkg426

Rouillard, J.-M., Lee, W., Truan, G., Gao, X., Zhou, X., & Gulari, E. (2004). Gene2Oligo: Oligonucleotide design for in vitro gene synthesis. *Nucleic Acids Research, 32,* W176-80. doi:10.1093/nar/gkh401

Rouchka, E. C., Khalyfa, A., & Cooper, N. G. F. (2005). MPrime: efficient large scale multiple primer and oligonucleotide design for customized gene microarrays. *BMC Bioinformatics, 6,* 175. doi:10.1186/1471-2105-6-175

Rozen, S., & Skaletsky, H. J. (2000). Primer3 on the WWW for general users and for biologist programmers. In Krawetz, S., & Misener, S. (Eds.), *Bioinformatics Methods and Protocols: Methods in Molecular Biology* (pp. 365–386). Totowa, NJ: Humana Press.

SantaLucia, J., Allawi, H. T., & Seneviratne, P. A. (1996). Improved nearest-neighbor parameters for predicting DNA duplex stability. *Biochemistry, 35*(11), 3555–3562. doi:10.1021/bi951907q

SantaLucia, J. (1998). A unified view of polymer, dumbbell, and oligonucleotide DNA nearest-neighbor thermodynamics. *Proceedings of the National Academy of Sciences of the United States of America, 95*(4), 1460–1465. doi:10.1073/pnas.95.4.1460

SantaLucia, J., & Hicks, D. (2004). The thermodynamics of DNA structural motifs. *Annual Review of Biophysics and Biomolecular Structure*, *3*, 415–440. doi:10.1146/annurev. biophys.32.110601.141800

Schena, M., Shalon, D., Davis, R. W., & Brown, P. O. (1995). Quantitative monitoring of gene expression patterns with a complementary DNA microarray. *Science*, *270*, 467–470. doi:10.1126/science.270.5235.467

Schretter, C., & Milinkovitch, M. C. (2006). OligoFaktory: a visual tool for interactive oligonucleotide design. *Bioinformatics (Oxford, England)*, *22*(1), 115–116. doi:10.1093/bioinformatics/bti728

Smith, D. H., Aboluion, N., Montemanni, R., & Perkins, S. (to appear). Linear and nonlinear constructions of DNA codes with constant GC-content. *Discrete Mathematics*.

Srivastava, G. P., Guo, J., Shi, H., & Xu, D. (2008). PRIMEGENS-v2: genome-wide primer design for analyzing DNA methylation pattern of CpG island. *Bioinformatics (Oxford, England)*, *24*(17), 1837–1842. doi:10.1093/bioinformatics/btn320

Stenberg, J., Nilsson, M., & Landegren, U. (2005). ProbeMaker: an extensible framework for design of sets of oligonucleotide probes. *BMC Bioinformatics*, *6*, 229. doi:10.1186/1471-2105-6-229

Sugimoto, N., Nakano, S., Yoneyama, M., & Honda, K. (1996). Improved thermodynamic parameters and helix initiation factor to predict stability of DNA duplexes. *Nucleic Acids Research*, *24*(22), 4501–4505. doi:10.1093/nar/24.22.4501

Talla, E., Tekaia, F., Brino, L., & Dujon, B. (2003). A novel design of whole-genome microarray probes for Saccharomyces cerevisiae which minimizes cross-hybridization. *BMC Genomics*, *4*, 38. doi:10.1186/1471-2164-4-38

Teletchea, F., Bernillon, J., Duffraisse, M., Laudet, V., & Hänni, C. (2008). Molecular identification of vertebrate species by oligonucleotide microarray in food and forensic samples. *Journal of Applied Ecology*, *45*(3), 967–975.

Tolstrup, N., Nielsen, P. S., Kolberg, J. G., Frankel, A. M., Vissing, H., & Kauppinen, S. (2003). OligoDesign: Optimal design of LNA (locked nucleic acid) oligonucleotide capture probes for gene expression profiling. *Nucleic Acids Research*, *31*(13), 3758–3762. doi:10.1093/nar/gkg580

Tulpan, D. C., Hoos, H. H., & Condon, A. E. (2002). Stochastic local search algorithms for DNA word design. *Lectures Notes in Computer Science*, Springer, Berlin, 2568, 229–241, 2002.

Tulpan, D. C., & Hoos, H. H. (2003). Hybrid randomised neighbourhoods improve stochastic local search for DNA code design. *Lectures Notes in Computer Science*, Springer, Berlin, 2671, 418–433.

Tulpan, D., Andronescu, M., Chang, S. B., Shortreed, M. R., Condon, A., Hoos, H. H., & Smith, L. M. (2005). Thermodynamically based DNA strand design. *Nucleic Acids Research*, *33*(15), 4951–4964. doi:10.1093/nar/gki773

Tulpan, D. C. (2006). Effective Heuristic Methods of DNA Strand Design. *Ph.D. thesis*, University of British Columbia, BC, Canada.

Tulpan, D., Andronescu, M., & Leger, S. (2010). Free energy estimation of short DNA duplex hybridizations. *BMC Bioinformatics*, *11*(1), 105. doi:10.1186/1471-2105-11-105

Vologodskii, A. V., Amirikyan, B. R., Lyubchenko, Y. L., & Frank-Kamenetskii, M. D. (1984). Allowance for heterogeneous stacking in the DNA helix-coil transition theory. *Journal of Biomolecular Structure & Dynamics*, *2*, 131–148.

Wang, X., & Seed, B. (2003). Selection of Oligonucleotide Probes for Protein Coding Sequences. *Bioinformatics (Oxford, England)*, *19*(7), 796–802. doi:10.1093/bioinformatics/btg086

Wang, Y., Miao, Z.-H., Pommier, Y., Kawasaki, E. S., & Player, A. (2007). Characterization of mismatch and high-signal intensity probes associated with Affymetrix genechips. *Bioinformatics (Oxford, England)*, *23*(16), 2088–2095. doi:10.1093/bioinformatics/btm306

Yang, Y. H., Dudoit, S., Luu, P., Lin, D. M., & Peng, V. (2002). Normalization for cDNA microarray data: a robust composite method addressing single and multiple systemic variation. *Nucleic Acids Research*, *30*, e15. doi:10.1093/nar/30.4.e15

Yano, K., Imai, K., Shimizu, A., & Hanashita, T. (2006)... *Nucleic Acids Research*, *34*(5), 1532–1539. doi:10.1093/nar/gkl058

Yee, J. C., Wlaschin, K. F., Chuah, S. H., Nissom, P. M., & Hu, W. S. (2008). Quality assessment of cross-species hybridization of CHO transcriptome on a mouse DNA oligo microarray. *Biotechnology and Bioengineering*, *101*(6), 1359–1365. doi:10.1002/bit.21984

Yoo, S. M., Choi, J. H., Lee, S. Y., & Yoo, N. C. (2009). Applications of DNA microarray in disease diagnostics. *Journal of Microbiology and Biotechnology*, *19*(7), 635–646.

Yurke, B., Turberfield, A. J., Mills, A. P., Simmel, F. C., & Neumann, J. L. (2000). A DNA-fuelled molecular machine made of DNA. *Nature*, *406*(6796), 605–608. doi:10.1038/35020524

Zhang, B.-T., & Shin, S.-Y. (1998). Molecular algorithms for efficient and reliable DNA computing. *Proceedings of the Third Annual Conference in Genetic Programming* (University of Wisconsin, Madison, Wiscon- sin, USA, 22-25 1998), J. R. Koza, W. Banzhaf, K. Chellapilla, K. Deb, M. Dorigo, D. B. Fogel, M. H. Garzon, D. E. Goldberg, H. Iba, and R. Ri- olo, Eds., Morgan Kaufmann, 735–744.

Zhao, Y., Li, M.-C., & Simon, R. (2005). An adaptive method for cDNA microarray normalization. *BMC Bioinformatics*, *6*, 28. doi:10.1186/1471-2105-6-28

Zheng, J., Svensson, J. T., Madishetty, K., Close, T. J., Jiang, T., & Lonardi, S. (2006). OligoSpawn: a software tool for the design of overgo probes from large unigene datasets. *BMC Bioinformatics*, *7*, 7. doi:10.1186/1471-2105-7-7

Zou, Y. Y., Yang, J., & Zhu, J. (2006). A robust statistical procedure to discover expression biomarkers using microarray genomic expression data. *Journal of Zhejiang University. Science*, *7*(8), 603 607. doi:10.1631/jzus.2006.B0603

Chapter 4
Promoter Structures Conserved between *Homo Sapiens, Mus Musculus* and *Drosophila Melanogaster*

Boris R. Jankovic
King Abdullah University of Science and Technology, Kingdom of Saudi Arabia

John A. C. Archer
King Abdullah University of Science and Technology, Kingdom of Saudi Arabia

Rajesh Chowdhary
Biomedical Informatics Research Center, USA

Ulf Schaefer
King Abdullah University of Science and Technology, Kingdom of Saudi Arabia

Vladimir B. Bajic
King Abdullah University of Science and Technology, Kingdom of Saudi Arabia

ABSTRACT

Some of the key processes in living organisms remain essentially unchanged even in evolutionarily very distant species. Transcriptional regulation is one such fundamental process that is essential for cell survival. Transcriptional control exerts great part of its effects at the level of transcription initiation mediated through protein-DNA interactions mainly at promoters but also at other control regions. In this chapter, the authors identify conserved families of motifs of promoter regulatory structures between Homo sapiens, Mus musculus and Drosophila melanogaster. By a promoter regulatory structure they consider here a combination of motifs from identified motif families. Conservation of promoter structure across these vertebrate and invertebrate genomes suggests the presence of a fundamental promoter architecture and provides the basis for deeper understanding of the necessary components of the transcription regulation machinery. The authors reveal the existence of families of DNA sequence motifs that are shared across all three species in upstream promoter regions. They further analyze the relevance of our findings for better understanding of preserved regulatory mechanisms and associated biology insights.

DOI: 10.4018/978-1-61350-435-2.ch004

Copyright © 2012, IGI Global. Copying or distributing in print or electronic forms without written permission of IGI Global is prohibited.

INTRODUCTION

Some of the key processes in living organisms remain essentially unchanged even in evolutionary very distant species. Transcription regulation is one of such fundamental processes that are necessary for cell survival. Promoters are considered the key regulatory regions of gene transcription initiation and therefore would have the potential to be conserved in cases of highly essential functions. However, conservation of transcription regulation machinery across different species is not well understood (Wray et al, 2003).

Transcription controls location, timing and extent of gene expression in living organisms (Carey et al., 2009). Transcription regulation is significantly responsible for the species-specific patterns of development specificities (Wittcopp, 2010). In that context, study of conserved areas of promoter regions across species at varying evolutionary distance may help our understanding of regulatory mechanisms at play.

Availability of data related to genomic sequences as well as experimentally confirmed transcription start sites (TSS) for a number of species allows for a thorough investigation of shared elements in promoter regions between species. With that objective in mind, we attempt to identify shared families of motifs (short DNA sequences) between promoters of orthologous genes of two mammals, *Homo sapiens* and *Mus musculus,* and promoters of an invertebrate *Drosophila melanogaster* (fruit fly). Our approach is conservative: a) We first find motif families (MFs) shared between the three species; although this is a crucial first step it does not imply that there is a preserved regulatory mechanism across these three species; b) We determined the genes in human and mouse, as well as in fruit fly, whose promoters share a sufficient number (6 to 10) of MFs; we investigated in more detail functional properties of those groups of genes identified by having promoters that share eight MFs. c) We matched the consensus sequences of identified MFs with

the known binding sites of transcription factors, to find out the most common transcription factors involved. Our study is based on inferring preserved promoter structure via shared MFs across three species, and study of bio-chemical significance of the genes that share these structures across three species.

BACKGROUND

The three species in our study were chosen primarily because their genomic sequences and TSSs are well studied and documented in addition to their evolutionary relationship. We would expect that the number of shared MFs would decrease with evolutionary distance, but the nature and dynamics of this process is another interesting aspect of our study.

Studying of promoter motifs for *D. melanogaster* is reported in (Down et al., 2007). This study reveals through statistical analysis 87 novel motifs putatively involved in transcription factor binding. These motifs are determined using only fruit fly promoters and need not be conserved in evolutionary remote species. However, one can look at the shared MFs in promoter regions of several species. The basic idea is that presence of same MFs in promoter regions may suggest conserved regulatory functionality. Clearly, the number of shared MFs, together with the lengths of motifs implies statistical significance of any such commonality.

Organisms that are well studied as well as being evolutionary distant are particularly good candidates for such an analysis. Because it satisfies these requirements, the comparison between human and *Fly* promoters is particularly convenient. Because of these properties, this combination has been studied before (FitzGerald et al, 2006). That study evaluates conserved regions by detecting presence and frequencies of all possible octamers on close to 11,000 *Fly* promoters and two sets of human promoters, approximately 12,000 – 15,000 records. Their study finds that *"Fly* and human promoters use different DNA sequences to regulate gene expression, supporting the idea that evolution occurs by modulation of gene expression" (FitzGerald et al, 2006, page 1).

We approached promoter conservation in a different manner. Firstly, availability of additional mammalian genomic data allowed for a broader opportunity to study conservation of regulatory mechanisms as a function of evolutionary distance. Therefore, the proposition that studying promoter structures in the considered three species would offer some more general inferences, seems reasonable. To establish a quantitative metric for measuring sequence similarity, the way of defining motif structure becomes crucial. Faced with that problem, one approach, utilized by FitzGerald et al. (2006) would be to fix the length of motifs as an 8-mer (octamer) and then investigate promoter sets for the presence of all octamers. Of course, the longer the motif the less likely that matching to promoter regions is a result of chance. Another important feature when comparing promoter regions of different species is the number of shared motifs that can be found. Intuitively, the more shared motifs found, the more likely that some regulatory mechanisms may be conserved.

In (Bajic et al, 2006) four different types of human promoters were identified based on the GC/AT richness of the upstream and downstream regions flanking transcription start sites (TSSs). It is interesting to note that the majority of Fly promoters belong to "AT-rich upstream: AT-rich downstream" type, whilst in the human genome such promoters however represent only a minority group (Bajic et al, 2006). Thus if there are shared MFs from promoters between these species it would be an interesting insight. The study of FitzGerald et al. (2006) shed some light onto this issue.

To derive the components of the promoter structures common to human, mouse and fly, we determined MFs that are shared between their promoters, but we restricted human and mouse promoters to those that correspond to pairs of orthologous genes. The MFs are determined *ab initio* by the Dragon Motif Builder (DMB) tool (Huang et al, 2005) that has been successfully applied across various studies (Mohanty et al, 2005; The FANTOM Consortium, 2005; Brahmachary et al, 2006; Chen et al, 2007; Meier et al, 2008; Yun et al, 2010, Park et al, 2010).

We discuss the results, link them to the regulatory proteins and make comparisons of the human and Fly transcription regulation. Our results represent a component of the computational systems biology approach for discovering parts of the transcriptional regulatory structures across different species.

METHODOLOGY

We used a set of orthologous human and mouse gene pairs derived from a recent work by (Ho et al, 2010). For each pair of orthologous genes (one from human and one from mouse) the genomic coordinates were extracted from the latest version of NCBI's mapview. For human, the 'Primary assembly' data was used. For mouse, the 'C57BL/6J' data was used, which is the reference assembly. The mapview files ('ftp://ftp.ncbi.nih.gov/genomes/H_sapiens/ mapview/seq_gene.md.gz'and'ftp://ftp.ncbi.nih. gov/genomes/M_musculus/mapview/seq_gene. md.gz') were downloaded on Sunday August 22nd 2010. The latest version of hg19 and mm9 were downloaded from UCSC (http://hgdownload.cse. ucsc.edu/downloads.html) on Sunday August 22nd 2010. There are 13,938 human and mouse ortholog pairs that we identified with our set of promoters.

From these sequences 1000 nucleotides regions upstream of TSSs were selected. We then downloaded a complete list of *Fly* promoters (http://hg-download.cse.ucsc.edu/goldenPath/dm3/bigZips/ upstream1000.fa.gz). This generated a dataset of 16,984 *Fly* promoters. The resulting set of 44,860 (13,938+13,938+16,984) promoters was submitted to DMB. We chose motif lengths of 9 bp. In addition, we limited the number of MFs to 200.

In the next step we annotated promoters by mapping MFs to promoter sequences. This is done using the position weight matrices generated by DMB for each MF. Mapping was done using the threshold that was set in DMB (0.9 of the scale from 0 to 1, where 1 is maximum). Using this annotation as a basis we determined several new MFs shared between promoters of *H. sapiens, M. musculus* and *D. melanogaster.*

We also compiled the list of orhtologous human, mouse and fly genes in order to compare this list with the list of those genes in the three species that share the same MF combinations of a given length. For all pairs of human and mouse orthologous genes as extracted from (Ho et al. 2010) the corresponding group of homologous genes in NCBI's Homologene (http://www.ncbi. nlm.nih.gov/homologene, accessed Oct. 9th 2010) was identified. If this group of orthologous genes also contained a gene from *D.melanogaster*, it was reported to be ortholog to both the human and the mouse gene in the pair in question. Of the 13,938 pairs of orthologous human and mouse genes we examined, 3,973 also have an orthologous gene in *D.melanogaster.*

The main challenge was to identify those promoters that have one or more motifs from shared MFs. Since this is computationally an NP-hard problem, we deployed a variant of Monte Carlo search methodology to this problem in order to: (a) find genes with the same promoter model (same number of shared MFs) such that there is at least one promoter from human, one from mouse and one from fly; (b) infer some statistical properties of motif distributions; and (c) establish some measure of conservation, expressed as a number of common motifs.

Since it is not possible to know *a priori* what is the maximum number of shared MFs between the species, we investigated values of between six and ten shared MFs. This computationally intensive approach was facilitated by the use of

multicore servers infrastructure in a parallelized processing approach. In order to better control the computational effort, individual processes would stop when the number of human, mouse and Fly promoters with N (= 6, 7, 8, 9, or 10) shared motifs would either reach 1,000 or a predetermined number of simulation runs has been accomplished.

RESULTS

We outline the results of our analysis as follows. We first report some statistics regarding the number and distribution of combinations of MFs of 6 to 10 that are found in at least one human, at least one mouse and at least one fly promoter region. We then list the genes that correspond to identified promoter regions that share MFs and make some comments on biological interpretation of our findings. Finally, we compare the group of genes sharing MF combinations with the set of orthologous genes between human, mouse and fly.

Identification of MF Combinations

Some basic statistical results of our search for shared MF combinations are summarized in Table 1.

When analyzing results from Table 1, it is important to keep in mind that the reported numbers of MF combinations found depend on the

Table 1. Number of motif combinations from N shared MFs

# of Shared MFs (N)	# of combinations found in Human-Mouse promoters	# of combinations found in Human-Mouse-Fly promoters
6	8564	2099
7	3866	454
8	242	14
9	2	0
10	0	0

number of simulation runs. Therefore, numbers reported in different rows are not directly comparable. For example, we are not inferring that there is 121 times more shared combinations when N = 8 than when N = 9.

However, the values compared in column 2 can be compared to some degree to the corresponding values reported in column 3. This is due to the fact that the same MF combination of a given size is tested for presence in all promoters available. Therefore, the values reported in columns 2 and 3 are derived from the same data set.

For example, when we looked for MF combinations composed of six MFs, we found 2099 such combinations so that there is at least one promoter containing motifs from all six MFs in human, mouse and Fly promoter sets. However, the same MF combinations resulted in 8564 cases when only human and mice were considered. We would expect that the ration 8564/2099 = 4.08 remain approximately the same regardless of the number of simulation runs. More generally, we would expect that the ratio of values in columns 2 and 3 for a given N is largely invariant with respect to computational methodology and that such represent an inherent property of evolutionary distance between the two mammals and *D.melanogaster*.

It is readily observable from Table 1 that such ratio tappers off very quickly with higher N. The essence of this relationship is plotted in Figure 1.

In Figure 1, the actual ratios of numbers of shared motifs between human/mouse and human/mouse/fly are shown for different combination lengths. The dynamics of the ratio implies fast reduction in numbers of shared MFs which is in line with expectations when evolutionary distance increases. A more comprehensive study might reveal the relationship of commonality in MFs of promoter regions with other phylogenetic measures of evolutionary distance.

Since there were 200 MFs identified by DMB, the natural question is whether some MFs are more commonly found as part of those MF combinations that were present in at least one human, one mouse and one fly promoter (successful combinations). This is illustrated in Figures 2-4 in form of a histogram of relative frequency of appearance of individual MFs under such conditions. Each MF is assigned a unique integer identifier and therefore a numbered entry in each of the histograms refers to the same MFs.

Figure 1. Schematic presentation between speciation and the ratio of MF commonality between human, mouse and fly for different combination lengths

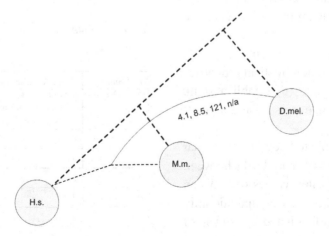

Figure 2. Relative frequency of individual MFs that are part of six-MFs combinations shared by human, mouse and fly promoter regions

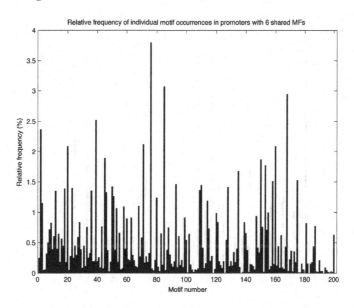

Figure 3. Relative frequency of individual MFs that are part of seven-MF combination shared by human, mouse and fly promoter regions

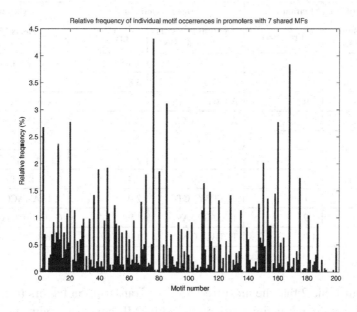

Review of Transcription Factors

In Table 2 we list top 10 individual MFs (each represented by its consensus motif) from successful MF combinations of 6, 7 and 8 MFs. The purpose of this list is to establish whether the MFs that are most frequently shared by human, mouse and fly are indicative of some regulatory or other biologically significant mechanism.

Figure 4. Relative frequency of individual MFs that are part of eight-MFs combination shared by human, mouse and fly promoter regions

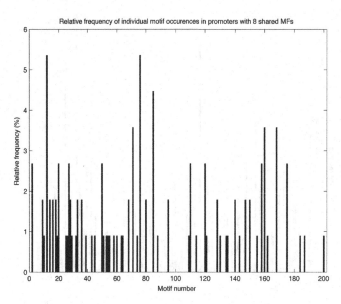

Table 2. Ranking of most frequent MFs in different successful MF combinations

Motif Rank	6-Motifs Combination		7-Motifs Combination		8-Motifs Combination	
	Consensus Motifs of shared MFs	Freq. (%)	Consensus Motifs of shared MFs	Freq. (%)	Consensus Motifs of shared MFs	Freq. (%)
1	WCTTTMTTT	3.8	WCTTTMTTT	4.3	WCTTTMTTT	5.4
2	AAAGRGAAA	3.1	TTTWATTTA	3.8	TTTAAAWTT	5.4
3	TTTWATTTA	2.9	AAAGRGAAA	3.1	AAAGRGAAA	4.5
4	TCTBCCCWC	2.5	ARAAAACCY	2.8	CAGCAAMAA	3.6
5	CTTTTTTTT	2.4	TTWATATTT	2.8	TTWATATTT	3.6
6	CAGCAAMAA	2.1	CTTTTTTTT	2.7	TTTWATTTA	3.6
7	ARAAAACCY	2.1	TTTAAAWTT	2.4	CTTTTTTTT	2.7
8	TTWATATTT	2.1	CTTTBYYCT	2.0	ARAAAACCY	2.7
9	TCCTGRAAV	1.9	TCCTGRAAV	1.9	GRGCAGCTG	2.7
10	CTTTBYYCT	1.9	TCTBCCCWC	1.9	CAGCTCAGH	2.7

It can be seen from Table 2 that the most frequent MF among all three combinations groups is MF characterized by WCTTTMTTT consensus motif. Table 3 lists transcription factors associated with this MF. This association is derived using PATCH program of Transfac Professional v11.4.

Transcription factors from Table 3 imply that this MF correlates with the HMG-box class of transcription factors, TCF/LEF, SOX and SRY. These proteins encode a conserved DNA binding domain (the HMG box) and *in vivo* control a wide range of development processes.

In addition to the most frequent MF, we also analyze another set of MFs that are present in

Table 3. Transcription factors associated with MF WCTTTMTTT

TF identifier	TF binding site	Binding sequence
AS$SRY_02	LEF-1	TCTTT-GTT
AS$SRY_57	Sox2	TCTTT-GTTT
AS$SRY_61	TCF-1	AATA-AAGT
AS$SRY_63	TCF-1	AATA-AAGT
HS$ADA_08	LEF-1	CTTTGTT
HS$ADA_08	SRY	CTTTGTT
HS$CD8A_04	SRY	CTTTGTT
HS$COL27A1_01	TCF-1(P)	CTTTGTT
HS$SRY_01	SRY	AACAAAG
HS$SRY_02	LEF-1	AACAAAG
HS$SRY_03	SoxP1	AACAAAG
MOUSE$FGF4_01	SoxLZ	AACAAAG
MOUSE$FGF4_03	Sox9:Sox9	AACAAAG
MOUSE$FGF4_05	SRY	AACAAAG
MOUSE$HBBY_01	SRY	AACAAAG
MOUSE$LY49A_01	SRY	AAGAAAG
MOUSE$MPZ_04	LEF-1	AACAAAG
MOUSE$OPN_07	c-Ets-1 c-Ets-2 c-Jun Erm, LEF-1	AACAAAG
MOUSE$POU5F1_08	SRY	AACAAAG
MOUSE$SRY_01	Sox-xbb1 Sox6-Iso-form1	AACAAAG
RAT$SPP1_04	Sox15 Sox2	AACAAAG
XENLA$ENGRAILED2_03	Sox-xbb1	TTTGTTT
XENLA$TWIN_02	Sox10	TTTGTTT

all three columns of Table 2, i.e. that are shared by human, mouse and fly in combinations of six, seven and eight MFs. Again, we investigate association of these MFs to known transcription factors binding sites. The associations listed in Table 4 are derived using PATCH program of Transfac Professional v11.4.

Table 4. MFs that are present in the list of top ten MFs for 6, 7 and 8 MF combinations

MF	Binding Factor	Sequence
CTTTTTTT	Sox-xbb1	TTTTTTT
ARAAAACCY	GR-beta	AGAAAA
TTWATATTT	TBP	TATAAA
	TFIID	TATAAA
	TBP	TATAAA
	TBP	TATAAA
	TBP	TATAAA
	HMG-Y	ATATTA
AAAGRGAAA	Ftz	AAAGCG
	Nkx2-5	AAAGTG
	PITX2A:Nkx2-5 PITX2B:Nkx2-5 PITX2C:Nkx2-5	AAAGTG
	IRF-1 IRF-2	AAGTGA
	IRF-1 IRF-2	AAGTGA
	IRF-1 IRF-2	AAGTGA
	VDR:RXR-alpha	AGTGAA
TTTWATTTA	POU2F1	TTAATT
	Pbx1	TTAATT
	NF-CLE0a NF-CLE0b	TCATTT
	Bcd	AAATTA

A total of 19 different transcription factor binding sites (Table 4) were identified in the five MF combinations described above. Notable among the group are the TFIID general transcription factor which recognizes the TATA box and initiates assembly of protein-DNA complexes on eukaryotic promoters, IRF1 and IRF2 interferon regulatory factors and HMG-Y transcription factors (see http://apps.sanbi.ac.za/ddoc/search.php for more information).

Review of Motif Conservation

At its greatest stringency, the screen identified significant base sequence conservation between fourteen combinations of eight 9-mer sequence strings in 50 promoter regions conserved across human, mouse and fly genomes. As would be expected, given their relatively close evolutionary distance, mammalian orthologs were always co-detected. Similarly, conservation with mammalian promoter regions was observed for those known Fly homologs within matched dataset (http://www.ncbi.nlm.nih.gov/homologene). However, the level of conservation between mammalian and non-orthologous fly genes was surprising (see Table 5 and Figures 5 through 8).

The conservation observed fell into four distinct classes: Significant motif conservation between the promoter regions of mammalian homologs and: (1) characterised Fly genes; (2)

Table 5. Genes associated with promoters sharing combinations of 8 MFs

Combination	Human	Mouse	Fly	Comment
1	TSHZ1	Tshz1	Tshz	Tissue patterning in human mouse, chicken and fly
2	TSHZ1	Tshz1	Rack1	Signalling, signal transduction and hormone response pathways
			PK61C CG9922	
3	PIGV	PigV	Tsh	Cell surface anchor protein, DNA and RNA binding protein
			Msi	
4	LRRTM3	Lrrtm3	CG5098	Mammalian CNS transmembrane protein.
5	SELL	Sell	CG31743	Cell surface adhesin
6	FAP	Fap	CG31624	Membrane protein
			CG13163	Inositol tris phosphate receptor.
			GlcAT-P	CG31624, CG13163, CG34451 have no defined function.
			CG34451	
			Itp-r83A	
7	NRAS	Nras	Chb	Oncogenes/ Spindle associated GTPase activity.
8	RPOS2	Rpos2	CG31554	Mammalian pattern development CG31554 has no defined function
9	LIPF	Lipf	Nplp2	Lipase, extracellular enzyme.
			CG5226 CG5384	CG5226, CG5384 have no defined function
			Stardust	membrane associated guanylate kinase
			STAT92E	STAT92E transcription factor
10	PRDM13	Prdm13	Ndae1 Olf186-F	CNS zinc finger protein in mammals
11	FEZF2	Fezf2	CG4409	Zinc finger; CG4409 has no defined function
12	ANGPTL1	Angptl1	CG8589	Angiogenesis
13	PIGV	PigV	CG11577	ibid
14	TMEM9B	Tmem9b	betaTub56D	Immune response

Figure 5. Relationship of genes associated with promoters sharing combinations of 8 MFs

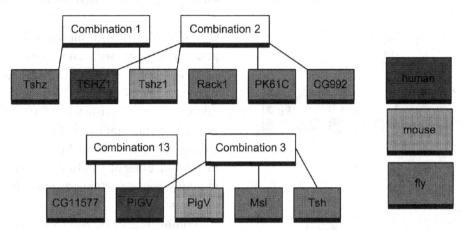

Figure 6. Relationship of genes associated with promoters sharing combinations of 8 MFs

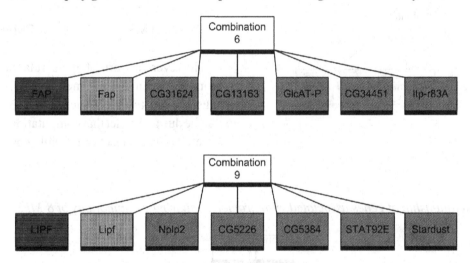

uncharacterised Fly genes with no known homologs in mammalian genomes (homologene database); (3) both characterised and uncharacterised Fly genes; and (4) linked conservation between two motif combinations and a subset of Fly promoter regions. Strikingly, all characterised classes but one involved regulatory factors. This may reflect a selection for complex multiligand promoter regions by stipulating matches to 8-motif family combinations. A wider analysis of 6-, 7- and 8-motif family combinations may help define this issue more clearly.

Five uncharacterised Fly gene promoters were associated with discrete homologous pairs of mammalian sequences (Rspo2, Fez, Angptl, Lrrtm3 and Sell). These conservations may indicate that the uncharacterised Fly genes may share some analogous function with their mammalian partners. Certainly these candidate relationships should be further investigated.

Cross acting conservation between combination 1 and 2 with the Tshz1 gene family suggests that there could be an underlying relationship between motifs of the two combination groups.

Figure 7. Relationship of genes associated with promoters sharing combinations of 8 MFs

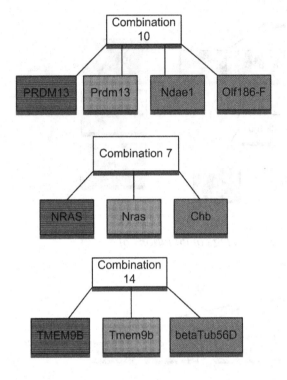

Analysis of Orthologous Genes

We identified 3,973 human-mouse orthologous gene pairs with an orthologous gene in D.melanogaster using the methodology described in Methodology section. What is of particular interest is to establish the relationship, if any, between human, mouse and fly genes that share combinations of a lot of MFs, in our case MFs in combinations of length 8, and clusters of orthologus genes containing genes from human, mouse and fly.

Within the genes sharing 8 MFs, the following human genes (and their mouse othologs) have orthologus genes in fly:

PIGV, LRRTM3, FAP, LIPF, TMEM9B.

However, no orthologous relationship was found between these genes and those sharing MFs; failure to detect such a relationship may also be due to the fact that computational methods covered only a subset of possible combinations.

Figure 8. Relationship of genes associated with promoters sharing combinations of 8 MFs

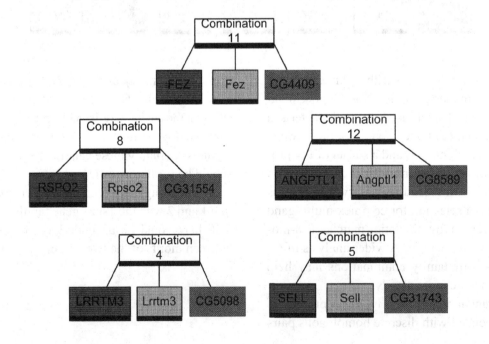

Significance Levels

One question that needs answering is whether MFs generated by DMB are random 9-mers or the MF selection process identified MF candidates that are highly present in the promoter data set. In order to do that, we test for the hypothesis that the generated MFs are by chance. The following, simplified analysis is adequate for this task. We first note that there are in total $4^9 = 262144$ possible 9-mers of nucleotides. Each upstream region of length L can be thought of containing $(L-9)$ 9-mer "slots". The probability of finding a given MF in any slot of the upstream region is $1/4^9$. Because of an extremely small probability of matching an MF to a slot, a simple analysis would show that the probability of finding at least one occurrence of the motif can be approximated with its upper bound to $p = (L-9)/4^9$. In this calculation we ignored that MFs are in fact consensus motifs and not just 9-mers that a more precise analysis would take into account. However, this difference in not crucial for our purposes. Given a combination of 8 different, independently drawn 9-mers, following the same argument it can be shown that the probability of all of them being present in a single upstream promoter region could be approximated to p^8. Therefore, the order of magnitude of the probability of finding a promoter with 8 shared MFs in the entire list of human promoters is 13938×10^{-20} or about $P_{Human} = 10^{-16}$. Using the same arguments for mouse and Fly, we estimate the probability of the same combination of 8 MFs being present also in mouse and Fly promoters to $P_{Human} P_{Mouse} P_{Dmel} = 10^{-48}$. This value is also an estimate of the p-value based on which we can reject the hypothesis that successful combinations of MFs that were selected by DMB are random.

CONCLUSION

This study has identified a number of shared MFs between human, mouse and fly upstream promoter regions. We note several conclusions: (a) It is possible to find MFs that are nine bp in length and shared between promoter regions of all three species; (b) We identified combinations of up to 8 MFs that are shared between the three species, whilst in orthologous pairs of human and mouse genes this number reaches nine; (c) We identified several transcription factor binding sites that correspond to shared MFs, and (d) For a number of fly genes that are not annotated yet, we provide possible links to other genes. This is of a particular interest for the fly genes that have no known orthologs.

Our genome wide analysis has identified significant sequence conservations among the promoter regions of orthologous human and mouse gene pairs and promoter regions within the fly genome expressed in terms of shared combinations of MFs. The most extensive and therefore most stringent conservation group consisted of 14 different groups of 8 MF combinations which correlated 14 human/mouse orthologous promoters with 24 Fly gene promoters. The majority of the characterised genes identified in this screen were members of well defined transcription factor families. Interestingly, several uncharacterised Fly gene promoters were correlated with highly conserved mammalian genes whose expression is tightly regulated suggesting that they too may be subject to similar genetic regulation. The predominance of regulatory factors in the 8 MF combination group may reflect an implicit selection for those conserved promoters encoding a more numerous and potentially more complex level of protein:DNA interactions in the transcriptional initiation process. A larger dataset based on 6 and 7 combination hits could be examined in future and may extend our understanding of this phenomenon. This bioinformatic approach is complementary to the experimental use of genome-wide techniques for the analysis of *in vivo* binding locations such as ChIP-array, ChIP-seq and DamID, thus a combined experimental-bioinformatic approach may again extend our understanding of transcriptional regulatory networks in animals.

REFERENCES

Bajic, V. B., Tan, S. L., Christoffels, A., Schönbach, C., Lipovich, L., & Yang, L. (2006, Apr). Mice and men: their promoter properties. *PLOS Genetics*, *2*(4), e54. doi:10.1371/journal.pgen.0020054

Brahmachary, M., Schönbach, C., Yang, L., Huang, E., Tan, S. L., & Chowdhary, R. (2006, Dec). Computational Promoter Analysis of Mouse, Rat and Human Antimicrobial Peptide-coding Genes. *BMC Bioinformatics*, *18*(7Suppl 5), S8. doi:10.1186/1471-2105-7-S5-S8

Carey, M. F., Peterson, C. L., & Smale, S. T. (2009). *Transcriptional Regulation in Eukaryotes: Concepts, Strategies, and Techniques*. CSHL Press.

Cheng, C., Yun, K-Y., Ressom, H., Mohanty, B., Bajic, V.B., Jia, Y., Yun, S.J. & de los Reyes, B.G. (2007, Jun). An early response regulatory cluster induced by low temperature and hydrogen peroxide in chilling tolerant japonica rice. *BMC Genomics*, 18, 8:175.

Down, T. A., Bergman, C. M., Su, J., & Hubbard, T. J. P. (2007). Large-Scale Discovery of Promoter Motifs in *Drosophila melanogaster*. *PLoS Computational Biology*, *3*(1), e7..doi:10.1371/journal.pcbi.0030007

FitzGerald, P. C., Sturgill, D., Shyakhtenko, A., Oliver, B., & Vinson, C. (2006). Comparative genomics of *Drosophila* and human core promoters. *Genome Biology*, 7, R53. doi:10.1186/gb-2006-7-7-r53

Ho, M. R., Chen, C. H., & Lin, W. C. (2010). Gene-oriented ortholog database: a functional comparison platform for orthologous loci. *Database (Oxford)*, *2010*, baq002. Epub 2010 Feb 10. doi:10.1093/database/baq002

Huang, E., Yang, L., Chowdhary, R., Kassim, A., & Bajic, V. B. (2005). *Information Processing and Living Systems*. World Scientific. An algorithm for *ab initio* DNA motif detection; pp. 611–614.

Meier, S., Gehring, C., MacPherson, C. R., Kaur, M., Maqungo, M., & Reuben, S. (2008). The promoter signatures in rice LEA genes can be used to build a co-expressing LEA gene network. *RICE*, *1*(2), 177. doi:10.1007/s12284-008-9017-4

Mohanty, B., Krishnan, S. P., Swarup, S., & Bajic, V. B. (2005). Detection and Preliminary Analysis of Motifs in Promoters of Anaerobically Induced Genes of Different Plant Species. *Annals of Botany*, *96*(4), 669–681. doi:10.1093/aob/mci219

Park, M. R., Yun, K. Y., Mohanty, B., Herath, V., Xu, F., & Wijaya, E. (2010). Supra-optimal expression of the cold-regulated OsMyb4 transcription factor in transgenic rice changes the complexity of transcriptional network with major effects on stress tolerance and panicle development. [Epub ahead of print]. *Plant, Cell & Environment*, *2010*(Aug), 27. doi:.doi:10.1111/j.1365-3040.2010.02221.x

The FANTOM Consortium. (2005, Sep 2). The transcriptional landscape of the mammalian genome. [*Erratum in: Science. 2006 Mar 24,311*] [5768] [:1713; www.sciencemag.org/content/309/5740/1559.long]. *Science*, *309*(5740), 1559–1563. doi:10.1126/science.1112014

Wittkopp, P. J. (2010). Variable Transcription Factor Binding: A Mechanism of Evolutionary Change. *PLoS Biology*, *8*(3), e1000342. doi:10.1371/journal.pbio.1000342

Wray, G. A., Hahn, M. W., Abouheif, E., Balhoff, J. P., Pizer, M., Rockman, M. V., & Romano, L. A. (2003, Sep). The evolution of transcriptional regulation in eukaryotes. *Molecular Biology and Evolution*, *20*(9), 1377–1419. doi:10.1093/molbev/msg140

Yun, K. Y., Park, M. R., Mohanty, B., Herath, V., Xu, F., & Mauleon, R. (2010). Transcriptional regulatory network triggered by oxidative signals configures the early response mechanisms of japonica rice to chilling stress. *BMC Plant Biology*, *10*(1), 16. doi:10.1186/1471-2229-10-16

Chapter 5
Recognition of Translation Initiation Sites in *Arabidopsis Thaliana*

Haitham Ashoor
King Abdullah University of Science and Technology, Saudi Arabia

Arturo M. Mora
King Abdullah University of Science and Technology, Saudi Arabia

Karim Awara
King Abdullah University of Science and Technology, Saudi Arabia

Boris R. Jankovic
King Abdullah University of Science and Technology, Saudi Arabia

Rajesh Chowdhary
Biomedical Informatics Research Center, USA

John A.C. Archer
King Abdullah University of Science and Technology, Saudi Arabia

Vladimir B. Bajic
King Abdullah University of Science and Technology, Saudi Arabia

ABSTRACT

Computational identification of translation initiation sites (TISs) has been of great importance in gene discovery and gene loci annotation because it predicts the start of protein coding regions. Many methods have been developed to identify TISs from cDNA and mRNA sequences, but much less work has considered TIS recognition directly from genomic DNA. In addition, to provide an insight into TIS signals conserved between distantly related eukaryotic species, the authors developed a human TIS recognition model that, when applied without modifications to TIS prediction in Arabidopsis thaliana genome, produced an accuracy of over 83 percent. When the model was trained on A. thaliana data, the resulting accuracy increased to 91 percent.

Their results suggest that in spite of the considerable evolutionary distance between Homo sapiens and A. thaliana, our approach successfully recognized deeply conserved genomic signals that characterize TIS. Moreover, they report the highest accuracy of TIS recognition in A. thaliana DNA genomic sequences.

DOI: 10.4018/978-1-61350-435-2.ch005

Copyright © 2012, IGI Global. Copying or distributing in print or electronic forms without written permission of IGI Global is prohibited.

INTRODUCTION

One of the objectives of bioinformatics is to identify important biological signals in various genomic sequences. The translation initiation site (TIS) is one such signal that denotes the start codon at which translation initiates. Accurate recognition of TIS signals can help in discovery of protein-coding genes and in better annotation of gene loci (Preiss & Hentze, 2003, Do & Choi, 2006). Annotation engines typically assign the TIS to the first ATG codon which generates a maximal Open Reading Frame (ORF), but this by no means is sufficiently accurate.

Canonical TISs consist of the ATG triplet nucleotides, but in rare cases may consist of ACG or CTG triplets. In this study, we focus on the canonical ATG sequences (Preiss & Hentze, 2003). However, an ATG triplet will occur, on average, every 64 nucleotides in random DNA. Thus, in higher eukaryotes with large genomes, there will be a plethora of false TIS signals. For instance, in the 3.3 billion base pairs (bp) human genome with an estimated coding capacity of ~30,000 genes and assuming all are protein coding and with no alternative TISs, there will be ~30,000 real TISs and 103,095,000 false TIS signals, i.e. ~3,436 fold excess of false to true signals. Thus, there is a clear need for accurate prediction of TIS signals contained in the DNA sequence.

The presence of introns within genes, makes the accurate prediction of the TIS signals from genomic DNA sequence much more difficult than from cDNA or mRNA sequences. Extensive research has been carried out to develop computational methods for recognition of TISs mainly in cDNA and mRNA sequences. Perhaps understandably, much less attention has been given to the more difficult problem of identifying computationally these signals within genomic DNA. The associated problem is determination of the best set of features that can be used to discriminate true form false genomic signals (Saeys et al., 2007), in our case TIS signals. In this study, we introduce several new global features to the pool of already studied TIS related features, and we select the set of relevant features using a wrapper method.

Most computational recognition approaches of TIS signals have used mRNA dataset for comparing results (Pedersen and Nielsen, 1997). This dataset contains a mix of mRNA sequences from different vertebrate genomes. They (Pedersen & Nielsen, 1997) implemented an Artificial Neural Network (ANN) to predict TISs and reported an accuracy of 85% on their dataset. Later, (Hatzigeorgiou, 2002) reported an accuracy of 94% on human cDNA sequences that contain complete ORFs. She also employed a combination of two ANNs as a prediction model. Ma and colleagues developed TISKey (Ma et al., 2006), which uses an ensemble of Support Vector Machines (SVMs) and with the Pedersen and Nelsen dataset reported accuracy of 93.7%. Zeng and AlHaj used multiple agent architecture with reinforcement learning and reported 96.72% accuracy(Zeng & AlHaj, 2008). Rajapakse and Ho implemented a hybrid approach of Markov model and ANN on the Pedersen and Nielsen dataset (Rajapakse & Ho, 2005) and reported 93.8% sensitivity and 96.9% specificity using 3-folds cross validation. Li et al. used the Hatzigeorgiou dataset of mRNA sequences with full ORFs, and by using a Gaussian mixture model reported sensitivity of 98.06% and specificity of 92.14% (Li et al., 2004).

Studies based on genomic DNA sequences exhibited lower levels of accuracy. Saeyes et al. reported on human genomic DNA sequences 80% sensitivity, and 87.5% specificity (Saeyes et al., 2007). Sparks and Brendel developed the MetWAMer system which uses a perceptron classification algorithm and clustering of data by the k-medoids algorithm and methionine-weight array matrices to achieve an accuracy of 85% on *A. thaliana* genomic DNA sequences dataset (Sparks & Brendel, 2008). Pertea and Salzberg demonstrated that GlimmerM achieved 84% accuracy on both *A. thaliana* and human genomic sequences (Pertea & Salzberg, 2002).

In our study, we developed implicit evidence of conservation of TIS recognition signals across distantly related species. Using our method, we report accuracy of 91.13% on *A. thaliana* genomic DNA data. This represents the best currently reported result for *A. thaliana* genomic TIS prediction. This improvement was obtained using the model structure from human genomic DNA sequences that were retrained on the *A. thaliana* data. Surprisingly, when we used the model trained on the human data and apply it to *A. thaliana* without any modification, we achieved 82.95% accuracy of TIS prediction on genomic DNA *A. thaliana* sequences. This result itself is at the level of the best previously reported results for TIS prediction in genomic DNA *A. thaliana* sequences. Our results suggest that there is a fundamental conservation of the key signals that characterize the TIS locations in both human and *A. thaliana* genomes. In our study, we have generated many features that characterize the TIS surroundings and we also used many of the previously studied features reported in (Li and Leong, 2005) and (Liu and Wong, 2003). Using a wrapper method based on Genetic Algorithm (GA) and ANN, out of all these features our methodology selected 92 and 93 features for human and *A. Thaliana* models, respectively, as the best set of features for the TIS recognition task. There have been other studies that dealt with the generation and selection of features for TIS recognition, such as, for example (Zeng et al., 2002).

BACKGROUND

The difference in recognition of the TIS signals in cDNA or mRNA sequences on one side and in genomic DNA sequences on the other is that the TIS surrounding has in general, different characteristics. In cDNA or mRNA the upstream region of TIS is represented by the 5'UTR sequence while the downstream sequences include the CDS region that contains that portion of the DNA that

encodes for protein and extends as long as the ORF. CDS exhibits specific properties reflected in the so called 'codon bias' such that there is a positional base bias with a weak periodicity of three. Contrary to this, the TIS in genomic DNA can have these upstream and downstream sequences interrupted by introns (Sleator, 2010). Moreover, the TIS triplet can be split between two different exons. Thus, it is obvious that (a) the recognition of TIS within the genomic sequence is much more difficult than the recognition of TIS in cDNA or mRNA and; (b) the features that characterize TIS surrounding in cDNA or mRNA and those in genomic DNA are different.

MATERIALS AND METHODS

Datasets

TIS human data was extracted directly from chromosomal genomic sequences using the corresponding consensus annotations (CCDS. current) in gff3 format. The latest data (reference sequence GRCh37) was downloaded from NCBI and we selected the list of 4,000 experimentally verified sequences for positive data and generated the same number of false TIS sequences from human chromosome 1, after ensuring that generated sequences are not present in the TIS positive list.

A. thaliana TIS data was also extracted directly from chromosome genomic sequences and the corresponding annotation were downloaded from www.arabidopsis.org. This yielded a total of 20,000 positive TIS data points. The same number of false TIS samples was generated from *A. thaliana* chromosome 1, after ensuring that such sequences were not already present in the TIS positive set. All extracted dataset sequences were 300 bp in length with the TIS covering positions 150-152 counted from the 5' end of sequence. For retraining TIS prediction model 5,000 positive and 5,000 negative sequences from *A. thaliana* data were randomly selected.

FEATURE GENERATION

In the context of TIS prediction, many useful features in sequences surrounding ATG signals we reported in literature. Prominent amongst these can be found in, for example (Ma et al., 2006; Tzanis & Vlahavas, 2006; Liu & Wong, 2003). Many of the reported features are local in the sense that they primarily characterize properties of the sequences immediately surrounding a candidate TIS. In addition to some local features that we used, we also supplemented this set of features with some that are more global in their reach. However, extending a set of proven features brings a principal problem in that a combination of features with good individual discriminating properties does not guarantee higher model accuracy. This is a well-known problem in machine learning and is due to several factors, such as correlation between feature values, decreased robustness, over-fitting, etc. For that reason, it is imperative that a strategy is put in place to select an optimal combination of features that yields the highest accuracy. Here, we first describe the feature selection strategy and then the resulting features used in the final model.

Since selection of optimal combination of candidate features is a combinatorial problem, we first reduce the size of search space by including a fixed subset of features into all model-building iterations. This subset consists of features that we believe play a significant role in TIS recognition, based on previously reported results. In addition, we considered a number of additional features and combined the fixed set with some of these additions to derive a candidate feature set. The core step in our feature selection process in the application of GA in search of an optimal features combination. Briefly, the process stipulates that all candidate features are numbered and assigned a value of 0 (not selected as a member of a feature set) or 1 (selected). In this way we form a "chromosome" in GA terms and the resulting model accuracy is deemed as the evaluation function. We then apply GA in a standard way, using a single point crossover together with mutation where each bit in a chromosome is subjected to 20 percent chance of having its value altered.

The features considered belong to several broad categories. These would include various frequency-based properties of the surrounding sequences of nucleotides or, more generally successive k-mers of nucleotides, position weight matrices (PWMs), etc. Another class of features was derived from statistics related to codon biases. In addition, information gain was also considered as a feature of the surrounding sequences. A brief description of major selected features is as follows.

K-mer frequencies: these represent frequencies of groups of nucleotides, equivalent to the Markov chain of order k. In this way, features such as frequencies of nucleotides and dinucleotides were derived, as well as positive (Pscore) and negative (Nscore) scores, representing the frequencies of 16 overlapping dinucleotides using a sliding window. For example, if we have the following sequence atgg we can identify three dinucleotides (at, tg, and gg). Such frequencies are then used to calculate the Pscores and Nscores for each ATG-surrounding sequences using PWM, thus generating two features for each sequence (sample).

Closely related to k-mer frequencies are nucleotide and dinucleotide frequencies separately reported for upstream and downstream regions from the ATG signal.

Kozak's feature: we utilized the Kozak's consensus sequence that was proposed in (Kozak, 1987). This feature is built on the observation that around the TIS it is highly probable to find an A or G in position -3 and a G in position +4. We check if our sample sequence conforms to GCC[A/G]CCatgG regular expression and if so we assign this binary feature a value of one. Otherwise, we assign the value of zero. Whilst useful, on its own it is not sufficiently discriminative for the accurate prediction of TIS (Ma et al., 2006). The analysis on our own data, summarized in Figures 1 and 2, confirms this finding. In addition to this binary

Kozak-derived feature, we also use the score based on the Kozak's consensus sequence that represents the number of positions that comply with the Kozak's rule. For example, if the example sequence is GCC**TC**A**atg**G, the consensus score would be 5, as those nucleotides that are underlined are not expected at their position according to the Kozak's rule.

ATG frequencies: we consider the following three features derived from ATG frequencies:

1. Number of ATG in the candidate in-frame-codons upstream
2. Number of ATG in the candidate out-of-frame codons downstream
3. Total number of ATG codons in the sequence

In its standard interpretation, in-frame codon characteristics represent one possible measure of coding potential. However, when working with genomic sequences that include introns as well, the standard definition cannot be applied. In our model, in-frame codons refer to the 3-mers in the genomic sequence that are aligned with the candidate TIS position with offsets of ...-6, -3, +4, +7..., etc. We refer to those ATG triplets that are not in-frame as out-of-frame.

Putative coding sequence length: this feature represents the number of nucleotides counted from the candidate TIS until the next in-frame stop codon (TAG, TAA or TGA). The idea behind this feature is that since most proteins are longer than 50 amino acids it is less likely that a positive sample would not contain a stop codon in-frame.

Figure 1. Nucleotide frequency distribution in positive samples

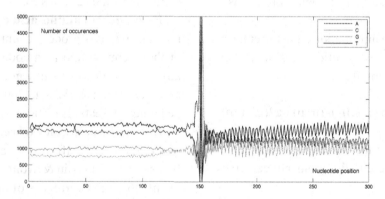

Figure 2. Nucleotide frequency distribution in negative samples

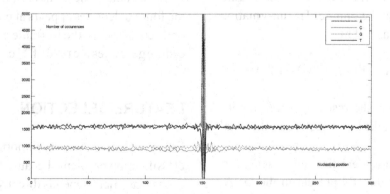

By the same reasoning, there is higher probability to find on the stop codons in negative samples.

C and G versus A and T frequencies: this feature arises from an observation that the frequency of nucleotides C and G is greater than that of A and T in the upstream part of the positive samples. In (Ma et al., 2006) a similar feature is proposed. In our study we compare C and G frequencies to A and T frequencies only in the twenty positions that have the highest information gain. In summary, this approach results in four features, i.e. ratios A/T, A/G, C/T and C/G. In doing so, we excluded some of the first ranked positions as they are already subsumed in the Kozak's feature.

Information gain: the nucleotide frequencies presented in Figures 1 and 2 suggest a generally higher level of entropy for negative sequences compared to the positive ones. Following this observation, we developed a more formal approach through utilization of information gain. The normalized value of the gain is taken as a model feature.

To calculate the information gain, the entropy level was used for the nucleotide's position, given by the following formula:

$$E = -p/(p+n) \log 2(p/(p+n)) - n/(n+p) \log 2(n/(n+p))$$

where p represents the number of positive sequences and n represents the number of negatives sequences.

After calculating the five entropy values (A, C, G, T entropies and the entropy of the system), it is then possible to calculate the information gain for each position in the sample. The information gain is calculated as follows:

$$\text{Gain} = E(S) - E(A) - E(C) - E(G) - E(T)$$

Once calculated, the resulting value for information gain is taken as a feature in the final classifier system.

Amino acid characteristics: amino acid characteristics are not directly present in the DNA.

We however artificially converted the in-frame and out-of-frame codons to the corresponding amino acids for generating a set of features we believe are contributing to better recognition of TIS. We used the characteristics of amino acids to classify the data. The following amino acids characteristics were considered: hydrophobic, hydrophilic, acidic, basic, aliphatic and aromatic (Liu and Wong, 2003). This process determines the in-frame and out-of-frame frequencies of each group of amino acids separately for the upstream and downstream regions. It is useful to separate the frequencies from the upstream and downstream regions because it has been proven that the difference between coding and non-coding region is one of the most relevant information we can get for TIS recognition. This process calculates the frequencies for the six amino acids properties for downstream and upstream, in-frame and out of frame independently, generating a total of 24 features (6 times 2 times 2).

Frequency of amino-acid coding triplets of nucleotides: this process counts the occurrence of the twenty amino acid-coding triplets in the upstream and downstream segments of the sample separately (Liu & Wong, 2003). This process generates 76 features (2 times 2 times 19).

In-frame nucleotides score: loosely inspired by the position-specific k-gram approach that was first suggested in (Liu & Wong, 2003), we count the number of occurrences of nucleotides in the in-frame codons in particular positions, for both upstream and downstream regions. The process works by noting the number of times that each of the four nucleotides appears at positions one, two or three in each of the in-frame codons. This procedure generates the total of 24 candidate features.

FEATURE SELECTION

Feature selection is a very important process in all classification problems because the performance of the classifiers depends directly on the selected features. Important features improve the capability of the classification algorithm to divide the classes more accurately. On the other hand, non-relevant features are those who do not contribute for distinguishing the classes and could be considered as "noise" for the classification algorithms. For example, having a large number of inputs/features increases the complexity of an ANN. It is also important to mention that the simpler the classifier is, the more robust it will be for classifying unseen samples, i.e. its generalization capability is usually better (Russell & Norvig, 2003; Mitchell T, 1997). Thus it is advisable to find a good combination of features for our TIS prediction task.

Individual Feature Ranking

There are many approaches for feature selection. Some authors (Li & Leong, 2005; Zeng et al., 2002) used Weka tool (Witten & Frank, 2000) by applying different measures, such as information gain ratio, Chi-square test, etc. to select features. The ranking of the features is done individually. This can give us an idea of the ability of individual features to discriminate between the classes. However, concentrating just on the top features may lead to missing other features that when considered individually are not highly ranked. This is that a feature by itself could be considered as non-relevant, but in some cases when the feature is combined with the other features it could provide ability to classify the samples in an optimal way. Figure 3 illustrates this idea. However, since there is no simple way to select the optimal combination of features, we applied GA for this purpose.

GA for FeatureSelection

A lot of research has been done in using GA to determine the ANN parameters (weights initialization, number of nodes in the hidden layer, number of hidden layers, etc). In the TIS prediction problem in particular we want to minimize

the misclassification or, in other words, maximize the accuracy of the system. In this study we focus on the feature selection using the ANN.

We now describe the four steps of the GA.

Initial Population

To generate the initial population, we have first to encode the solution into chromosomes. In this implementation the chromosomes are the set of features to be considered in the ANN. To generate these chromosomes, a random binary value (either zero or one) will be assigned to each feature, and only those features assigned the value of one will be considered for the evaluation.

Fitness Function

The evaluation or fitness function is used to rank the chromosomes in the population. For this problem, the ANN trains and tests the data based on the features generated in the previous step (initial population) using a k-fold cross validation.

Figure 3. Two features that individually result in poor classification together make perfect classification by a linear classifier

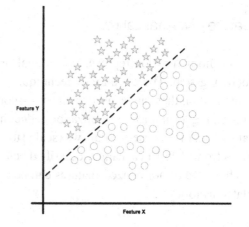

Selection and Crossover

When the whole population is evaluated, individuals with best fitness are ranked and the crossover is performed between them in order to generate a new offspring. In this way, the new generation will have in most cases a higher fitness than the previous one. However, if only individuals with the highest fitness values are consideredfor crossover, GA may get confined to a non-optimal local extremum. To avoid this, individuals with lower fitness values can also be considered as possible parents with some probability. In our implementation, chromosomes with the highest fitness are selected for crossover with probability of 80% whilst those with lowest fitness values are selected with probability of 20%.

The crossover is done in a one-point crossover manner, meaning that a crossover point is randomly selected in the chromosomes to generate two new offsprings.

Mutation

The optional mutation process provides an element of randomness in the population to avoid descent into a suboptimal local minimum. It allows GA to explore a wider area in the solution space. In our implementation, we selected the probability of altering each bit (gene) in the chromosome of 20% as the value that has resulted in the best convergence in our testing.

Features Normalization

Feature normalization represents a crucial pre-processing step. There are many techniques for normalization that can be used such as: Z-score, data-scaling (minmax normalization), decimal scaling, etc. In our case, the data was scaled to the values from -1 to 1 in a manner described below.

The value of normalized features can be calculated as follows:

Normalized value = (Normal value − range)/bases,

where range and bases can be given by the following equations:

range = (max value − min value)/2

bases = (max value + min value)/2.

Data scaling tends to be very useful for the neural network because it can increase the speed of training of the network (Han & Kamber, 2006). Another point is that data value before normalization are distributed in different ranges which can make the decision of the neural network biased for some attributes rather than others, for example, in the case of an attribute which is less important than others, but it has a much larger value than all other attributes. These higher values may give a wrong indicator for the decision of the neural network. So to avoid this problem, normalization is applied where it places all the values in the same range.

MAIN CLASSIFIER

Our classifier is implemented as an ANN. Based on the TIS prediction literature, one can see that many previous systems, such those described in (Tikole & Sankararamakrishnan, 2008; Rajapakse et al., 2005; Pedersen & Nielsen, 1997), used ANN with good results. In general, ANNs learning algorithms are considered to be straightforward and efficient. For a more detailed description of the ANN, an abundant literature available should be consulted, such as (Mitchell, 1997).

The structure of our ANN follows a standard design with input, one hidden, and output layers. The input layer accepts the features selected by GA (92 features for human and 93 for *A. thaliana*), the hidden layer consists of 29 neurons with sigmoid activation function, and the output layer consists of two neurons with sigmoid activation functions. The number of neurons in the hidden layer was determined based on empirical tests. In this study we use the backpropagation algorithm for training of weights.

In the training process, the two output neurons represent the two classes, so in case of positive samples (C1), the target value output of the first neuron (O1) is set to 1, and the target value for the second output neuron (O2) is set to -1, whereas in the case of negative samples (C2) the target value of O1 is set to -1 and the target value of O2 is set to 1.

The modeling process consists of two phases. In the first one, we use both GA and backpropagation algorithms to select the best set of candidate features. After these features are selected, in the second phase, we train the ANN classifier using only those features with varying sizes of training sets in hope of finding a model that retains high accuracy with minimal training set size, as described below.

In the first phase, ANN weights are optimized (through the back propagation algorithm) for a given set of features (that are selected by GA) and the resulting model error is used by GA to select another, possibly more optimal set of features and for which a new ANN is trained. This iterative process is repeated until the number of GA iterations exceeds a predefined threshold. The model error is represented as the error of 3-fold cross-validation. Within each fold, two third of data are used for training set. We found that the best results were achieved when 75 percent of the training set is used for ANN weights training and the remaining 25 percent of the training set is used as validation set.

To create a model that generalizes well with unseen samples, we trained our classifier under different training and testing conditions. We tried to reduce the size of the training set as much as possible without compromising the accuracy of the system. By reducing the size of the training set, one can avoid over-fitting problem. This comes from the fact that when using a large training set than required, the samples contained in it might be redundant, forcing the system to learn idiosyncrasies of training samples (Mitchell, 1997). After trying different splits of the data, the best model was obtained by splitting data into 65 percent training and 35 percent test data. Furthermore, five percent of training data was used as validation test during the training phase. The purpose of validation test is to prevent model over-fitting by evaluating model performance on its samples during training (Prechelt, 1998).

Where an inflection point in model output error on validation samples is reached, i.e. when error increases with number of training iterations, this becomes an indicator that further training iterations will likely lead to over-fitting and therefore the model training process should stop at that point. Since estimating the direction of validation error by comparing errors of a two subsequent iterations is prone to transient effects, we compare errors between two epochs, where any such effects would cancel out for a suitable length of an epoch.

We evaluate the model in terms of:

Accuracy: (true positives + true negatives)/total number of samples
Sensitivity: true positives/(true positives + false negatives)
Specificity: true negatives/(true negatives + false positives)

The higher the values for accuracy, sensitivity and specificity, the more confident we are in the model's validity.

Testing set is always unseen for the model during the training phase. In a complete dataset, the validation set is derived from the training set and Figure 4 illustrates this process. The training phase should stop when the error is at an inflection point, i.e. when model error on validation set starts increasing or fails do decrease after a predefined number of epochs.

Figure 5 shows the behavior of the model error curve on the validation set during the training process. As we can observe from the last figure,

Figure 4. Splitting of the data. A portion of the training set is reserved as validation set.

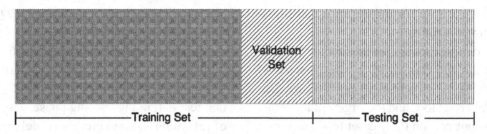

Training Set   Testing Set

Figure 5. Training and validation error curves

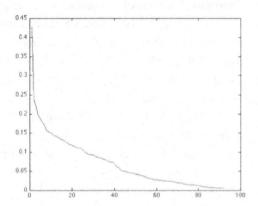

the error keeps decreasing till almost reaching 0. Using validation methodology considerably improved the results and helped reduce the amount of computational effort. The X-axis represents the number of epochs and the Y-axis the error after each epoch.

Weights Initialization

The last enhancement done to the ANN is by initializing the weights to a specific range close to 0. By initializing the weights to values close to zero the back propagation algorithm will leave values close to 0 for all those features that are non-relevant for the classification. This method increases the performance of the system in the condition of the variable normalization, where initializing the weights could be randomly but limited to a specific range which tend to be a small range of weights.

In summary, in the process of determining the best combination of features, GA was used as a wrapper in combination with the ANN.

RESULTS

We summarize the performance of our human model developed from the corresponding human DNA data and tested on human data in Table 1.

Table 1. Performance of human TIS model

Method	Accuracy (%)	Sensitivity (%)	Specificity (%)
3-fold cross-validation	94.27	94.10	94.80
60/5/35 partition	93.28	90.85	95.71

Table 2. Performance of human TIS classifier on A. Thaliana Dataset

Accuracy (%)	Sensitivity (%)	Specificity (%)
82.95	82.45	83.45

Table 3. Performance of A. Thaliana TIS classifier on A. Thaliana Dataset

Accuracy (%)	Sensitivity (%)	Specificity (%)
91.13	90.64	91.61

Table 2 summarizes results of testing the original human TIS recognition model on the *A. thaliana* data. These results showed a surprisingly high level of accuracy achieved that is very close to the best reported accuracy results for *A. thaliana* genomic sequences 85%, (Sparks & Brendel, 2008) despite the absence of *A. thaliana* training dataset.

Table 3 summarizes the performance of *A. Thaliana* model, derived from A. Thaliana dataset.

CONCLUSION

In this study, we build TIS prediction models from human and arabidopsis genomic sequences. Our model is an ANN-based binary classifier using a selected subset of the originally considered features. Feature selection was done utilizing GA, whilst the classifier is implemented as a single hidden-layer ANN. Both human and *A. thaliana* models exhibit, to the best of our knowledge, a higher accuracy in prediction of TIS in respective genomic sequences than any other TIS prediction models reported in literature. Furthermore, the model derived on human data produced surprisingly high accuracy when applied to TIS prediction on *A. thaliana* genomic sequence thus providing an implicit evidence of a conserved TIS architecture between plants and mammals. This suggests that the model derived from human data conserves key features in other organisms like *A. thaliana*. These results may provide a starting point for developing more generic models for TIS prediction in eukaryotes.

REFERENCES

Do, J.H & Choi, D.K. (2006). Computational approaches to gene prediction. *J Microbiol. Apr; 44*(2),137-44.

Han, J., & Kamber, M. (2006). *Data Mining: Concepts and Techniques* (2nd ed.). San Francisco: Morgan Kaufmann.

Hatzigeorgiou, A (2002). Translation initiation start prediction in human cDNAs with high accuracy. *Bioinformatics. Feb;18*(2),343-50.

Kozak, M. (1987). An analysis of 5'-noncoding sequences from 699 vertebrates messenger RNA. *Nucleic Acids Research, 15*, 8125–8148. doi:10.1093/nar/15.20.8125

Li G, L & Leong, T.Y. (2005). Feature Selection for the Prediction of Translation Initiation Sites. *Genomics Proteomics Bioinformatics. May,3*(2),73-83.

Li G, Leong TY,& Zhang L (2004). Translation Initiation Sites Prediction wit Mixture Gaussian Models. *Algorithms in Bioinformatics (2004),* 338-349.

Liu, H., & Wong, L. (2003). Data Mining Tools for Biological Sequences. *Journal of Bioinformatics and Computational Biology, 1*(1), 139–167. doi:10.1142/S0219720003000216

Ma, C., Zhou, D., & Zhou, Y. (2006). *Feature Mining Integration for Improving the Prediction Accuracy of Translation Initiation Sites in Eukaryotic mRNAs.* gccw, 349-356. Fifth International Conference on Grid and Cooperative Computing Workshops.

Mitchell, T. (1997). *Machine Learning* (*International Edition*). New York: McGraw Hill.

Pedersen, A. G., & Nielsen, H. (1997). *Neural network prediction of translation initiation sites in eukaryotes: Perspectives for EST and genome analysis.* Proc. 5th International Conference on Intelligent Systems for Molecular Biology, 226–233.

Pertea, M., & Salzberg, S. (2002). A Method to Improve the Performance of Translation Start Site Detection and Its Application for Gene Finding. In R. Guigo & D. Gusfield (Eds.) *WABI 2002, LNCS 2452*. pp. 210–219, (2002). Springer-Verlag Berlin Heidelberg.

Prechelt, L. (1998). Early stopping – but when? In G.B. Orr, K.–R. Müller (Eds.),*Neural Networks: Tricks of the Trade*. LNCS 1524, pp. 55–69, 1998. Ó Springer–Verlag Berlin Heidelberg (1998)

Preiss, T., & Hentze, M. (2003). Starting the protein synthesis machine: eukaryotic translation initiation. *BioEssays*, *25*(12), 1201–1211. doi:10.1002/bies.10362

Rajapakse, J. C., & Ho, L. S. (2005, Apr-Jun). Markov encoding for detecting signals in genomic sequences. *IEEE/ACM Transactions on Computational Biology and Bioinformatics*, *2*(2), 131–142. doi:10.1109/TCBB.2005.27

Russell, S., & Norvig, P. (2003). *Artificial Intelligence A Modern Approach* (2nd ed.). New York: Prentice Hall.

Saeys, Y., Abeel, T., Degroeve, S., & Van de Peer, Y. (2007). Translation Initiation Site Prediction on a Genomic Scale: Beauty of Simplicity. *Bioinformatics (Oxford, England)*, *23*, i418–i423. doi:10.1093/bioinformatics/btm177

Saeys, Y., Inza, I. & Larrañaga, P. (2007). A review of feature selection techniques in bioinformatics. *Bioinformatics. Oct 1;23(*19), 2507-17. Epub 2007 Aug 24.

Sleator, R. D. (2010, Aug 1). An overview of the current status of eukaryote gene prediction strategies. *Gene*, *461*(1-2), 1–4. Epub 2010 Apr 27. doi:10.1016/j.gene.2010.04.008

Sparks, M.E. & Brendel, V. (2008). MetWAMer: eukaryotic translation initiation site prediction. *BMC Bioinformatics. Sep 18*(9),381.

Tikole, S., & Sankararamakrishnan, R. (2008). Prediction of Translation Initiation Sites in Human mRNA sequences with AUG Start Codon.*Weak Kozak Context: A Neural Network Approach, BBRC*, 1166-1168.

Tzanis, G., & Vlahavas, I. (2006). *Prediction of Translation Initiation Sites Using Classifier Selection.* Chapter in Advances in Artificial Intelligence. [Springer-Verlag]. *Lecture Notes in Computer Science*, *3955*, 367–377. doi:10.1007/11752912_37

Witten, I. H., & Frank, E. (2000). *Data Mining: Practical Machine Learning Tools with Java Implementations*. San Francisco: Morgan Kaufmann.

Zeng, F., Yap, R. H., & Wong, L. (2002). Using feature generation and feature selection for accurate prediction of translation initiation sites. *Genome Inform.*, *13*, 192–200.

Zeng, J., & Alhajj, R. (2008). Predicting translation initiation sites using a multi-agent architecture empowered with reinforcement learning. *CIBCB, 2008*, 241–248.

Section 2

Chapter 6
The Present and the Future Perspectives of Biological Network Inference

Paola Lecca
The Microsoft Research – University of Trento, Centre for Computational and Systems Biology

Alida Palmisano
The Microsoft Research – University of Trento, Centre for Computational and Systems Biology

ABSTRACT

Biological network inference is based on a series of studies and computational approaches to the deduction of the connectivity of chemical species, the reaction pathway, and the reaction kinetics of complex reaction systems from experimental measurements. Inference for network structure and reaction kinetics parameters governing the dynamics of a biological system is currently an active area of research. In the era of post-genomic biology, it is a common opinion among scientists that living systems (cells, tissues, organs and organisms) can be understood in terms of their network structure as well as in term of the evolution in time of this network structure. In this chapter, the authors make a survey of the recent methodologies proposed for the structure inference and for the parameter estimation of a system of interacting biological entities. Furthermore, they present the recent works of the authors about model identification and calibration.

DOI: 10.4018/978-1-61350-435-2.ch006

Copyright © 2012, IGI Global. Copying or distributing in print or electronic forms without written permission of IGI Global is prohibited.

1. NETWORK INFERENCE: GOALS AND METHODOLOGICAL APPROACHES

To define the network structure of a biological system, network biology researchers use data generated by experimental methods, including high-throughput proteomic, genomic, and metabolomic data, as well as computational capabilities to identify and infer the topology and the causality of the interactions. It is beneficial to conceptualize a cell or higher units of biological organization as systems of interacting elements, i. e. as networks of influences, physical or statistical, between components. High-throughput experimental methods enable the measurement of expression levels for thousands of genes and the determination of thousands of protein–protein or protein–DNA interactions. It is increasingly recognized that theoretical and computational network inference methods are needed to make sense of this abundance of information. Viewing biological systems in terms of their underlying network structure is a powerful concept. All networks share common characteristics, and, consequently, common mathematical frameworks can be developed to understand their structure and how they can be regulated. For such conceptual framework, that is the basis for a systems-level description, one needs to know (i) the identity of the components that constitute the biological system; (ii) the dynamic behavior of the abundance or activity of these components; and (iii) the interactions among these components (Kitano, 2002). Ultimately, this information can be combined into a network that, if it is validated and revealed to be consistent with current knowledge, provides new insights and predictions, such as the behavior of the system in conditions that were previously unexplored.

Currently methodological approaches and algorithms have been proposed to determine reaction mechanisms from time series data which are collected for gene and protein interactions and for metabolic pathways and networks. The aim of these techniques is to infer the system of biochemical reaction mechanisms from time series data on the concentration or abundance of different reacting components of a network, with little prior information about the pathways involved. The great majority of these methods belongs to the class of the mechanistic approaches to the network inference knowledge. Crampin et al. (Crampin, Schnell, & McSharry, 2004) provide a survey of mathematical and computational mechanistic techniques proposed to deduce complex biochemical reaction networks. The majority of the reviewed techniques require the generation and analysis of significant quantities of experimental data in terms of composition and concentration time series.

The mechanistic view of a system of biochemical reactions is widespread among the modelers. It is considered important for several reasons: (i) an improved understanding of the functional role of different molecules can be achieved only with the knowledge of the mechanism of specific reactions and the nature of key intermediates; (ii) the control (or regulation) of different biochemical pathways can best be understood if some hypothesis for the reaction mechanism is available; (iii) kinetic modelling, which forms the basis for understanding reaction dynamics, is based on comprehensive information about the reaction mechanism. Kinetic models allow simulation of complicated pathways, and even whole-cell dynamics, which is proving to be an increasingly important predictive tool (Noble, 2002; Crampin, Schnell, & McSharry, 2004).

The data required for kinetic modelling are typically time series data of the response of a biochemical system to different conditions and stimuli. The reason why these data are used is that time series data reveal transient behavior, away from chemical equilibrium, and contain information on the dynamic interactions among reacting components. From time resolved data of reagent concentration, the mechanistic inference methods deduce the nature of reagents and their interactions (how they react with, or transform into, each other) and determine the rates of these transformations. Mechanistic inference can be broken down into two tasks: first, a connectivity or 'wiring diagram' has to be established and second, the individual interactions are assigned appropriate kinetics, or rate laws. In fact, in a topological sense, a network is a set of nodes and a set of directed or undirected edges between the nodes. Various experimental methods allow determining such networks. These methods include whole genome sequencing and annotation (genomics), the measurements of the messenger RNA molecules that are synthesized under a given condition (transcriptomics), the protein abundance, interactions and functional state (proteomics), measurements of the presence and concentration of metabolites (metabolomics), and metabolic fluxes (fluxomics) (Palsson B., 2006). There also exist methods, based on the use of fluorescent reporting molecules, to determine the binding sites of protein to the DNA and to measure fluxes through reactions inside a cell. All these methods can be used to generate the experimental observations that computational methodologies and algorithms can organize in network of interactions (Palsson, 2006; Sprite, Glymour, & Scheines, 2000; Hayete, Garden, & Collins, 2007; Ideker, 2004).

Before dealing with the computational methods for systems identification, we recall the main biological networks currently under study. They can be classified as follows.

1. *Transcriptional regulatory networks*. Genes are the nodes and the edges are directed. If the gene is an activator, then it is the source of a positive regulatory connection; if an inhibitor, then it is the source of a negative regulatory connection. Computational algorithms used to infer the topology take as primary input the data from a set of microarray runs measuring the mRNA expression levels of the genes under consideration for inclusion in the network.

2. *Signal transduction networks*. Proteins are the nodes and the edges are directed. Primary input into the inference algorithm would be data from a set of experiments measuring protein activation / inactivation (e.g., phosphorylation / dephosphorylation) across a set of proteins.

3. *Metabolite networks*. Metabolites are the nodes and the edges are directed. Primary input into an algorithm would be data from a set of experiments measuring metabolite levels.

4. *Intraspecies or interspecies communication networks*. Nodes are excreted organic compounds and the edges are directed. Input into an inference algorithm is data from a set of experiments measuring levels of excreted molecules.

5. *Protein-protein interaction networks*. The study of these networks demands a detailed physical chemistry/thermodynamic understanding of intermolecular forces.

Among these five categories of networks, the protein-protein interaction networks are currently attracting the attention of experimentalists and modelers. While the inference of gene regulatory networks has a longer tradition in computational systems biology, the inference of protein-protein network is only recently approached with mathematical and algorithmic approaches. In the meantime, various experimental methods contribute to support the theoretical investigation of systems of protein-protein interactions. We here recall the most popular and recent: dual polarization interferometry (DPI), static (and dynamics) light scattering (SLS and DLS), surface plasmon resonance, fluorescence polarization anisotropy, fluorescence resonance energy transfer (FRET), Nuclear Magnetic Resonance (NMR), multicellular relaxation experiments.

Usually network inference aims to use time-course data of the reagents abundance to infer topology and dynamics of the network. In this context, the inference faces particular problems due to the quality and the quantity of the experimental data of time course data that are available for biological processes (Lawrence, Girolami, Rattray, & Sanguinetti, 2010). First, data are often available only for a subset of the network components. Second, the number of time points in a dataset is often small, and the time points are separated by large time intervals between successive measurements. A third challenge is given by the high variability in measurements of each variable due both to experimental errors and random fluctuation of the cellular environment. Finally, another big challenge is to determine what the information content is in the various omics data types since they address different layers of complexity and function in the hierarchical structure of living systems (Palsson B., 2006). Thus, at present, network inference is at an early stage of development not only because of the inherent complexity of the chemical pathways governing the cell dynamics or the dynamics of ecosystems. It is also a demanding work because it requires the design of new experimental protocols in the framework of already established experimental techniques. These protocols have to be tailored to the acquisition of those types of data from which the present mathematical and the algorithmic models of inference can deduce the interaction pathway. In this context the development of inference models and algorithms could play an important role in aiding the design of new experimental protocols.

1.1 Perturbation Methods

The most direct approach to build a wiring diagram consists in evaluating the Jacobian matrix. The (i, j)-th entry of the Jacobian matrix corresponds to the magnitude of change in the time behavior of species i in response to an infinitesimal change in the level of species j. The experimental method to build this matrix for a biochemical network consists in perturbing one or more of the concentra-

tions from steady state and monitor the response of each of the chemical species as the system relaxes. The biggest hurdle to this method is that the response of each of the biochemical species in the network must be monitored in order to determine the Jacobian: even if recent advances of the experimental technologies allow to record simultaneous measurements of the concentration of several species, for practical reasons it may not be possible to measure many concentrations concurrently. Rather than to deduce connectivity from observations on the response to perturbations of arbitrary small amplitude made at different locations in the network, more feasible experiments can be made to deduce connectivity from the order and magnitude of the responses of different species to stimuli perturbing the network at different points.

If the concentration of one or more species of a network at steady state is increased by some arbitrary amount, unlike the previous methods for determining the Jacobian which relied on small amplitude perturbations, the responses in the concentrations of the other species will reveal qualitative properties of the network (Vance, Arkin, & Ross, 2002). As the concentrations increase and decrease following the initial impulse, the order of the appearance of peaks and troughs in the time courses for the different species reveals information about their ordering in a pathway. For example, consider an unbranched chain of reactions as in Figure 1.

Suppose at the beginning the concentration of species A and B are both equal to 100, in arbitrary units (a. u.), and assume without loss of generality that the ks are all equal to 0.1 a. u.. If we perturb the reaction chain of Figure 1 at one end, for instance by applying pulses to A we will be able to see the propagation of the pulse along the chain. Figure 2 (A) shows that changing the concentration of A to 200 and keeping the concentration of B equal to 100, the response of C follows the response of B. Non-null derivatives in the initial dynamics of B indicate direct connection

Figure 1. A didactic example of chain of reactions adapted from (Crampin, Schnell, & McSharry, 2004)

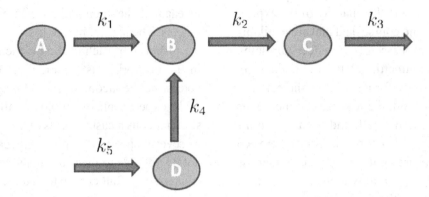

of A to B. If we repeat this experiment by perturbing D, by changing its concentration to 200 and keeping the concentration of A equal to 100, we obtain the dynamics showed in Figure 2 (c).

Vance et al. (Vance, Arkin, & Ross, 2002) motivated this approach arguing that, by perturbing the components of the network, sufficient information can be collected to infer the causal order of the responses. One year later this method has been successfully used by Torralba et al. (Torralba, Yu, Shen, Oefner, & Ross, 2003) in an experimental study to determine a part of the

glycolysis pathway in vitro. However, for complicated networks the interpretation of the responses is usually difficult and the network will be more difficult to reconstruct. Moreover, in general the pulse propagates dissipatively through the network, so the highest intensities of the responses, i. e. the best information, can be recovered on those species closest in a pathway to the point of perturbation. On the contrary, on species placed far from the point of disturbance the responses will have less intensity.

Figure 2. Time behavior of the species A, B, C, D, for three different set of initial quantities

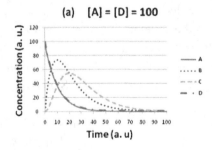

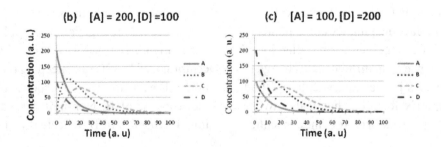

1.2 Correlation-Based Methods

Due to the difficulty of interpreting the response time-series on complex biochemical networks, the perturbation methods can be regarded as semi-quantitative approaches used to guide further experimental investigations devoted to grasp biological insights about the underlying mechanisms, rather than as methods to deduce quantitative connectivity between species. More quantitative approaches to network identification are the so-called correlation-based methods. These methods are used especially for inferring gene networks from microarray data (Faith, et al., 2007; Schmitt, Raab, & Stephanopoulos, 2004; Hayete, Garden, & Collins, 2007).

The key-idea of correlation-based inference method is to group together species with similar dynamic profiles using a data clustering approaches. In order to perform a clustering analysis the similarity between two time series must be quantified. Consider N species, $X_i(t)$ for $i=1,\ldots,N$ the correlation matrix of the $N(N-1)/2$ independent pairwise correlation coefficients can be used to cluster the data set into groups of species within which correlations between species are high, when compared to pair-wise correlations between different groups. These groupings can most easily be discerned by calculating a matrix of pair-wise distances, d_{ij} from the correlation matrix, whereby $d_{ij}=0$ for two species which are completely positively correlated.

The distance matrix can subsequently be analyzed to find clusters in the data, for example, using clustering techniques (Chipman, Hastie, & Tibshirani, 2008; Arkin, Shen, & Ross, 1997).

Very often in practical situations the influence of one species on another takes some finite amount of time to propagate through the network, so that two time series which have a low correlation may in fact be strongly correlated if a time lag is allowed for between the data points for the two species. In this case the ordering of responses to impulse stimuli reveals information about

network connectivity. In particular, this will be evident in the time series if the time interval Δt between concentration measurements is smaller than the characteristic response timescales for the network. Time-lagged correlations extend this technique by determining the best correlations among profiles shifted in time. For a transcription profile represented by a series of n measurements taken at equally spaced time points, the correlation between species i and j with a time lag, τ, is $\mathbf{R}(\tau)=(r_{ij}(\tau))$, defined by

$$r_{ij}(\tau) = \frac{S_{ij}(\tau)}{\sqrt{S_{ii}(\tau)S_{jj}(\tau)}} \tag{1}$$

and

$$S_{ij}(\tau) = \left\langle \left(X_i(t) - \bar{X}_i\right)\left(X_j(t+\tau) - \bar{X}_j\right)\right\rangle \tag{2}$$

where $X_i(t)$ denotes the concentration of species i at time t, $\bar{X}_i$ is the concentration of species i averaged across all time points, and the angled brackets represent a time average over all of the measurements. The matrix of lagged correlations $\mathbf{R}(\tau)$ can be used to rank the correlation and anticorrelation between species through conversion to a Euclidean distance metric, d_{ij}:

$$\begin{aligned} d_{ij} &= \sqrt{c_{ii} - 2c_{ij} + c_{jj}} \\ &= c_{ij}\sqrt{2(1 - c_{ij})} = \max_\tau \left|r_{ij}(\tau)\right| \end{aligned} \tag{3}$$

where, c_{ij} is the maximum absolute value of the correlation between two genes with a time lag τ. If the value of τ that gives the maximum correlation is 0, then the two species are best correlated with no time lag. The matrix $\mathbf{D}=(d_{ij})$ describes the correlation between two species, i and j, in terms of "distance" by making species that are least correlated (for any τ) the "farthest" apart (Arkin & Ross, 1995). A network of potential interactions, as well as cause and effect relationships, can be inferred by finding species that are closely related and then examining the corresponding value of τ.

The determination of a range of values for the time lag τ, and, more importantly, the possibility to estimate it automatically in the course of the inference procedure are crucial. In fact, the range of values for τ affetcs the number of false positive, if it is too large; while it affects the number of false negatives if it is too small. Let us deepen this point by developing the main steps of the correlation-based formalism. The linear correlation coefficient between two time-series $X_i(t)$ and $X_j(t)$ is defined by:

$$r_{ij} = \frac{1}{m} \sum_{k=1}^{m} \left(\frac{X_i(t_k) - \bar{X}_i}{\sigma_i} \right) \left(\frac{X_j(t_k) - \bar{X}_j}{\sigma_j} \right)$$

where $\bar{X}_i$ is the mean value of the time-series $X_i(t)$ and σ_i is the sample standard deviation.

According to Arkin et. al. (Arkin, Shen, & Ross, 1997) and Samoilov et. al. (Samoilov, Arkin, & Ross, 2001), the covariance function between X_i and X_j is shown in Box 1 where $\hat{X}_i$ is the measured value of the concentration of the species i-th, and:

$$\hat{X}_i^{\min(\max)} = \min(\max)_{t_k} \left\{ \hat{X}_i(t_k), \ k = 1, ..., m \right\}$$

$p(X_i)(t), X_j(t+\tau)$ is the pair distribution function, corresponding to the density of points on a scatter plot of $X_i(t)$ and $X_j(t+\tau)$, and m is the number of measurements. The pair distribution function gives the density of points in the a rectangle $dX_i \times dX_j$ on the plot (X_i, X_j). τ is a delay (*time lag*)

introduced to detect correlations that otherwise could be non-detectable. The delay τ is usually an input parameter chosen by the user, and the time behavior of the correlation between species is explored in the rage from $-\tau$ to $+\tau$ (Samoilov, Arkin, & Ross, 2001). However, here we propose two methods with which it can be automatically calculated within the computational framework of a network inference algorithm.

Consider:

$$\tau_i(t_k) \approx s_i^{-1}(t_k) = \left. \frac{dX_i}{dt} \right|_{t=t_k}$$

where $s_i(t_k)$ is the slope of the curve interpolating experimental time-series of species i at time point t_k.

Then, given τ_{ij} for each couple of species (X_i, X_j) as in the following

$$\tau_{ij} = \max \left\{ \max_k \{ \tau_i(t_k) \}, \ \max_k \{ \tau_j(t_k) \} \right\}$$

three possible estimates for τ can be taken into account

$$\tau = \min_{i,j}(\tau_{ij})$$

$$\tau = \max_{i,j}(\tau_{ij})$$

$$\tau = \text{average}_{ij}(\tau_{ij})$$

The second and third options are recommended. In fact, the value obtained by the first

Box 1.

$$C_{ij}(t) = \int_{\hat{X}_i^{\min}}^{\hat{X}_i^{\max}} \int_{\hat{X}_j^{\min}}^{\hat{X}_j^{\max}} \left(X_i(t) - \bar{X}_i \right) \left(X_j(t+\tau) - \bar{X}_j \right) p\left(X_i(t), X_j(t+\tau) \right) dX_i dX_j \qquad (4)$$

Box 2.

$$C_{ij}(t_k) = \sum_{\mu} \sum_{v} \left\{ \left(X_i(t_k) - \bar{X}_i \right)\left(X_j(t_k + \tau) - \bar{X}_j \right) p_{\mu v} \right\} \tag{5}$$

estimation could be not large enough to detect possible long-term correlations.

Since, generally, the analytical expression of $p(X_i(t), X_j(t+\tau))$ cannot be obtained, the calculation of the integral in Equation (4) can be performed only switching from a continuous to a discrete domain, so that the integral can be approximated by a sum shown in Box 2.

In order to estimate the pair distribution function $p_{\mu v}$, Samoilov et al. (Samoilov, Arkin, & Ross, 2001) proposed to divide the space of the phase plane into rectangles of varying size so that the distribution of points is uniform in each rectangle to within a given accuracy. The algorithm developed by A. Fraser et. al (Fraser & Swinney, 1986) is the most used procedure to perform such a partition of the phase plane X_i - X_j. The pair distribution density can then be estimated as:

$$p_{\mu v} = \frac{N_{\mu v}}{N_{tot} A_{\mu v}} \tag{6}$$

where $N_{\mu v}$ is the number of points in the particular rectangle labeled μ, v, N_{tot} is the total number of points and $A_{\mu v}$ is the area of the rectangle.

In Lecca et al. (Lecca, Palmisano, & Ihekwaba, 2010) we proposed a different solution to the problem of the pair distribution function. Instead of dividing the phase plane into rectangle of variable size, we propose a Voronoi tessellation of the space, following the results of the recent study of Browne (Browne, 2007) and Du et al. (Du & Grunzburger, 2002).

This division of the space according to point proximity leads to region boundaries being straight lines, bisecting and running perpendicular to the line connecting the Delaunay neighbors. Boundary points are equidistant to exactly two sites, and vertices are equidistant to at least 3. Neighboring points are points whose associated Voronoi regions share a common boundary. Thus, Voronoi tessellation generates a clustering of the points in the phase plane that in a good approximation satisfies the requirement of homogeneity for the distribution of points inside a cell, and $p_{\mu v}$ (5) can be calculated as follows

$$p_{\mu v} = 1/\text{Area}(V_{\mu v}) \tag{7}$$

where $V_{\mu v}$ is the Voronoi cell μv.

Once the covariance matrix has been calculated, the time-lagged correlation matrix $\mathbf{R}(\tau)$ can be built according to the definition in Equation (1) (Arkin, Shen, & Ross, 1997; Samoilov, Arkin, & Ross, 2001).

Finally, from the correlation matrix we calculate a distance matrix, whose elements are defined as in Equation (3). The distance matrix can subsequently be analyzed to find clusters in the data, for example, using hierarchical clustering techniques, or the K-means clustering algorithm (Chipman, Hastie, & Tibshirani, 2008), or multidimensional scaling algorithm (Arkin, Shen, & Ross, 1997). In fact, the information contained in the distance matrix can be extracted and interpreted graphically. A projection of the distances onto the plane can be exploited to represent the stronger connections (shorter distances) between species as a connected graph, while weaker interactions (longer distances) are collapsed, and can be ignored (Arkin, Shen, & Ross, 1997). The multidimensional scaling technique finds the optimum projection, for a given distance matrix, to give the best separation of the data (Samoilov, Arkin, & Ross, 2001). Graphical interpretation of the projected data can reveal not only the ordering of species in pathways, but also some clues as to the type of interaction. For instance, species which are strongly localized may form a subsystem which is weakly coupled to the rest of the network, or may represent reversible conversion of reaction intermediates at quasi-steady state.

The time-lagged correlation method ensures good performances if species with high correlation have been chosen using enough data points to give statistical significance, otherwise all of the τ values used will merely overfit the data. Such errors may occur if values for τ are unreasonably long from a biological standpoint. Finally, it is worthy to say that the strength point of the correlation-based approaches is that information can be extracted from experimental time series data with little *a priori* knowledge of the underlying mechanisms. Moreover, to some degree, these methods can deal with the effects of unobserved species on the network inference problem. This is because correlation between X_i and X_j will still be observed in the data even if their interaction is mediated via some intermediate, or intermediates, which are not measured.

A word of caution: often the inferred correlation graphs presents false edges, e.g. edges that do not correspond to a real biological interaction between the nodes. The cutting of false correlations from the graph is obtained with the calibration of network models. Each edge of the graph representing the interaction network is weighted by the value of the putative kinetic rate constant. Edges weighted by a kinetic constant of zero represent no dynamics and are cut. To calibrate the network, i.e. to detect null dynamics or nonplausible correlations, we developed an innovative probabilistic model of inference of the rate coefficients. The tool implementing this model is called *KInfer* (Knowledge Inference) (Lecca, Palmisano, & Ihekwaba, 2010) that is based on the theoretical model of inference described in

Section 2.2. In the following section we report an example of application of correlation-based approaches joint to calibration methods for the determination of an interaction sub-network of NF-kB signaling pathway (Lecca, Palmisano, & Ihekwaba, 2010).

1.2.1 Example: NF-kB Signaling Pathway

Activation of the NF-kB transcription factor can be triggered by exposing cells to a multitude of external stimuli such as tumor necrosis factor and interleukin 1. These cytokines initiate numerous and diverse intracellular signaling cascades, most of which activate the IKK complex. This IKK complex regulates the activity of the NF-kB transcription factor positively by phosphorylating the inhibitor, IkB. The IKK complex catalyses the transfer of the terminal phosphoryl group of ATP to the I-kB protein substrate, thereby tagging the inhibitor protein for ubiquitination subsequently leading to degradation. The previously inactive NF-kB is thus activated and available for regulating gene expression. This crucial component in the NF-kB activation cascade typically consists of two catalytic subunits, IKK1 and IKK2, and the regulatory unit IKK. The cytoplasmic inhibitors of NF-kB are phosphorylated by activated IKK at specific N-terminal residues, tagging them for poly-ubiquitination and rapid proteasomal degradation. This allows NF-kB to be released upon activation where it then translocates to the nucleus to induce the transcription of genes encoding regulators of immune and inflammatory responses, as well as of genes involved in apoptosis signaling and cell proliferation. Since recombinant human IKK2 (rhIKK2) phosphorylates IkBa in vitro, we examined its activity on IkBa, followed by the association and dissociation reactions, as shown in the chemical reaction system in Table 1, where, for simplicity, IKK2 is indicated by E.

For this example the time series of the reactant concentrations are taken from Ihekwaba et al.

Table 1. Second order reactions rate constants of the currently understood phosphorylation pathway (Ihekwaba, Wilkinson, Broomhead, Waithe, Grimpley, & Benson, 2007)

Reactants	Rate constant	Error of estimate	Units
E, ATP	1.2308	0.0008	1/(nM min)
E·ATP	0.9306	0.00018	1/min
E·ATP, IkBα	2.8506	0.0003	1/(nM min)
E·ATPIkBα	0.692538	0.000018	1/min
E·IkBα, ATP	1.351	0.004	1/(nM min)
E, ATP, IkBα	0.4345	0.0004	1/(nM min)

(Ihekwaba, Wilkinson, Broomhead, Waithe, Grimpley, & Benson, 2007) and from Lecca et al. (Lecca, Palmisano, & Ihekwaba, 2010). The time series are taken as the input of the network inference procedure; the output is a weighted distance matrix: The weights are the rate constants inferred by KInfer (Kinetics Inference). KInfer is a software tool that we recently developed for parameter inference. The weighted distances between species are represented as solid circles with different colors and different sizes, corresponding to the intensities of the correlation between the species (Figure 3 and Figure 4). Table 1 shows the set of non-null rate coefficients that are used as weights in calculating the distances among the species. The distance matrix reflects the experimentally observed dynamics (Figure 5), and the model of interaction is in agreement with the experimentally observed dynamics.

1.3 Bayesian Methods

Bayesian methods aim to find a directed, acyclic graph describing the causal dependency relationships among components of a system and a set of local joint probability distributions that statistically model these relationships (Friedman, 2004; Yu, Smith, Wang, Hartemink, & Jarvis, 2004; Friedman N., Linial, Nacjman, & Pe'er, 2000). Three mathematical models are traditionally used to infer and validate a biological interaction network from the experimentally observed dynamics

of the system: graph inference, graph analysis, and dynamic network modeling. Graph inference refers to the problem in which the information on the identity and the state of system elements is used to infer interactions or functional relationships among these elements and to construct the interaction graph underlying the system. Graph analysis means the use of graph theory to analyze a known (complete or incomplete) interaction graph and to extract new biological insights and predictions from the results. Dynamic network modeling aims to describe how known interactions among defined elements determine the time course of the state of the elements, and of the whole system, under different conditions. A dynamic model that correctly captures experimentally observed normal behavior allows researchers to track the changes in the system behavior due to perturbations. These three models for inference, validation and analysis are often combined in the literature since they provide three facets of the same objective: to understand, predict, and if possible control the dynamic behavior of biological interacting systems.

We provide in this section a brief introduction to the ideas behind Bayesian inference, and refer the reader to Friedman et al. for a more comprehensive treatment (Friedman N., Linial, Nacjman, & Pe'er, 2000). The Bayesian framework for inference is associated with the usage of the Bayes theorem that relates the conditional and marginal

Figure 3. Visualization of the correlation matrix for IKa phosporilation pathway. Each entry of the correlation matrix has been weighted on the value of the kinetic rate constant of the corresponding reaction between the two reagents.

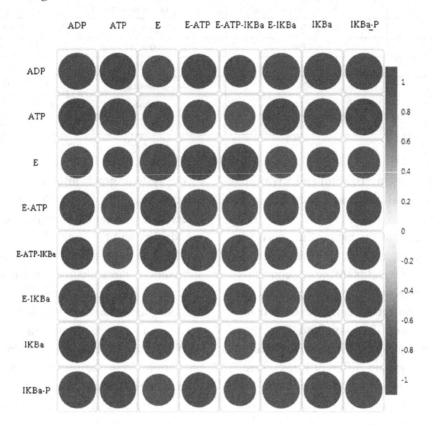

probabilities of events X and Y, provided that the probability of Y does not equal zero:

$$p(X|Y)\,p(Y) = p(Y|X)\,p(X)$$

Figure 4. Weighted correlation matrix visualized as network

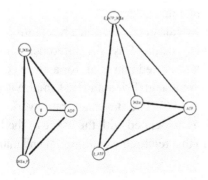

where

- $p(X)$ is the *prior probability* or *marginal probability* of X. It is "prior" in the sense that it does not take into account any information about Y.
- $p(X|Y)$ is the *conditional probability* of X, given Y. It is also called the *posterior probability* because it is derived from or depends upon the specified value of Y.
- $p(Y|X)$ is the conditional probability of Y given X. It is also called the *likelihood*.
- $p(Y)$ is the prior or marginal probability of Y, and acts as a normalizing constant.

The graphs inferred with Bayesian methods are often referred as *Bayesian networks*. A Bayesian

Figure 5. Inferred dynamics for the components of the system in Table 1

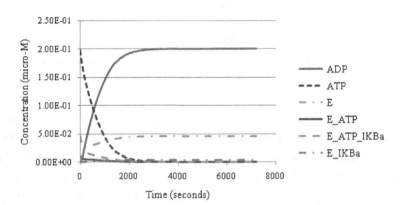

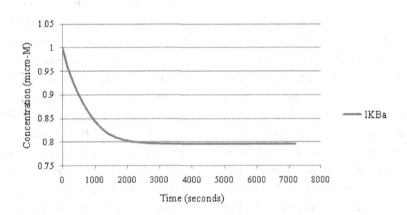

network is a graphical model for probabilistic relationships among a set of random variables X_i, where $i=1,…,N$. These relationships are encoded in the structure of a directed acyclic graph G, whose nodes are the random variables X_i The relationships between the variables are described by a joint probability distribution $p(X1…,XN)$ as shown in Box 3 where the $m+1$ variables, on which the probability is conditioned, are called the parents of the variable i in G and represent its regulators; the joint probability density $p(X1, ,XN)$ is expressed as a product of conditional probabilities by applying the chain rule of probabilities and independence (this rule is based on the Bayes theorem). The joint probability distribution can be decomposed as the product of conditional probabilities as in Equation (8) only if the Markov assumption holds, that is, each variable X_i is independent of its non

descendants, given its parent in the directed acyclic graph G. In order to reverse-engineer a Bayesian network model of an interaction network, we should find the directed acyclic graph G that best describes the experimental observations O. This is performed by choosing a scoring function that evaluates each graph G (i.e. a possible network topology) with respect to the experimental data, and then searching for the graph G that maximizes the score.

The score can be defined using the Bayes rule:

$$p\left(G|O\right) = \frac{p(G|O)p(G)}{p(O)}$$

where $p(G)$ can either contain some a priori knowledge on network structure, if available, or can be a constant non-informative prior, and $p(O|G)$

Box 3.

$$p(X_1,...,X_N) = \prod_{i=1}^{N} p\left(X_i = x_i \middle| X_j = x_j,...,X_{j+m} = x_{j+m}\right) \tag{8}$$

is a function, to be chosen by the algorithm that evaluates the probability that the data $\mathcal{O}$ has been generated by the graph $\mathcal{G}$. A popular score is the Bayesian Information Criterion (BIC) defined as follows:

$$BIC = 2\ln(L) + k\ln(n)$$

where n is the sample size, L is the maximized value of the likelihood function for the estimated model, and k is the number of free parameters. In Bayesian inference methods for graph inference, the starting edges are established heuristically based on an initial assessment of the experimental data and are refined by an iterative search-and-score algorithm until the causal network and posterior probability distribution best describing the observed state of each node are found. Trying out all possible combinations of interaction among entities, that is, all possible graphs G, and choosing the G with the maximum Bayesian score is an NP-hard problem. Therefore, a heuristic search method is used, like the greedy hill climbing approach, the Markov Chain Monte Carlo method or simulated annealing.

Bayesian networks model probabilistic dependencies among variables and not causality, that is, the parents of a node are not necessarily also the direct causes of its behaviour. However, an edge can be interpreted as a causal link if we assume that the Causal Markov Condition holds. This can be stated simply as: a variable X is independent of every other variable conditional on all its direct causes. A word of caution: it is not known whether this assumption is a good approximation of what happens in real biological networks (Bansal, Belcastro, Ambesi-Impiombato, & di Bernardo, 2007).

Today, the literature reports various network inference algorithms inspired to Bayesian methods most of them applied to graph inference of gene networks, as consequence of the collection of genomic scale snapshots of gene expressions in the last decade (Rogers, Khanin, & Girolami, 2007; Yu, Smith, Wang, Hartemink, & Jarvis, 2004; Friedman, Inferring cellular networks using probabilistic graphical models, 2004; Wilkinson, 2007). Bayesian inference was recently used also to infer the signaling network responsible for embryonic stem cell fate responses to external cues (Woolf, Prudhomme, Daheron, Daley, & Lauffebberger, 2005). A comprehensive report of the current state of the art can be found in Lecca et al. (Lecca, Nguyen, Priami, & Quaglia, 2010), Albert (Albert, 2007) and Crampin et al. (Crampin, Schnell, & McSharry, 2004). However, nowadays, in the biological sciences it is becoming increasingly common to collect data in high-throughput experiments also on proteomic and metabolomic scales. Protein-protein interaction networks, metabolite networks and, very recently also signal transduction networks are at the moment poorly explored fields in the context of network inference.

Bayesian network inference algorithms are able to capture linear, non-linear, combinatorial, stochastic and other types of relationships among variables across multiple levels of biological organization. However, there are still limitations in using Bayesian inference algorithms to network inference. First, it is well known that inference algorithms perform better with highly time-resolved data - and Bayesian algorithms are no exception - but in molecular biology the quantity of data that can be collected is often sparse and with a low time-resolution. Second, discrete Bayesian networks typically use combinatorial interaction models, making it difficult to determine the sign and relative magnitude of interactions between variables. On the contrary, Bayesian networks typically use additive interaction models, making it easy to deduce the sign and relative magnitude of interactions between variables, but they are not able to handle inherently combinatorial interactions between the variable (for instance, transcriptional regulators are known to often be combinatorial rather than additive). Finally, Bayesian probabilistic inference needs a detail of a *priori k*nowledge that often is not possible to have from experiments.

Correlation-based approaches to network inference hold the promise to handle these situations, and some few investigations about the applicability of these methods to specific type of data and biological processes can be found in the literature (Samoilov, Arkin, & Ross, 2001). However, this methodology needs to be advanced and generalized, and combined with causal inference algorithms in order to make it capable to treat different type of data and biological processes, and to determine not only the topology but also the causal structure of the network.

2. PARAMETER INFERENCE

A model of a biological system consists in its topological and causal structure as well as in the quantitative information contained in its parameters. The estimation of parameter values (model calibration) is the bottleneck of the computational analysis of biological systems. Modeling approaches are central in systems biology, as they provide a rational framework to guide systematic strategies for key issues in medicine as well as the pharmaceutical and biotechnological industries. Inter- and intra-cellular processes require dynamic models that contain the rate constants of the biochemical reactions. These kinetic parameters are often not accessible directly through experiments.

Therefore methods that estimate rate constants with the maximum precision and accuracy are needed. We first report a brief state of the art of this topic, and then we review a method for estimating rate coefficients of biochemical networks from noisy observations of concentration levels at discrete time points. The method has been developed by the authors and recently published in Lecca et al. (Lecca P., Palmisano, Ihekwaba, & Priami, 2010).

2.1 The State of the Art

The relation between the instantaneous rate of reaction and the concentrations of the reactants at any moment is given by the law of mass action, i.e. the rate at which a substance takes part in a reaction is proportional to the concentration of the substance raised to the order of the reaction. Such formulation is made for simultaneous as well as isolated reactions, and for heterogeneous as well as homogeneous systems. The ability to infer these constants of proportionality for a system of biochemical reactions is crucial in systems biology, yet their direct measurement is a challenging experimental problem.

Parameter estimation is commonly achieved by the best fit of numerical simulations to experimental observations. The fitting procedure is based on optimization techniques where a measure of the distance between model prediction and experimental data (the cost function) is used as the optimality criterion to be minimized. In most approaches dealing with parameter estimation the cost function is the likelihood function, also known as joint transitional density. It expresses the probability of obtaining the observed outcomes in terms of measured systems variables and parameters. Thus it can be used to determine unknown parameters based on known outcomes. The optimal values of the parameters can be estimated by maximizing the likelihood function (maximun likelihood criterion) or, equivalently, by minimizing the log-likelihood function. However, when estimating parameters of dynamical systems with optimization methods, a number of difficulties may arise, the most important being convergence to local solutions, very flat objective function in the neighborhood of the solution, over-determined models, and non-differentiable terms in the systems dynamics. Due to the non-linear nature of the dynamics of the biological processes, these problems are often multimodal, so that traditional gradient based methods fail to identify the global solution and may converge to a local minimum. Moreover, in the case in which a bad fit has been performed, there is no way of knowing if it is due to a wrong model structure or if it is consequent to a local convergence.

The recent literature reports many examples of new effective methods attempting either to work out these difficulties or to develop new methodologies of parameter estimation both in deterministic and stochastic models. Here we briefly mention the most recent ones. Wang et al. proposed an algorithm for inference of kinetic rate parameters based upon maximum likelihood using stochastic gradient descent method (Wang, Scott, Mjolsness, & Xie, 2010). Polisetty et al. (Polisetty, Voit, & Gatzke, 2006) suggested global optimization techniques as alternative to traditional local methods.

Rodrigez-Fernandez et al. (Rodrigez-Fernandez, Mendes, & Banga, 2006) developed a hybrid stochastic-deterministic global optimization method. Moles et al. in (Moles, Mendes, & Banga, 2003) explored several state-of-the-art deterministic and stochastic global optimization techniques and compared their accuracy and effectiveness on nonlinear biochemical dynamic models. Tian et al. (Tian, Xu, & Burrage, 2007) presented a simulated maximum likelihood method to evaluate parameters in stochastic models described by stochastic differential equations. They propose different types of transitional probability and a genetic optimization algorithm to search for optimal reaction rates. Chou et al. (Chou, Martens, & Voit, 2006) developed an alternate regression method, that dissects the parameter inference problem into iterative steps of linear regression. Sugimoto et al. (Sugimoto, Kikuchi, & Tomita, 2005) provided a computational technique based on genetic programming that simultaneously generates biochemical equations and their parameters from time series data. Reinker et al. (Reinker, Altman, & Timmer, 2006) are the authors of the approximate maximum likelihood method and the singular value decomposition likelihhod method that estimate stochastic reaction constants from molecule count data measured with errors at discrete time points. Wang et al. (Wang, Scott, Mjolsness, & Xie, 2010) also developed a method for parameter inference for discretely observed stochastic kientic models. Unlike Reinker et al. Wang et al. used a stochastic gradient descendent. Tools for parameter fitting through regression or maximum likelihood methods can be found as integral part of simulation tools (e. g. Copasi (Hoops, Sahle, Gauges, Lee, Pahle, & Simus, 2006)), but there exist also "stand-alone" software exclusively designed for that purpose, like Splindid (Bashi, Forrest, & Ramanathan, 2005) and PET (Zwolak, 2007). Finally we mention the works of Boys et al. (Boys, Wilkinson, & Kirkwood, 2008), Golitki (Golightly & Wilkinson, 2008) and Wilkinson (Wilkinson, 2006; Wilkinson, 2007), that developed Bayesian model-based inference techniques. Baysesian schemes depart from the approaches previously mentioned. They offer some advantages over the maximum likelihood methods, for instance when the volume of data is limited or the analytic form of the kinetic model makes the maximization of the likelihood not straightforward. Nevertheless, Bayesian approaches require to specify a prior distribution for all unknown parameters, but, in problems of calibration of biochemical models, prior knowledge is either vague, or non-existent, and that makes it very difficult to specify a unique prior distribution. The prior information can come from preliminary experiments and reference data. Sometimes parameters related to physical properties are reported in the form of means and standard deviations or are bounded by physical conditions. Unfortunately it is not that simple in systems biology: experiments for the collection of in vivo time-series data are expensive, hence they are not repeatable. Data are seldom complete and they typically contain noise that consists of a mixture of natural variability among cells, uncertainties about the particular experimental conditions at the time of the observation; none of these sources of variation is truly and a priori quantifiable.

The need of robustness against the noise affecting the data is still a challenge for most of the current tools for parameter estimation. Experimental uncertainties on parameters propagate from the measurements of the concentrations of the species. Inferring the parameters with an estimate of their uncertainty, even pessimistic as the variance, is essential if we want to use these tools in the context of optimal experimental design.

2.2 KInfer: The Model of Inference

In this section, we report the theoretical framework of the software KInfer (Lecca P., Palmisano, Ihekwaba, & Priami, 2010) that we developed for estimating parameters of biochemical networks from time course data. KInfer is a free downloadable software for non- commercial purposes (KInfer, 2009).

Consider N reactant species, $S_1, S_2,...,S_N$ with concentrations $X_1, X_2,...,X_N$, that evolve according to a system of rate equations:

$$\frac{dX_i}{dt} = f_i\left(X^{(i)}(t); \theta_i\right) \tag{9}$$

where θ_i, $i=1,2,...,N$, is the vector of the rate coefficients, which are present in the expression of the function f_i. We wish to estimate the set of parameters $\Theta = \cup \theta_i$ ($i=1,2,...,N$), whose element θ_i is the set of rate coefficients appearing in the rate equations of i-th species, therefore:

$$\theta_1 = \left\{\theta_{11}, \theta_{12},...,\theta_{1N_1}\right\}$$
$$\theta_2 = \left\{\theta_{21}, \theta_{22},...,\theta_{2N_2}\right\}$$
$$\cdots \qquad \cdots$$
$$\theta_i = \left\{\theta_{i1}, \theta_{i2},...,\theta_{iN_i}\right\}$$
$$\cdots \qquad \cdots$$
$$\theta_N = \left\{\theta_{N1}, \theta_{N2},...,\theta_{NN_N}\right\}$$

$X^{(i)}$ is the vector of concentrations of chemicals that are present in the expression of the function f_i for the species i.

According to the law of mass action, the functions f_i have the general form shown in Box 4.

In this equation $X^{(ij)}$, with $i=1,2,...N$, $j=1,2,...,N_i$, is a vector whose set of elements is a subset of the set of elements of the vector $X^{(i)}$.

The function g_{ij} is the product of reactant concentrations, and varies according to the empirical law of rate equation as follows:

$$g_{i1}\left(X^{(i1)}(t)\right) = \prod_{w \in S_1 \subseteq [1,N]} X_w^{\alpha_w}$$
$$g_{i2}\left(X^{(i2)}(t)\right) = \prod_{w \in S2 \subseteq [1,N]} X_w^{\alpha_w}$$
$$\cdots \qquad \cdots$$
$$g_{iN_i}\left(X^{(iN_i)}(t)\right) = \prod_{w \in S_{N_i} \subseteq [1,N]} X_w^{\alpha_w}$$

Box 4.

$$f_i(t) = \theta_{i1} g_{i1}\left(X^{(i1)}(t)\right) + \theta_{i2} g_{i2}\left(X^{(i2)}(t)\right) + ... + \theta_{iN_i} g_{iN_i}\left(X^{(iN_i)}(t)\right). \tag{10}$$

where $\alpha_w \in \mathbf{R}$ denotes the partial order of reaction with respect to the reactant having concentration X_w. Substituting these expressions in Equation (10) gives Equation (11) in Box 5.

We assume we have noisy observations $\hat{X}_i = X_i + \mathrm{T}$ at times $t_0, \ldots, t_M$, where $\square \sim \mathcal{N}(0, \sigma 2)$ is a Gaussian noise term with mean zero and variance $\sigma 2$. We also assume a number M of concentration measurements for each considered species.

We approximate the rate Equation (9) as a finite difference equation between the observation times,

$$X_i(t_k) = X_i(t_{k-1}) + (t_k - t_{k-1}) f_i(\mathrm{X}^{(i)}; \theta_i, \sigma) \qquad (12)$$

where $k=1,\ldots,M$. In Equation (12) the rate equation is viewed as a model of increments/decrements of reactant concentrations; i.e., given a value of the variables at time t, the model can be used to predict the value at the next time point. Increments/decrements between different time points are conditionally independent by the Markov nature of the model (12). Therefore, given the Gaussian model for the noise, it is possible to estimate the probability to observe the value $\hat{X}_i(t_k)$ given the model at time $t_{k-1}, X_i(t_{k-1})$, and the set of parameters θ_i, as:

$$
\begin{aligned}
& p\left(\hat{X}_i(t_k) \big| X_i(t_{k-1}), \theta_i, \sigma\right) \\
& = \mathcal{N}\left(X_i(t_{k-1}) + f_i(\mathrm{X}(t_{k-1}), \theta_i, \sigma), \sigma^2\right)
\end{aligned}
\qquad (13)
$$

Moreover, by symmetry, the true value of $X_i(t_k)$ is normally distributed around the observed value $\hat{X}_i(t_k)$, so that we get Equation (14) in Box 6.

Therefore, the probability to observe a variation D_i for the concentration of the i-*th* species between the time t_{k-1} and t_k, given the parameter vector θ_i is:

$$p(D_i(t_k)|\theta_i, \sigma = \mathcal{N}(E[fi_(\mathrm{X}(tk_{-1}), \theta i \ \sigma)], 2\sigma 2) \qquad (15)$$

and Equation (16) in Box 7 where K_i is the number of chemical species in the expression for f_i.

Box 5.

$$f_i(t) = \theta_{i1} \prod_{w \in S_1 \subseteq [1,N]} X_w^{\alpha_w} + \theta_{i2} \prod_{w \in S_2 \subseteq [1,N]} X_w^{\alpha_w} + \cdots + \theta_{iN_i} \prod_{w \in S_{N_i} \subseteq [1,N]} X_w^{\alpha_w} \qquad (11)$$

Box 6.

$$p\left(X_i(t_k), \theta_i, \sigma \big| \hat{X}_i(t_k)\right) = \mathcal{N}\left(X_i(t_{k-1}) \big| \hat{X}_i(t_{k-1}), \sigma^2\right) = \frac{1}{\sqrt{2\pi}\sigma} \exp\left[-\frac{\left(X_i(t_{k-1}) - \hat{X}_i(t_{k-1})\right)^2}{2\sigma^2}\right] \qquad (14)$$

Box 7.

$$E\left[f_i\left(\mathrm{X}^{(i)}(t_{k-1}), \theta_i, \sigma\right)\right] = \int f_i\left(\mathrm{X}^{(i)}, \theta_i, \sigma\right) \prod_{i=1}^{K_i} \left[p_i\left(X_i(t_k), \theta_i, \sigma \big| \hat{X}_i(t_k)\right)\right] d\mathrm{X}^{(i)} \qquad (16)$$

While the increments/decrements are conditionally independent given the starting point $X_i(t_k)$, the random variables $D_i(t_k)$ are not independent of each other. Intuitively, if $X_i(t_k)$ happens to be below its expected value because of random fluctuations, then the following increment $D_i(t_{k+1})$ can be expected to be bigger as a result, while the previous one $D_i(t_k)$ will be smaller. A simple calculation allows us to obtain the covariance matrix of the vector of increments for the i-*th* species.

This is a banded matrix $\mathbf{C}_i \equiv \mathbf{C} = \text{Cov}(\mathbf{D}_i)$ with diagonal elements given by:

$$E\left[D_i^2(t_k) - E\left[D_i^2(t_k)\right]\right] = 2\sigma^2$$

and a non-zero band above and below the diagonal given by the equation in Box 8 with all other entries zero. The likelihood for the observed increments/decrements therefore will be Equation (17) in Box 9 where:

$$\mathbf{D} = \{\mathbf{D}_1, \mathbf{D}_2, \ldots, \mathbf{D}_N\}$$

and:

$$\mathrm{m}_i(t_k) \equiv E\left[f_i(\mathrm{X}(t_{k-1}), \theta_i, \sigma)\right]$$

The Equation (17) can be optimized w. r. t. the parameters $\Theta = (\theta_1, \theta_2, \ldots, \theta_S)$ of the model to yield estimates of the parameters themselves and of the noise level.

The main numerical problem of this approach is the computation of the expectations of the rate functions given by Equation (16). Non-integer values of the coefficients α can make estimating the integral analytically difficult. We propose an approximate method in which the Gaussian noise is replaced by an approximate uniform (white) noise, with the amplitude of the uniform noise being obtained as a sample from the Gaussian cumulative distribution function.

At the first order, for small σ we can approximate the Gaussian with zero mean and variance σ with an uniform distribution defined on the interval $\left[-\dfrac{\sqrt{2\pi\sigma}}{4}, \dfrac{\sqrt{2\pi\sigma}}{4}\right]$, so that:

$$\prod_{i=1}^{K_i} p_i = \prod_{i=1}^{K_i} \mathcal{X}_i \qquad (18)$$

where:

$$\mathcal{X}_i(X_i) = \begin{cases} \dfrac{2}{\sqrt{2\pi\sigma}} & \text{if } -\dfrac{\sqrt{2\pi\sigma}}{4} \leq X_i \leq \dfrac{\sqrt{2\pi\sigma}}{4} \\ 0 & \text{otherwise} \end{cases}$$

Box 8.

$$E\left[\left(D_i(t_k) - E\left[D_i(t_k)\right]\right)\left(D_i(t_k) - E\left[D_i(t_{k-1})\right]\right)\right] = -\sigma^2$$

Box 9.

$$p(\mathrm{D}|\Theta) = \prod_{i=1}^{N} \mathcal{N}(\mathrm{D}_i | \mathrm{m}_i(\Theta), \mathrm{C}) = \left(\frac{1}{\sqrt{2\pi \ \det(\mathrm{C})}}\right)^N \exp\left[\sum_{i=1}^{N} -\frac{1}{2}(\mathrm{D}_i - \mathrm{m}_i)^T \mathrm{C}^{-1}(\mathrm{D}_i - \mathrm{m}_i)\right] \qquad (17)$$

Therefore we get Equation (19) in Box 10. Now, since:

$$f_i\left(X^{(i)}(t_{k-1}, \theta_i, \sigma)\right) = \sum_{h=1}^{N_i}\left(\theta_{ih}\prod_{w\in S_h} X_w^{\alpha_w}\right)$$

we have Equation (20) in Box 11.

If in the Equation (17), $\mathbf{m}_i$ is substituted with the expression (20), Equation (17) becomes more tractable and can be optimized w. r. t. the parameters $\Theta=(\theta_1, \theta_2,...,\theta_S)$ and σ. The values of the model's parameter for which $p(\mathbf{D}|\Theta)$ has a maximum are the most likely values giving the observed kinetics.

This procedure has been successfully applied to many synthetic and real case studies. Most important ones are: glucose metabolism of L. lactis, gene regulatory networks, NF-kB signaling pathway, SERCA pump mechanisms. We refer the reader to Lecca et al. (Lecca P., Palmisano, Ihekwaba, & Priami, 2010) for a detailed description of each case study.

In fact, our method approximates the law of mass action and provides a tool to predict the values of the variables X_i at time t, conditioned on their values at the previous time point. The variations of the concentration of the species at different time points are conditionally independent by the Markov nature of the discrete model of the law of mass action. Assuming the observation noise to be Gaussian with variance σ^2, the probability of observing a variation D_i for the concentration X_i of species i between time t_{k-1} and t_k is a Gaussian with variance depending on σ and with mean the

Box 10.

$$E\left[f_i\left(X^{(i)}(t_{k-1}, \theta_i, \sigma)\right)\right] = \left(\frac{2}{\sqrt{2\pi\sigma}}\right)^{K_i} \int_{\hat{X}-\frac{\sqrt{2\pi\sigma}}{4}}^{\hat{X}+\frac{\sqrt{2\pi\sigma}}{4}} f_i\left(X^{(i)}(t_{k-1}, \theta_i, \sigma)\right)dX^{(i)} \tag{19}$$

Box 11.

$$
\begin{aligned}
E\left[f_i\left(X^{(i)}(t_{k-1}, \theta_i, \sigma)\right)\right] &= \left(\frac{2}{\sqrt{2\pi\sigma}}\right)^{K_i} \int_{\hat{X}-\frac{\sqrt{2\pi\sigma}}{4}}^{\hat{X}+\frac{\sqrt{2\pi\sigma}}{4}} \sum_{h=1}^{N_i}\left(\theta_{ih}\prod_{w\in S_h} X_w^{\alpha_w}\right)dX^{(i)} \\
&= \left(\frac{2}{\sqrt{2\pi\sigma}}\right)^{K_i} \left\{\sum_{h=1}^{N_i}\theta_{ih}\int_{\hat{X}-\frac{\sqrt{2\pi\sigma}}{4}}^{\hat{X}+\frac{\sqrt{2\pi\sigma}}{4}}\left(\prod_{w\in S_h} X_w^{\alpha_w}\right)dX^{(i)}\right\} \\
&= \left(\frac{2}{\sqrt{2\pi\sigma}}\right)^{K_i} \left\{\sum_{h=1}^{N_i}\theta_{ih}\left[\left(\prod_{w\in(S-S_h)}\left(X_w\Big|_{\hat{X}-\frac{\sqrt{2\pi\sigma}}{4}}^{\hat{X}+\frac{\sqrt{2\pi\sigma}}{4}}\right)\right)\cdot\prod_{w\in S_h}\int_{\hat{X}-\frac{\sqrt{2\pi\sigma}}{4}}^{\hat{X}+\frac{\sqrt{2\pi\sigma}}{4}} X_w^{\alpha_w}dX_w^{(i)}\right]\right\} \\
&= \left(\frac{2}{\sqrt{2\pi\sigma}}\right)^{K_i} \left\{\sum_{h=1}^{N_i}\theta_{ih}\left[\left(\prod_{w\in(S-S_h)}\left(X_w\Big|_{\hat{X}-\frac{\sqrt{2\pi\sigma}}{4}}^{\hat{X}+\frac{\sqrt{2\pi\sigma}}{4}}\right)\right)\cdot\prod_{w\in S_h}\frac{1}{\alpha_w+1}X_w^{\alpha_w+1}\Big|_{\hat{X}-\frac{\sqrt{2\pi\sigma}}{4}}^{\hat{X}+\frac{\sqrt{2\pi\sigma}}{4}}\right]\right\} \\
&= \left(\frac{2}{\sqrt{2\pi\sigma}}\right)^{K_i} \left\{\sum_{h=1}^{N_i}\theta_{ih}\left[\left(\frac{\sqrt{2\pi\sigma}}{2}\right)^{\#(S-S_h)}\times\prod_{w\in S_h}\frac{1}{\alpha_w+1}\left(\left(\hat{X}_w+\frac{\sqrt{2\pi\sigma}}{4}\right)^{\alpha_w+1}-\left(\hat{X}_w-\frac{\sqrt{2\pi\sigma}}{4}\right)^{\alpha_w+1}\right)\right]\right\}
\end{aligned}
\tag{20}
$$

expectation value of the law of mass action under the noise distribution.

Our approximation of the law of mass action provides a model for the variations of the species concentration, rather than a model for the time-trajectory of the species concentrations. This makes the evaluation of the expectation value of law mass action function (the integral of the transitional probability) simpler and analytically tractable. The rate coefficients and the level of noise σ are then obtained by maximizing the likelihood function defined by the observed variations. The probabilistic formulation of the inference model handles the noise inherent in biological data, and it enables further extensions, such as a fully Bayesian treatment of the parameter inference and automated model selection strategies based on the comparison between marginal likelihoods of different models. This method has been successfully applied to many relevant case studies: we refer the reader to (Lecca P., Palmisano, Ihekwaba, & Priami, 2010).

The need of robustness against the noise affecting the data is still a challenge for the most of the current tools for parameter estimation. Experimental uncertainties on parameters propagate from the measurements of the concentrations of the species. Inferring the parameters with an estimate of their uncertainty, even pessimistic as the variance, is essential if we want to use these tools in the context of optimal experimental design.

KInfer is part of the software platform CoS-BiLab (CoSBiLab, 2010) that implements a new conceptual modeling, analysis and simulation approach - primarily inspired by *algorithmic systems biology* (Priami, 2009) - to biological processes. Algorithmic systems biology grounds on the belief that algorithms can help in coherently extracting the key biological principles that underlie the experimental observations, especially those data collected by high-throughput experiments. In making advances within algorithmic systems biology there is an acknowledged need for the ongoing development of both probabilistic

and mechanistic models of complex biological processes. In addition to such models the development of appropriate and efficient inferential methodology to identify and reason over such models is necessary.

3. CONCLUSION

The advent of high-throughput experimental technologies forced biologists, modelers, and computer scientists to view the biological entities as systems. Moreover, the ability to generate detailed lists of biological components, determine their interactions, and generate genome-wide datasets has led to the birth of systems biology. The recent advent of algorithmic systems biology forced biologists and modelers to think of a biological process in terms of its mechanistic interactions. The execution of the algorithm produces the simulation of the behavior of the system in question. Network inference is preliminary to the simulation of the system, because it identifies the system that we are going to simulate and analyze. Its input are the experimental data, static or dynamic data, coming from different experiments and protocols. Therefore data quality assessment methods and data integration methods are preliminary to network inference. The output of the inference is generally a set of models of networks, among which a discrimination is necessary to eliminate the less biological plausible models or those models that are mathematically inconsistent (i. e. over- or under- determined parametric models). Network inference is thus the link between the *in vivo* and *in vitro* systems biology and the *in silico* systems biology.

REFERENCES

Albert, R. (2007). Network Inference, Analysis, and Modeling in Systems Biology. *The Plant Cell, 19*, 3327–3338. doi:10.1105/tpc.107.054700

Arkin, A., & Ross, J. (1995). Statistical construction of chemical reaction mechanisms from measured time-series. *Journal of Physical Chemistry*, *99*, 970–979. doi:10.1021/j100003a020

Arkin, A., Shen, P., & Ross, J. (1997). A Test Case of Correlation Metric Construction of a Reaction Pathway from Measurements. *Science*, *277*(29), 1275–1279. doi:10.1126/science.277.5330.1275

Bansal, M., Belcastro, V., Ambesi-Impiombato, A., & di Bernardo, D. (2007). How to infer gene networks from expression profiles. *Molecular Systems Biology*, *3*(78).

Bashi, K., Forrest, A., & Ramanathan, M. (2005). SPLINDID: a semi-paramteric, model based method for obtaining transcription rates and gene regulation paramters from genomic and proteomic expression profiles. *Bioinformatics (Oxford, England)*, *21*(20), 3873–3879. doi:10.1093/bioinformatics/bti624

Boys, R. J., Wilkinson, D. J., & Kirkwood, T. B. (2008). *Bayesian inference fora discretely observed stochastic kinetic model*. Springer Netherlands.

Browne, M. (2007). A geometric approach to non-paramteric density estimation. *Pattern Recognition*, *40*, 134–140. doi:10.1016/j.patcog.2006.05.012

Chipman, H., Hastie, T. J., & Tibshirani, R. (2008). *Clustering microarray data of Gene Expression Microarray Dat. (T. P. Speed, A cura di)*. Chapman & Hall.

Chou, I. C., Martens, H., & Voit, E. O. (2006). Paramter estimation in biochemical systems models with alternating regression. *Theoretical Biology & Medical Modelling*, *3*(25).

CoSBiLab. (2010). Retrieved from http://www.cosbi.eu.

Crampin, E. J., Schnell, S., & McSharry, P. E. (2004). Mathematical and computational techniques to deduce complex biochemical reaction mechanisms. *Progress in Biophysics and Molecular Biology*, *86*, 72–112. doi:10.1016/j.pbiomolbio.2004.04.002

Du, Q., & Grunzburger, M. (2002). Grid generation and optimization based on centroidal Voronoi tessellations. *Math. Comp.*, *133* (2-3).

Faith, J. J., Hayete, B., Thaden, J. T., Mogno, I., Wierzbowski, J., & Cottarel, G. (2007). Large-scale mapping and validation of Escherichia coli transcriptional regulation from a compendium of expression profiles. *PLoS Biology*, *5*(1), 54–66. doi:10.1371/journal.pbio.0050008

Fraser, A. M., & Swinney, H. L. (1986). Independent coordinates for strange attractors from mutual information. *Physical Review A.*, *33*(2), 1134–1140. doi:10.1103/PhysRevA.33.1134

Friedman, N. (2004). Inferring cellular networks using probabilistic graphical models. *Science*, *303*, 799–805. doi:10.1126/science.1094068

Friedman, N., Linial, M., Nacjman, I., & Pe'er, D. (2000). Using Bayesian networks to analyze expression data. *Journal of Computational Biology*, *7*, 601–620. doi:10.1089/106652700750050961

Golightly, A., & Wilkinson, D. (2008). Bayesian inference for nonlinear multivariate diffusion models observed with error. *Computational Statistics & Data Analysis*, *52*(3), 1674–1693. doi:10.1016/j.csda.2007.05.019

Hayete, B., Garden, T. S., & Collins, J. J. (2007). Size matters: network inference tackles the genome scale. *Molecular Systems Biology*, *3*(77).

Hoops, S., Sahle, S., Gauges, R., Lee, C., Pahle, J., & Simus, N. (2006). COPASI - a COmplex PAthway SImulator. *Bioinformatics (Oxford, England)*, *22*, 3067–3074. doi:10.1093/bioinformatics/btl485

Ideker, T. (2004). A Systems Approach to Discovering Signaling and Regulatory Pathways – or, How to Digest Large Interaction Networks Into Relevant Pieces. *Advances in Experimental Medicine and Biology, 547*, 21–30. doi:10.1007/978-1-4419-8861-4_3

Ihekwaba, A. E., Wilkinson, S. J., Broomhead, D. S., Waithe, D., Grimpley, R., & Benson, N. (2007). Bridging the gap between in silico and cell based analysis of the NF-kB signalling pathway by in vitro studies of IKK2. *The FEBS Journal, 90*, 1678–1690. doi:10.1111/j.1742-4658.2007.05713.x

KInfer. (2009). Tratto da. Retrieved from http://www.cosbi.eu/index.php/research/prototypes/kinfer.

Kitano, H. (2002). Systems biology: A brief overview. *Science, 295*, 1662–1666. doi:10.1126/science.1069492

Lawrence, N. D., Girolami, M., Rattray, M., & Sanguinetti, G. (2010). *Learning and Inference in Computational and Systenms Biology*. Cambridge, MA: The MIT Press.

Lecca, P., Nguyen, P., Priami, C., & Quaglia, P. (2010). Network inference from Time-Dependent Omics Data. In B. Mayer. Humana Press Springer Science+Businnes Media, LLC.

Lecca, P., Palmisano, A., Ihekwaba, A. E., & Priami, C. (2010). Calibration of dynamic models of biological systems with KInfer. *European Journal of Biophysics, 39*(6), 1019. doi:10.1007/s00249-009-0520-3

Lecca, P., Palmisano, P., & Ihekwaba, A. E. (2010). Correlation-based network inference and modelling in systems biology: the NF-κB signalling network case study. *Int. Conf. on Intelligent Systems, Modelling and Simulation* (p. 170-175). Liverpool: IEEE Computer Society.

Moles, G. C., Mendes, P., & Banga, J. R. (2003). paramter estimation in biochemical pathways: a comparison of global optimiztion methods. *Genome Research, 13*, 2467–2474. doi:10.1101/gr.1262503

Noble, D. (2002). The rise of computational biology. *Nat. Rev. Mol. Biol.* (3), 459-463.

Palsson, B. (2006). *Systems biology. Properties of reconstructed networks*. Cambridge, UK: Cambridge University Press. doi:10.1017/CBO9780511790515

Polisetty, P. K., Voit, E. O., & Gatzke, E. P. (2006). Identification of metabolic system parameters usign global optimization methods. *Theoretical Biology & Medical Modelling, 3*(4).

Priami, C. (2009). Algorithmic Systems Biology. An opportunity for computer science. *Communications of the ACM, ACM, 52*(5), 80–88. doi:10.1145/1506409.1506427

Reinker, S., Altman, R. M., & Timmer, J. (2006). Parameter estimation in stochastic biochemical reactions. *153* (4), 168-178.

Rodrigez-Fernandez, M., Mendes, P., & Banga, J. (2006). A hybrid apporach for efficient and robust parameter estimation in biochemical pathways. *Bio Systems, 83*, 248–265. doi:10.1016/j.biosystems.2005.06.016

Rogers, S., Khanin, R., & Girolami, M. (2007). Bayesian model-based inference of transcription factor activity. *BMC Bioinformatics, 8*, 52. doi:10.1186/1471-2105-8-S2-S2

Samoilov, M., Arkin, A., & Ross, J. (2001). On the deduction of chemical reaction pathways from measurements of time series of concentrations. *Chaos (Woodbury, N.Y.), 11*(1), 108. doi:10.1063/1.1336499

Schmitt, W. A., Raab, R. M., & Stephanopoulos, G. (2004). Elucidation of gene interaction networks through time-lagged correlation analysis of transcriptional data. *Genome Research, 14,* 1654–1663. doi:10.1101/gr.2439804

Sprite, P., Glymour, C., & Scheines, R. (2000). *Causation, Prediction and Search Adaptive Computation and Machine Learning.* MIT Press.

Sugimoto, M., Kikuchi, S., & Tomita, M. (2005). Reverse engineering of biochemical equations from time-course data by means of genetic programming. *Bio Systems, 80,* 155–164. doi:10.1016/j.biosystems.2004.11.003

Tian, T., Xu, S., & Burrage, K. (2007). Simulated maximum likelihoodmethod for estimating kinetic rates in gene expression. *Bioinformatics (Oxford, England), 23*(1), 84–91. doi:10.1093/bioinformatics/btl552

Torralba, A. S., Yu, K., Shen, P. D., Oefner, P. J., & Ross, J. (2003). Experimental test of a method for determining causal connectivity of species in reactions. *Proceedings of the National Academy of Sciences of the United States of America, 100,* 1494–1498. doi:10.1073/pnas.262790699

Vance, W., Arkin, A., & Ross, J. (2002). Determination of causal connectivities of species in reaction network. *Proceedings of the National Academy of Sciences of the United States of America, 99,* 5816–5821. doi:10.1073/pnas.022049699

Wang, Y., Scott, C., Mjolsness, E., & Xie, X. (2010). Parameter inference for discretely observed stochastic kinetic models using stochastic gradient descendent. *BMC Systems Biology, 4*(99).

Wilkinson, D. J. (2006). *Stochastic modelling for systems biology.* London: Chapman and Hall/CRC Taylor & Francis Group.

Wilkinson, D. J. (2007). Bayesian methods in bioinformatics and computational systems biology. *Briefings in Bioinformatics, 2*(8), 109–116.

Woolf, P. J., Prudhomme, W., Daheron, W., Daley, G. Q., & Lauffebberger, D. A. (2005). Bayesian analysis of signaling networks governing embryonic stem cell fate decisions. *Bioinfromatics, 21,* 741–753. doi:10.1093/bioinformatics/bti056

Xia, Y., Yu, H., Jansen, R., Seringhaus, M., Baxter, S., & Greenbaum, D. (2004). Analyzing cellular biochemistry in temrs of molecualr networks. *Annual Review of Biochemistry, 73,* 1051–1087. doi:10.1146/annurev.biochem.73.011303.073950

Yu, J., Smith, V. A., Wang, P. P., Hartemink, A. J., & Jarvis, E. D. (2004). Advances to Bayesian network inference for generating causal networks from observational biological data. *Bioinfromatics, 20*(18), 3594–3603. doi:10.1093/bioinformatics/bth448

Yu, J., Smith, V. A., Wang, P. P., Hartemink, A. J., & Jarvis, E. D. (2004). Advances to Bayesian network inference for generating causal networks from observational data. *Bioinformatics (Oxford, England), 20*(18), 3594–3603. doi:10.1093/bioinformatics/bth448

Zwolak, J. (2007). *PET- Parameter Estimation toolkit.* Retrieved from http://mpf.biol.vt.edu/pet/contact.php.

Chapter 7
Structural and Dynamical Heterogeneity in Ecological Networks

Ferenc Jordán
The Microsoft Research – University of Trento, Centre for Computational and Systems Biology, Trento, Italy

Carmen Maria Livi
The Microsoft Research – University of Trento, Centre for Computational and Systems Biology, Trento, Italy

Paola Lecca
The Microsoft Research – University of Trento, Centre for Computational and Systems Biology, Trento, Italy

ABSTRACT

Diversity is a key feature of biological systems. In complex ecological systems, which are composed of several components and multiple parallel interactions among them, it is increasingly needed to precisely understand structural and dynamical variability among components. This variability is the basis of adaptability and evolvability in nature, as well as adaptive management-based applications. The authors discuss how to quantify and characterize the structural and dynamical variability in ecological networks. They perform network analysis in order to quantify structure and we provide a process algebra-based stochastic simulation model and sensitivity analysis for better understanding the dynamics of the studied ecological system. They use a large, data-rich, real ecological network for illustration.

INTRODUCTION

Diversity is one of the few concepts of biology that are familiar also to politicians and laymen. There is a common belief that diversity is "good" and should be maintained at several levels of biological organization, from genes to ecosystems. In order to decide whether it is true, we need to understand diversity much better, and not only at a descriptive (mostly structural) level but also, and much more, from a functional and more dynamical point of view.

DOI: 10.4018/978-1-61350-435-2.ch007

Copyright © 2012, IGI Global. Copying or distributing in print or electronic forms without written permission of IGI Global is prohibited.

Since the diversity of biological objects is valuable primarily in the context of their populations, it may be useful to ask these questions in a systems biology context. The hierarchical organization of life means that most biological systems are composed of subsystems and compose supersystems, for example populations are composed of individuals and compose an ecological community. Interactions are of key importance in connecting lower-level systems and, thus, interactions themselves determine the subsystem-system or system-supersystem relationships (Allen & Starr, 1982). Without relevant interactions, lower-level components remain only a set of components, instead of being subsystems forming a system. The explicit study of hierarchy is a key issue but frequently missed in modern systems biology, that normally focuses on the huge amount of components without considering the relationship with the lower and higher levels. On the contrary, classical systems biology was unable to analyze huge amounts of components but was more sensitive to hierarchy.

If we aim to understand the diversity of some biological components from this systems view, we cannot neglect the composition and topology of the system they build up. Heterogeneity of positions in anisotropic networks is a key to understand diverse roles of components. If we aim to understand a human social group, we need some information on the number of individuals, on their sex ratio and age distribution, but the key information is whether they form a social system (e.g. a classroom) or they are only a set of people (e.g. travelling on the same bus). The same applies for social animals, where the paradigm of group size is recently being exchanged with the paradigm of the social network. As we know more about the global topology of animal social networks as well as we identify their key players based on local network indices, we begin to understand the relevance and limits of group size and network-independent attributes of individuals. The same question here is not only how many

species we have and what are their abundance distributions, but also how are they connected to each other and how does their network position determine what roles they play in the ecological community. Here, the big challenge is to translate taxonomical knowledge (identities) to ecological language (roles).

In this chapter, we present a real network to illustrate how structural and dynamical heterogeneity can be studied. We discuss some novel approaches to systems ecology and systems-based conservation, based on stochastic dynamical modeling of ecosystems.

A SYSTEMS VIEW ON VARIABILITY: COMPUTATIONAL CHALLENGES

Systems Biology and Systems Ecology

Both real databases and computational power are growing continuously in biological research. Still, what we call systems biology today is mostly based on collecting huge amounts of information without a hierarchical perspective and coherent integration. However, real integration needs also qualitative, not only quantitative changes in dynamical systems models. A major qualitative change could be the parallel analysis of multiple hierarchical organizational levels (e.g. genes in individuals, individuals in ecosystems). In order to improve the predictive power of biological models, novel computational tools would be important. Apart from managing huge databases and visualising complex systems, new types of algorithms could link community and systems ecology by providing tools for process-based approaches. The solution to these problems will become computable by increasing computer power and introducing novel conceptual and computational tools (Levin et al., 1997; Pascual, 2005; Green et al., 2005; Seth, 2007).

The relatively old field of systems ecology views ecosystems from a holistic perspective, as an extension of general systems theory. Early research aimed to describe ecosystems by rigorous, quantitative ways, for example, characterizing the state of an ecosystem by single, macroscopic indicators (e.g. ascendency: Ulanowicz, 1986). Besides of this primarily global interest, the local and mesoscale heterogeneity was also clear (anisotropic networks: Margalef, 1991; indirect effects: Elton, 1927). Especially in systems ecology, there is recently increasing interest in novel approaches providing new information with the hope of making ecological models more predictive. As opposed to molecular and cellular systems biology, the major challenge in ecology is not necessarily the large number of components but the number and multiplicity of parallel interactions and processes and the resulting complexity of systems behavior (Olff, 2009). Computational approaches may turn out to be even more useful here.

As a dominant field of systems ecology, food web modelling focuses either on the structural analysis of complex trophic networks (Martinez, 1991; Dunne et al., 2002; Jordán et al., 2007) or on dynamic simulations of smaller, mostly hypothetical, networks (Abrams, 1999; Jordán et al., 2002). It is only recently that dynamic simulation of large food webs has become feasible (Christensen & Walters, 2004; Okey, 2004), due to growth in computational capacity and available methodology. Dynamic simulations enable new kinds of quantitative measures of the relative importance of species, following the relatively large set of topological importance indices that mostly focus on node centrality (Harary, 1961; Jordán & Scheuring, 2004; Estrada, 2007). These measures are based on dynamic sensitivity analyses: relative responses of the biological community to simulated perturbations on particular species, whether or not keystones (which have large effects relative to their proportional biomass; Power et al., 1996; Hurlbert, 1997). The development of increasingly useful indices is a key to improving

(1) general understanding of ecosystem functioning, (2) prediction of secondary extinctions and (3) ranking of conservation priorities. Stochastic food web modelling can be more appropriate than deterministic modelling based on ODEs (ordinary differential equations, see EwE models: Christensen & Walters, 2004; Libralato et al., 2006), especially under certain circumstances (e.g. when there are some species in the system with very small populations). However, the deterministic approach aims to provide more general results (Montoya et al., 2009). A stochastic dynamic framework for food web analysis could be used to simulate ecodynamics and provide dynamic importance metrics adapted to this modelling framework.

Variability and Stochasticity in Hierarchical Biosystems

At each level of hierarchical organization, variability is the key to adaptability and evolvability. Thus, diversity is an essential feature of evolutionary systems. However, static and typical information is much easier to collect and to study. Only some fields of biology are dedicated explicitly to investigating variability. Quantitative genetics is an example, where phenotypic variability is decomposed into genetic and environmental components (Roff, 1997). Also in ecology, much work is still to be done in order to better map and understand variation, as well as to give a proper functional meaning to "diversity".

Although many works already suggested to focus more on ecological processes than on ecological structures (e.g. Thompson, 1982; Ulanowicz, 1986), there is still the need for better representations of these functionalities. A number of studies are still focused on static patterns, while dynamics is only inferred from certain static properties (like degree distribution used as a proxy for vulnerability or robustness: Solé & Montoya, 2001). Considering environmental noise may also be important for modelling ecodynamics. The sensitivity of genotypes (reaction norm: Roff, 1997) and interspecific interactions (interaction norm: Thompson, 1988) to environmental variation is well known. Environmental stochasticity and contingency provides the freedom of choice for individual organisms within various constraints. Because of these reasons, the need for improving stochastic modelling is increasing. For future conservation management, noise and variability will be studied for the sake of providing a pool of solutions for adaptive management, rather than looking for strategies to minimize their impacts.

If the size of a population is relatively small, its temporal behaviour is noisy. For example, the actual number of sexually mature individuals depends on time as a kind of demographic noise. Birth and death also contribute to this kind of stochasticity: differential equations describing the biomass of phytoplankton or herring can be quite accurate, however, the living biomass of killer whales in a small area changes in a characteristically step-wise manner (as the number of individuals is an integer). Spatial heterogeneity (e.g. lekking), individual-level differences among conspecifics (e.g. different strategies), local rules instead of global determination (Okuyama, 2009), priority effect in competition (Doak & Marvier, 2003), and the multiplicity of interactions all typically increase the stochastic component of population dynamics.

Moreover, while the average of several stochastic simulations is generally similar to the outcome of deterministic simulations, the former also describes the variability of different runs. In analysing the states of a dynamic system, the "width" of the possible trajectories can be at least as important as the shape of the average trajectory. In conservation biology, there is emerging interest in using variability as an indicator for evaluating biodiversity (Feest et al., 2010). In fact, variability can be the key to adaptability and evolvability. For example, during climate change, successful species are characterized by phenotypes that are not necessarily "good" but flexible enough. Fi-

nally, stochastic simulation makes it possible to explicitly model extinction. In the typically used continuous, deterministic models, extinction is impossible (the population can always recover also from very low densities). It can only be modelled as population size decreasing below a certain critical threshold value. In case of small populations, local extinction (and possible recolonization) is a realistic scenario.

Beyond the interactive complexity of ecological processes, another major challenge here is the weak generality of rules. Several ecological processes are best modeled by individual, agent or event-based models, where local rules govern macroscopic systems behavior. Generalities and universal rules may be so weak that their analysis essentially does not provide predictive power. One component of this local regime is the high variability of components: ecological systems are heterogeneous, anisotropic, and this is the very key to adaptability and future success. Thus, understanding the local rules-based variability and stochastic behavior of ecological systems components is a key to the understanding and management of several natural systems.

A key property of ecological processes is stochasticity, caused by external (abiotic environmental noise, climate change) or internal (demography, individual-level variability) factors. It is important to explicitly study this inherent noise, either at individual level or at the population level. Certain sources of noise are much more important in small populations. Individual-based modeling (IBM) (DeAngelis & Mooij, 2005; DeAngelis & Gross, 1992; Grimm, 1992) offers tools for both, and sets the stage for understanding complex adaptive systems (CASs) (Levin, 1998). In case of CASs, a key aim is to understand how can global patterns emerge out of local rules and interactions. As opposed to deterministic population-level models, stochastic IBMs make it possible to model actual extinction events. While the extinction of rare species is at the frontier of applied ecological research and conservation biology, it is strange that deterministic population-level modeling is limited in both handling the noisy behavior of small populations and modeling extinction. For example, the same amount of living biomass can behave in a more stochastic way if it corresponds to two whale individuals, and in a more deterministic way if it corresponds to millions of organisms in the zooplankton. On the other side, it is clear that stochastic IBMs are of limited generality, as opposed to (sometimes analytically solvable) deterministic models (Judson, 1984). To discover general laws and to mechanistically understand particular situations are different research strategies (Simberloff, 2003). Although standardization and evaluation of IBMs are difficult (e.g., because of the extensive lack of published computer codes), and their generality is poor, they provide powerful solutions for particular case studies. The great challenge here is to find which relevant local mechanisms can really trigger macroscopic patterns, as this is the way to link population biology to communities and ecosystems. In particular, novel conceptual tools and algorithms are needed to model concurrent, multiple effects. IBMs provide a bottom-up approach based on sophisticated local mechanisms. Another virtue of IBMs is their ability to supply detailed predictions on real systems (e.g., modelling the effects of 5 killer whale individuals on sea otters, see Williams et al., 2008), although this goal is fulfilled at the price of generality. This approach makes it possible to consider molecular level or trait-based information or aggregating individuals to larger groups (e.g. superindividuals: Scheffer et al., 1995). If a given amount of biomass is consumed, deterministic models clearly cannot show the difference whether it is a single tuna individual, hundreds of small pelagic animals or millions of meso-zooplankton organisms. In CASs, bottom-level variability leads to adaptability and evolvability. The bottom-up, local rules-based view seems to be also more intuitive in biology, as opposed to top-down descriptions. This different attitude mirrors the difference between the basic methodology of physics as opposed to computer science.

QUANTIFYING STRUCTURAL AND DYNAMICAL DIVERSITY IN ECOSYSTEMS

Structural Diversity

Structural heterogeneity of nodes in networks can be quantified by topological indices in network analysis. The variety of indices considers direct and indirect, binary and weighted as well as directed and symmetrical interactions in the ecological networks. Based on each index, we can provide a ranking of components based on importance. Some indices quantify the similarity of these positions (Luczkovich et al., 2003; Jordán et al., 2009) and the similarity of the indices themselves, based on ranking (Jordán et al., 2007) and distribution (Bauer et al., 2010). Furthermore, there are methods for quantifying the position (e.g. centrality) of sets of nodes.

The relationship between network position and community role may be best exemplified in the case of top-predators and producers. In a directed graph representing material fluxes in ecosystems, they are the graph nodes with zero out-degree (D_{out}) and zero in-degree (D_{in}), respectively (degree, D is the number of neighbors; D_{in} is the number of neighbors sending a link to a focal node, while D_{out} is the number of neighbors the focal node sends links to). The role of these groups is characteristic, and we can identify them in food webs at the first glance. The classification of basic ecological roles include also specialist and generalist consumers (with $D_{in} = 1$ and $D_{out} >> 1$, respectively), omnivores (with fractional trophic level) and wasp-waist species (with $D_{in} >> 1$ and $D_{out} >> 1$). More sophisticated network metrics may reveal more special ecological roles (e.g. keystone predators, like *Pisaster*, may be characterized by $D_{out} = 0$,

$D_{in} = 1$ and a large indirect neighbourhood not measured by degree, see Paine, 1966).

This may be modified in several ways. For example, adding detritus to the inter-specific interaction network will result in (1) a dramatic increase in directed loops that are otherwise rare in food webs, (2) increasing the out-degree of each node by one, and (3) increasing the in-degree of detritivores by one. In some representations, detritus and all other kinds of non-living material form the same group, thus, the in-degree of producers may also be increased. Also, the direction of links can be neglected in some cases. Consumers clearly have population dynamical effects on preys (in top-down direction), so if inter-specific interactions are studied in a broad sense, instead of focusing only on bottom-up material flows, undirected networks represent ecosystems better.

Apart from the above extreme nodes in directed food webs, there are more interesting (less trivial) particular network positions. In several marine food webs, we may speak of wasp-waist structure and wasp-waist position. This means one or a few intermediate species in the middle of the food web, for example, small pelagics like sardine and anchovy, jellyfish or copepods. These intermediate species may be responsible for a very large proportion of bottom-up material transport. The topological consequences of such food web structure has been analyzed. For example, the interaction between two wasp waist species can be extremely strong even if they interact with each other only indirectly in the system (while, at the same time, they have several direct partners in weaker relationships). Earlier studies on these strange network positions raised questions like how variable food web positions can be, how different the structural roles are that species play in communities. Two major approaches focused on regular equivalence (Luczkovich et al., 2003) and redundancy (Jordán et al., 2009).

Figure 1 illustrates that this function-based problem is totally different from the traditional, taxonomy-based sense of diversity. Figures 1a, 1b

and 1c show three toy food webs, while Figures 1d, 1e and 1f show their degree ranks (degree of a graph node is the number of its neighbors, i.e. the number of links it has). Graph 1c is the smallest in terms of the number of species but the positional variation of nodes is the highest here (coefficient of variation for nodal degree values in the networks 1a, 1b and 1c are $CV^D_A=0,156$, $CV^D_B=0,119$ and $CV^D_C=0,727$, respectively). By adding two new species to graph 1a, we gain graph 1b with more or less the same topological diversity of nodes. These two species are likely to have no essentially novel functions. However, graph 1c shows a topologically and functionally more diverse community, even if it is less rich in species.

It must be noted here that, for a constant number of species, topological diversity can be increased only at the price of structural redundancy. This leads to the problem of aggregating food webs. All food webs are aggregations of field data in some sense. The question is how to aggregate, whether based on biological intuition or rigorous rules. Community ecologists typically prefer the mixture, by aggregating a lot of species into "trivial groups" and then aggregating the graph nodes with similar neighborhood (trophospecies: Yodzis and Winemiller, 1999). The aggregation procedure may strongly influence topology and positional diversity. Since food webs aim to represent functionality (as they are ecological models), it is reasonable to make them structurally variable: redundancy within trophospecies may be expressed in terms of biomass or abundance, even if topologically hidden.

There are several examples for food webs where reasonable resolution is not at the species level. One is the aggregation of desert spiders into size classes, since individuals of all species can eat the individuals of all other species, provided that their body size is larger (so, the species-level description would provide a directed complete graph, while the size-based description provides a less dense, more informative graph. Another

Figure 1. Three toy food webs (a, b and c) with different number of species (diversity) and different community structure (topology). The ranks of node degree are shown in d, e and f.

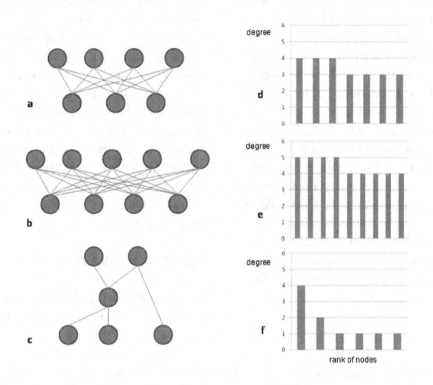

one is the aggregation of marine predatory fish into age classes (see juvenile and adult herring separated already in Elton, 1927), since adults of all species can eat the larvae of all other species. In both cases, species-based food webs provide uninformative, homogeneous networks, poorly representing functional aspects. However, topological analysis of the aggregated versions provides some information about ecosystem functioning: in these, more heterogeneous networks, the diversity of positions reflects the diversity of ecological roles.

The applicability of some network measures is presented on a case study. The Ecopath with Ecosim (EwE) model of the Prince William Sound (Alaska) food web has been described and analysed in detail (Okey and Pauly, 1999; Okey, 2004; Okey and Wright, 2004). The model contains 48 living components (Okey, 2004).

The simplest way to quantify the network position of a node is counting the number of its neighbors (i.e. node degree, D), however it has been shown to be less robust than other measures. Ecological networks may be characterized by different degree distributions, depending on aggregation level. Some results support scale-free like distribution with a diversity of hubs and low-connectance nodes, while other results (based on more aggregated webs) suggest also uniform and unimodal distributions. Thus, both nodes and networks themselves can show a diversity of degrees and degree distributions respectively.

While degree is the most local measure, by considering only neighbors, other indices can consider also the neighborhood of neighbors, i.e. indirect interactions up to n steps (TI^n index: Jordán et al., 2003). Typically, the distribution of this index is also unimodal.

While the previous indices characterized direct and indirect centrality in networks, it may also be considered that some nodes are in important positions, not because of being central, but because of having a unique, non-redundant, non-replaceable position. This can be quantified by the topological overlap index ($TO^3_{0,6}$) developed in Jordán et al. (2009). Based on this, several nodes are of zero importance and only a few seem to play key roles. This community-pattern is more similar to the keystone pattern suggested by Mills et al. (1993).

Finally, we use another index already introduced in ecology to characterize the similarity of network positions and neighborhoods, based on regular equivalence (REGE: Luczkovich et al., 2003). This index also suggests a uniform distribution, even if key nodes are different from those of the previous indices.

Figure 2 shows the relative importance of network nodes, based on these four measurements. Node size is proportional to index value in each case. Figure 3 shows the ranking of nodes based on index values. We see that the use of multiple topological indices provides complementary information on positional importance. Different indices provide different ranks and different value distributions, but what is more interesting here is the overall variability, the community-wide diversity of positions. Some ranks reflect more heterogeneous networks (Figure 3c), where the relative importance of species is closer to the keystone pattern.

Dynamical Diversity

All of the static indices described above, the toolkit of network analysis, are used as proxy for better

Figure 2. The Prince Williams Sound food web. The size of nodes is proportional to different topological indices: D (a), TI³ (b), TO³$_{0,6}$ (c) and REGE (d). Larger nodes are positionally more important in maintaining network structure, according to the particular indices. Networks are drawn by CoSBiLab Graph (Valentini and Jordán, 2010).

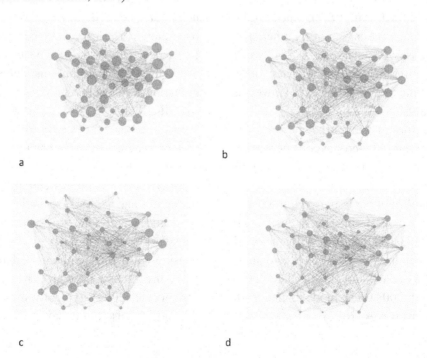

a

b

c

d

Figure 3. Ranking the nodes of the Prince Williams Sound food web, based on different topological indices: D (a), TI³ (b), TO³$_{0,6}$ (c) and REGE (d). Different indices suggest different variability of relative positional importance. Whether the identity of the leading nodes differs is seen in Figure 2.

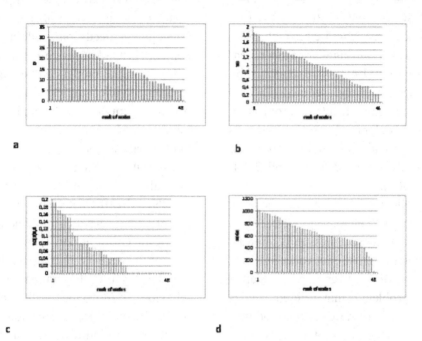

understanding network dynamics, the behavior of individual components and the whole network itself (Jordán et al., 2008). The structural diversity of genes and organisms goes hand in hand with the functional diversity of behavioral strategies and ecological roles. Since the former is easier to understand, measure and classify, we have much more information on gene sequences and species lists than on redundancy and organization in social and ecological systems. However, understanding structure and function in parallel is the only way: a list of species, for example, is informative only if we know how similar the coexisting species are to each other, to what extent their functions overlap and how redundant ecosystem functioning is. These issues are intimately related to the stability properties of ecosystems, for example, how do ecosystems react to species loss. From this perspective, the identity (taxonomic position) of species is much less important than their participation in ecological processes and community

patterns (for example, what kind of pathways they maintain). The ecological role of a species can be defined as being an energy gate that can switch between alternative pathways. Stability properties of ecosystems (e.g. resistance, resilience) are linked to systems topology and functional redundancy (Lawton & Brown, 1994), not only to the properties of particular species.

The multiplicity of system components and interactions, as well as the large number of parameters in ecosystems, pose huge computational problems. Apart of using larger computers of increased computational power, the alternative strategy is to develop novel kinds of tools. Beyond the recently introduced various algorithms (e.g., cellular automata, genetic algorithms, formal logic, particle tracking, Petri nets and swarm intelligence), a new stream of computational techniques is based on quantitative extensions of process algebra, that has been already used in molecular computational and systems biology

(Priami, 2009). Several process algebra-based programming languages have been developed to explicitly model interactions of biological entities (e.g. WSCCS, CMDL, BlenX). The first ecological applications addressed social insect colonies. The WSCCS language-based theoretical investigations of Tofts (1993) were supported by experiments. Process algebra-based models helped also understanding colony-level synchronization processes in insect colonies. Extensions towards population biology and epidemiology are being quickly developed (Norman & Shankland, 2004; McCaig et al., 2009).

A major challenge in community ecology is how to integrate our increasing databases on various interaction types (Bertness and Callaway, 1994). Food webs, mutualistic networks and competitive interactions are just very rarely modelled in parallel. One problem is that different studies do not overlap (e.g., they describe the food web of community A and the plant-pollinator network of community B). The larger problem consists of using different currencies to characterize different interaction networks, under a unique framework (e.g. carbon flow for food webs and visitation frequency for plant-pollinator webs). These biological issues cannot be fully addressed by process algebraic models, but efficient and simple solutions can help and contribute to model development.

BlenX is a process algebra-based programming language (Dematté et al., 2007), supported by the Beta Workbench environment (Dematté et al., 2008). The internal dynamics are processes and boxes communicating with each other through channels, also known as binders. The rate of communication is quantified by the affinity (rate) which is defined between the different types of binders, measuring interaction strength (see Figure 4). An important feature of process algebras is composability: the meaning of the model depends on the features of its components and the way how they depend on each other (how it is composed). Wise composition has several advantages: model

development can be modular, standardization is relatively easy and the evaluation can be rigorous. Over a certain level of model complexity, developing the model is not complicate anymore. Model development needs only adding some simple elements instead of rewriting major parts of the code. An initial model can be easily fine-tuned according to pilot studies or sensitivity analyses, or can be simply extended and modified. These features are advantageous for recurrent application and standardization.

Since it is an event-based description, combinatorial explosion in parameter-rich, complex models can be efficiently reduced by its use. BlenX is an efficient tool which implements the Gillespie algorithm (Gillespie, 1977) for stochastic simulations of biosystems. In biology, this has already been heavily used for simulating the stochastic behaviour of molecules in the cell (Dematté et al., 2008). Ecological applications were also suggested recently: indirect effects and cycling (Finn, 1976) were measured by the particle tracking method of Kazanci et al. (2009), while hypothetical food webs were generated and studied by Powell and Boland (2009). We note that here we use an inherently stochastic model, instead of an inherently deterministic system with some added stochastic component (e.g. Jordán et al., 2003b).

For any practical use, simulation and sensitivity analysis are of highest importance, regardless of the modeling tool being used. Stochastic, individual-based or event-based simulations make it possible to study the variability of system behaviour. Apart of responses of the mean, responses of the variance can also be measurable after disturbance.

A notorious problem in systems ecology is how to model various interaction types in parallel. Figure 5 shows an example of how to use the compositional feature of the BlenX modeling framework. Figure 5a shows a simple toy food web with top predators T and C, consumers A and B as well as producers D, E, F and G. One can be interested in the simulated population dynamics of

Figure 4. Following kinetic models in molecular biology (illustrated in a), some simple ecological situations can also be implemented (illustrated in b). Frequency of prey-predator interactions may be considered as the product of prey density, predator density and interaction rate (following mass action kinetics). In some situations it is quite realistic. Multiple, parallel interactions can also be modelled this way (c): different rates (k_n) describe different interactions among boxes representing individual organisms (belonging to different species labelled by A, B and C). Each box has internal (P_n, e.g. birth, reproduction) and external (t_n, predation, pollination, cooperation) dynamics. The latter is realized through binders and communication channels visualized by different colors.

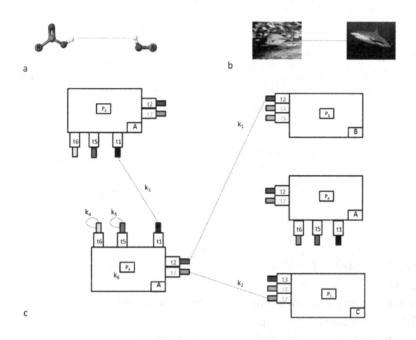

species B, especially if it is involved also in other kinds of interspecific interactions (mutualism, competition, facilitation, see Figures 5b, 5c and 5d, respectively). A final question is what is the outcome of considering all of these added interactions (Figure 5e). The population size of species B is shown by the solid black curve in Figure 5f. Positive effects (mutualism in red and facilitation in green) increase, while negative effects (competition in blue) decrease its population size, while everything else is unchanged. The composition of all kinds of interactions results in the highly unpredictable dashed black line. Note also that this is a stochastic simulation (with more or less typical outcome). By very simple modifications of the initial BlenX model we can flexibly combine these interactions. Composability ensures that

increasing model complexity does not require linearly increasing program size. Instead, the relationship is saturating: after some point, several new parameters, functions and variables can be added by only slightly increasing the size of the computer program. These features also offer new ways of explicitly studying additivity and non-linearity. The stochastic simulation outcome shown in Figure 5f is intuitively understandable, concrete results depending on real parameters. Different interaction intensities (currencies) are all expressed in terms of reproduction rate, allowing to consider several concurrent relations under a single, integrative framework.

We have translated the EwE-model of the Prince William Sound (Okey, 2004) into BlenX (Livi, 2009). Biomass values of trophic groups

Figure 5. A toy food web of only prey-predator interactions (a), and its more complicated versions with adding mutualism (b), competition (c), facilitation (d) and all three together (e), Figure 5f shows the simulated population size of species B in each five cases.

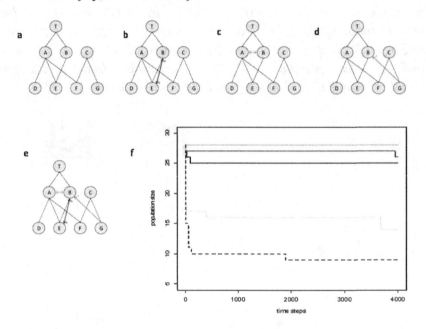

have been translated to numbers of individuals, based on species-specific body size data. For simplicity, we have used the logarithm of number of individuals and then multiplied by 10. Trophic flows were directly translated into interaction rates. See Figure 6 for illustrating a subnetwork of the whole community food web. We excluded all external effects (e.g. material flows) and supposed that the system is close to equilibrium. Thus, death rates were chosen from a realistic range (from 0.001 to 0.1, typically 0.01) to fine-tune the model to quasi-equilibrium (note here that some authors use mortality as a sum of natural mortality and predation, like Okey, 2004, and it is not easy to separate them).

We describe the dynamics in a way that is similar to modelling molecular kinetics in the cell. Simple rates are assigned to single-individual interactions (like reproduction, birth, death), while the kinetics of pairwise interactions follow mass-action:

$$A + B \rightarrow A$$

with rate k_1, and

$$A + B \rightarrow A^*$$

with rate k_2, where A^* is an individual of species A reproducing immediately with the infinite k_3 rate:

$$A^* \rightarrow A + A.$$

The ratio of k_1 to k_2 determines how much B must be consumed by A before being able to reproduce. It is somewhat similar to the hungry and well-fed states of individuals in the model of Powell and Boland (2009). They assume that only sated individuals (A^*) can reproduce and only hungry individuals (A') can be eaten. One challenge here is to integrate ecological stoichiometry (Sterner & Elser, 2002) with our model. It needs to specify how many feeding events, of exactly which prey, is enough for reproduction

Figure 6. A subnetwork of the Prince William Sound food web. The size of fish is roughly proportional to population size (number of individuals), while arrow width roughly indicates interaction rates (based on field measurements, expressed in t * km^{-2} * year^{-1}). Data from Okey (2004).

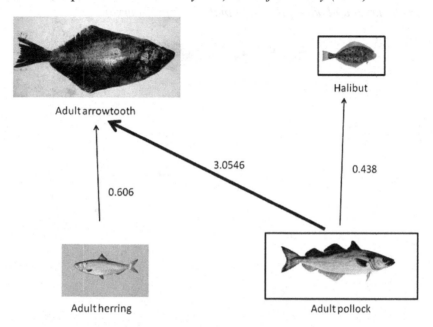

(this could also be expressed in rates). This is a very simplistic description of a prey-predator interaction but simple kinetic rules seem to apply quite well in several ecological situations: for example, the number of shark-bitten pinnipeds is proportional to shark and pinniped abundance, while community shift in exploitative competition is proportional to prey availability, relative competitive abilities and the relative densities of consumers (Stevens et al., 2000). These parameters correspond to kinetic rates and concentrations in simple chemical reactions: if two molecules A and B have compatible functional groups, they may react and the probability of the reaction depends on the concentration of both molecules and the reaction rate (also on the concentration of products if the reaction is reversible). The simplest kinetics for an interspecific interaction may follow the same logic: prey density, predator density and the prey preference of the predator are three parameters describing the probability of feeding. As reference, 20 simulations were run in 40000 steps, corresponding to a 30 years period

(see Figure 7 for illustrating the simulated time-series). Based on these runs with the same initial conditions and parameters, we can measure the variability of system behaviour.

For sensitivity analysis, we performed pulse perturbations, reducing the population size of each functional group by half, one by one, in different runs. We also made perturbations where population sizes were divided by 4, multiplied by 2 and multiplied by 4. The chosen mode of perturbation is comparable with the one in deterministic sensitivity analysis conducted by Okey (2004), but note that a variety of perturbation techniques have been used in the study of other systems (e.g. halving reproduction rates, Okey, 2004). Here we have not performed sensitivity analysis where combinations of parameters have been changed simultaneously.

We used several response functions but, for simplicity, present only results based on a metric very similar to the Hurlbert response index (Hurlbert, 1997), the only difference is that we compare the population sizes in the reference in-

Figure 7. The simulated dynamics of the four interacting fish species shown in Figure 6. Note that the four curves are extracted from a whole-community simulation. Positions in the whole food web are also shown: adult arrowtooth in black (light pink curve), halibut in yellow (light green curve), adult herring in green (dark green curve) and adult pollock in pink (dark pink curve).

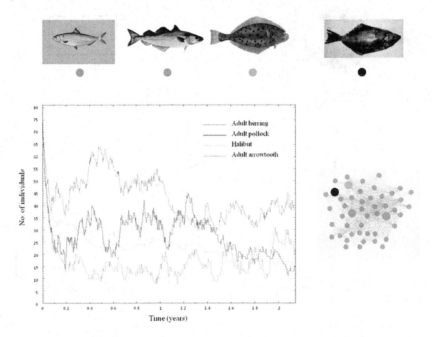

terval for the control and the perturbed simulation runs instead of two states in the same simulation, before and after perturbation. The mean-based, Hurlbert response-based importance of a species i ($I_H(M)$) is defined as the summed effect on all other j species ($j = 1...n$, i does not equal j) when i is disturbed, where the effect on j is the absolute value of the difference between its reference population size (p) and the mean population size over $n=20$ simulations where i is disturbed (p^*, Hurlbert, 1997; Livi et al. in press). In both the reference and the disturbance simulations, population sizes were measured at the same t time point. A variance-based measure is the same but considering the variance of population sizes over the n simulations instead of the mean ($I_H(V)$). This measures how large is the effect of disturbing i on the other members of the community. Variance was divided by the mean values (used before) and the Hurlbert response measure was calculated for the coefficient of variation. Thus, the focus here is not on changed population size but, instead, on changed variability in population size (for several stochastic simulations). This variance-based approach may tell less about actual effects but more about control. Similarly, it can be calculated how large is the effect of disturbing any j species of the community on species i, and this can be also measured based on mean ($I_H^*(M)$) and variance ($I_H^*(V)$). These measures describe how sensitive is species i to disturbing others in the community. Thus, we quantify the importance of species by four ways, community effect and community sensitivity, both based on either mean or variance. In the matrix of $|p - p^*|$ response values (where perturbation in row x will result in a response in column y), I_H corresponds to row sums and I_H^* corresponds to column sums. We note that the real advantage of stochastic simulation is the ability to consider and explicitly study variability in the simulation runs. Notice that I_H quantifies global response to local change, while I_H^* quantifies local response to global change.

The community remained close to equilibrium during the simulations, even if some minor extinction events occurred (just like in EwE models, see the extinction of pepino in Okey, 2004).

In Figure 8, the size of graph nodes is proportional to their stochastic dynamic importance (measured as the effect on the mean population size of other species, i.e. mean-based $I_H(M)$). Based on this sensitivity analysis, the importance rank of species is led by nearshore demersals (component number 23), followed by adult arrowtooth (#9) and herbivorous zooplankton (#45). Apart of this ranking, based on effects on others (I_H), we also provide the ranking of species based on how much they are influenced by disturbing other members

of the community (I_H^*): here, halibut (#5) is of outstanding importance, followed by juvenile herring (#34) and adult salmon (#10) as the three most sensitive species.

Different indices suggest somewhat different distributions for importance values of species (Mills et al., 1993). Figure 9 shows that in some cases a keystone pattern-like distribution (i.e. a few species with outstanding importance values and the majority with much lower ones) appears, while in other cases the distribution is closer to uniform or unimodal.

In this modelling exercise, deep demersal fish (#18) and sandlance (#32) frequently went extinct, but their survival depends on which other species is perturbed. For example, perturbing the sablefish (#12) by dividing its population size by two helps the deep demersals (#18) to survive (however

Figure 8. The Prince Williams Sound food web. The size of nodes is proportional to different community importance indices, based on stochastic dynamical sensitivity analysis: $I_H(M)$ (a), $I_H^*(M)$ (b), $I_H(V)$ (c) and $I_H^*(V)$ (d). Larger nodes are dynamically more important in effecting others or being influenced by others (in terms of changes in either the mean or the variance). Networks are drawn by CoSBiLab Graph (Valentini and Jordán, 2010).

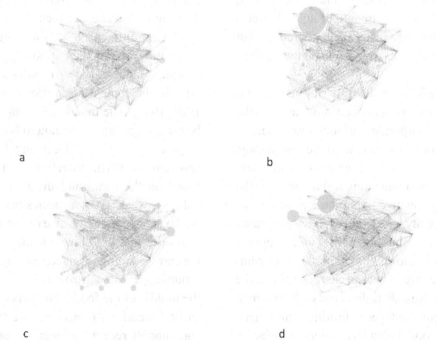

a

b

c

d

Figure 9. Ranking the nodes of the Prince Williams Sound food web, based on different community importance indices: $I_H(M)$ (a), $I_H{}^*(M)$ (b), $I_H(V)$ (c) and $I_H{}^*(V)$ (d). Different indices suggest different variability of relative dynamical importance. Whether the identity of the leading nodes differs is seen in Figure 8.

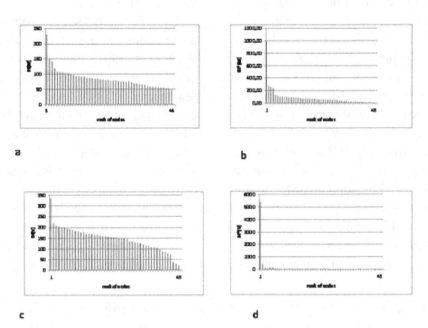

their population size remains very small) but not the sandlance (#32). Another particular interaction between jellics (#35) and juvenile pollock (#30) was also studied. The strength of mutual effects between them is around the average strength (but see Purcell et al., 2000, reporting on their strong interactions).

The sensitivity analysis performed in our simulation framework provided information on the behaviour and importance of individual species, pairwise interactions, and the whole community. Moreover, we have gained some insight also into the comparison of modelling techniques. For the distribution of relative importance values in the whole community, most indices show a keystone pattern-like distribution, while some support unimodal or close to uniform importance distributions. The identity of key species depends on the index chosen. Nearshore demersals (#23) seem to be the most important species in influencing others, both in mean population size and in its variance.

The result is totally different if we quantify which species are most sensitive to changes in others. Halibut (#5) leads both lists, with huge advantage. The big difference between "influence others" and "being influenced" in the same simulations raises big questions about how to measure species importance and how to understand sensitivity (also in the context of environ analysis, Patten, 1981, 1991). The functional group that seems to be most important according to both approaches is juvenile herring (#34, being both effective and sensitive). The correlation between indices based on the mean and the variance of effect values is weak, i.e. if a species has a large effect on the mean population size of others, it does not guarantee that it will have a large effect also on the corresponding variances. Strongly interacting groups appear at each trophic level, mostly around the middle of the food web. This may refine the earliest paradigm (keystones are top predators) and support recent findings on species of high importance in the middle of the trophic scale (Cury et al., 2000; Stibor et al., 2004) or at least below the highest top-predators (like bonito, Coll et al., 2009). All deterministic dynamic importance indices suggest either top-predators or producers to be of highest importance (Okey, 2004; Libralato et al., 2006). Static topology was relatively poor in predicting the identity of dynamic key species in these simulations. Degree shows some weak positive correlation.

The effect of sablefish (#12) on deep demersals (#18) and sandlance (#32) can be explained by looking at the weights on network links: sablefish (#12) feeds on both preys to a different extent. Trophic flow from deep demersals (#18) to sablefish (#12) is 0.0903, while it is only 0.0019 to sandlance (#32; for mass transfer data, see Okey, 2004). Larger flows are responsible for stronger effects in this case. In case of the relationship between jellies (#35) and juvenile pollock (#30) their well-documented strong interaction is not seen in our simulation, probably because the dominant effect is of non-trophic or spatial nature (like amensalism or aggregation, see also Purcell et al., 2000).

SOLUTIONS AND RECOMMENDATIONS

Comparing the structural and dynamical importance ranks (i.e., the structural and dynamical heterogeneity of the ecosystem) provides essential information on (1) how to predict the global effects of local changes, (2) how to predict the local effects of global changes and (3) how to predict the interspecific effects within the context of the whole ecosystem. This information can be of high importance in outlining scenarios for better understanding of: (1) species extinctions, (2) climate change and (3) biological control.

Studying structural and dynamical variability of system components makes it possible to outline adaptive management frameworks (Holling, 2001; Sagarin & Taylor, 2008). The precise understanding on position-dependent behavior is a prerequisite for predicting dynamical variability instead of trying to focus on average values and typical behaviors expressed by equations of deterministic models. Novel tools provided by computer science may fill these gaps of traditional ecological modeling. Especially the multiplicity and concurrency of processes, the variability of components and the weakness of universal laws are the major challenges conventional methods face. Generally, the most important problems of conservation practice call for individual-based, stochastic modelling (considering the rarity and noisy behaviour of the smallest populations to protect). Here, there is a need for better integrating theory and empirical data.

FUTURE RESEARCH DIRECTIONS

Directions of future research may include building hybrid models describing abundant species (zooplankton) in a deterministic and rare ones (orca) in a stochastic way. Also, considering spatial dynamics would be an important extension (Ciocchetta & Jordán, 2010), just like studying demographical details (size-overfishing, Okey et al., 2004) and refining the basic structure of the model (in order to model diverse functional responses and kinetics). Finally, more research is needed on comparing the same simulation outcomes analysed by different response measures (see Harley, 2003). As a further complication, higher-order interactions (the effect of species i on the effect of species j on species k) could also be analysed (Yodzis, 2000).

CONCLUSION

The application perspectives of compositional process algebras in ecology are manifold. Creating a general modeling framework for systems-based conservation is urgent, as species-level conservation programs are conflicting (see May et al., 1979, or Yodzis, 2001, for the need of multispecies fisheries). Moreover, the variability of both forms and processes need to be considered, as variability is the key to adaptability. The importance of variation has been recognized both in the past (Simberloff, 1980) and also recently (Berkes, 2004) but it is still out of the mainstream. Finally, as process algebras are efficient in modeling several interacting processes, they may open new ways for building integrative modeling frameworks of complex socio-ecological problems (e.g. sustainable agroecosystems).

ACKNOWLEDGMENT

We thank Thomas A. Okey for collaboration. We are also grateful to Roberto Valentini, Paola Quaglia, Marco Scotti, James Lynch, Ozan Kahramanoğullari, Federica Ciocchetta, Sean Sedwards, Barbara Bauer, Simone Libralato and Wei-chung Liu for discussions and comments.

REFERENCES

Abrams, P. A. (1999). Is predator-mediated coexistence possible in unstable systems? *Ecology*, *80*, 608–621.

Allen, T. F. H., & Starr, T. B. (1982). *Hierarchy: Perspectives for Ecological Complexity*. Chicago, IL: University of Chicago Press.

Bauer, B., Jordán, F., & Podani, J. (in press). Node centrality indices in food webs: rank orders versus distributions. *Ecological Complexity*.

Berkes, F. (2004). Rethinking community-based conservation. *Conservation Biology*, *18*, 621–630. doi:10.1111/j.1523-1739.2004.00077.x

Bertness, M. D., & Callaway, R. (1994). Positive interaction in communities. *Trends in Ecology & Evolution*, *9*, 191–193. doi:10.1016/0169-5347(94)90088-4

Christensen, V., & Walters, C. J. (2004). Ecopath with Ecosim: methods, capabilities and limitations. *Ecological Modelling*, *172*, 109–139. doi:10.1016/j.ecolmodel.2003.09.003

Ciocchetta, F., & Jordán, F. (2010). Modelling and analysing hierarchical ecological systems in BlenX. *Technical Report TR-1-2010*, CoSBi, Trento.

Cury, P., Bakun, A., Crawford, R. J. M., Jarre, A., Quiñones, R. A., Shannon, L. J., & Verheye, H. M. (2000). Small pelagics in upwelling systems: patterns of interaction and structural changes in "wasp-waist" ecosystems. *Journal of Marine Science*, *57*, 603–618.

DeAngelis, D. L., & Gross, L. J. (1992). *Individual-based Models and Approaches in Ecology*. New York, NY: Chapman and Hall.

DeAngelis, D. L., & Mooij, W. M. (2005). Individual-based modeling of ecological and evolutionary processes. *Annual Review of Ecology Evolution and Systematics*, *36*, 147–168. doi:10.1146/annurev.ecolsys.36.102003.152644

Dematté, L., Priami, C., & Romanel, A. (2007). BetaWB: modelling and simulating biological processes. In G.A. Wainer, & H. Vakilzadian (Eds.), *Proceedings of Summer Computer Simulation Conference (SCSC 2007)* (pp. 777-784). San Diego: Society for Computer Simulation International.

Dematté, L., Priami, C., & Romanel, A. (2008). The Beta Workbench: a computational tool to study the dynamics of biological systems. *Briefings in Bioinformatics*, *9*, 437–449. doi:10.1093/bib/bbn023

Doak, D., & Marvier, M. (2003). Predicting the effects of species loss on community stability. In Kareiva, P., & Levin, S. A. (Eds.), *The Importance of Species* (pp. 140–160). Princeton, NJ: Princeton University Press.

Dunne, J. A. (2002). Network structure and biodiversity loss in food webs: robustness increases with connectance. *Ecology Letters, 5*, 558–567. doi:10.1046/j.1461-0248.2002.00354.x

Elton, C. (1927). *Animal Ecology*. Chicago, IL: The University of Chicago Press.

Estrada, E. (2007). Characterisation of topological keystone species: local, global and "meso-scale" centralities in food webs. *Ecological Complexity, 4*, 48–57. doi:10.1016/j.ecocom.2007.02.018

Feest, A., Aldred, T. D., & Jedamzik, K. (2010). Biodiversity quality: a paradigm for biodiversity. *Ecological Indicators, 10*, 1077–1082. doi:10.1016/j.ecolind.2010.04.002

Finn, J. T. (1976). Measures of ecosystem structure and function derived from analysis of flows. *Journal of Theoretical Biology, 56*, 363–380. doi:10.1016/S0022-5193(76)80080-X

Gillespie, D. T. (1977). Exact stochastic simulation of coupled chemical reactions. *Journal of Physical Chemistry, 81*, 2340–2361. doi:10.1021/j100540a008

Green, J. L. (2005). Complexity in ecology and conservation: mathematical, statistical, and computational challenges. *Bioscience, 55*, 501–510. doi:10.1641/0006-3568(2005)055[0501:CIEACM]2.0.CO;2

Grimm, V. (1999). Ten years of individual-based modelling in ecology: what have we learned and what could we learn in the future? *Ecological Modelling, 115*, 129–148. doi:10.1016/S0304-3800(98)00188-4

Harary, F. (1961). Who eats whom? *General Systems, 6*, 41–44.

Harley, C. D. G. (2003). Species importance and context: spatial and temporal variation in species interactions. In Kareiva, P., & Levin, S. A. (Eds.), *The Importance of Species* (pp. 44–68). Princeton, NJ: Princeton University Press.

Holling, C. S. (2001). Understanding the complexity of economic, ecological and social systems. *Ecosystems (New York, N.Y.), 4*, 390–405. doi:10.1007/s10021-001-0101-5

Hurlbert, S. H. (1997). Functional importance vs keystoneness: reformulating some questions in theoretical biocenology. *Australian Journal of Ecology, 22*, 369–382. doi:10.1111/j.1442-9993.1997.tb00687.x

Jordán, F., Benedek, Zs., & Podani, J. (2007). Quantifying positional importance in food webs: a comparison of centrality indices. *Ecological Modelling, 205*, 270–275. doi:10.1016/j.ecolmodel.2007.02.032

Jordán, F., Liu, W. C., & Mike, Á. (2009). Trophic field overlap: a new approach to quantify keystone species. *Ecological Modelling, 220*, 2899–2907. doi:10.1016/j.ecolmodel.2008.12.003

Jordán, F., Liu, W. C., & van Veen, F. J. F. (2003). Quantifying the importance of species and their interactions in a host-parasitoid community. *Community Ecology, 4*, 79–88. doi:10.1556/ComEc.4.2003.1.12

Jordán, F., Okey, T. A., Bauer, B., & Libralato, S. (2008). Identifying important species: a comparison of structural and functional indices. *Ecological Modelling, 216*, 75–80.

Jordán, F., & Scheuring, I. (2004). Network Ecology: topological constraints on ecosystems dynamics. *Physics of Life Reviews, 1*, 139–172. doi:10.1016/j.plrev.2004.08.001

Jordán, F., Scheuring, I., & Molnár, I. (2003). Persistence and flow reliability in simple food webs. *Ecological Modelling, 161*, 117–124. doi:10.1016/S0304-3800(02)00296-X

Jordán, F., Scheuring, I., & Vida, G. (2002). Species positions and extinction dynamics in simple food webs. *Journal of Theoretical Biology, 215,* 441–448. doi:10.1006/jtbi.2001.2523

Judson, O. P. (1994). The rise of the individual-based model in ecology. *Trends in Ecology & Evolution, 9,* 9–14. doi:10.1016/0169-5347(94)90225-9

Kazanci, C. (2009). Cycling in ecosystems: an individual based approach. *Ecological Modelling, 220,* 2908–2914. doi:10.1016/j.ecolmodel.2008.09.013

Lawton, J. H., & Brown, V. K. (1994). Redundancy in ecosystems. In Schulze, E. D., & Mooney, H. A. (Eds.), *Biodiversity and Ecosystem Function* (pp. 255–270). Berlin: Springer Verlag.

Levin, S. A. (1998). Ecosystems and the biosphere as complex adaptive systems. *Ecosystems (New York, N.Y.), 1,* 431–436. doi:10.1007/s100219900037

Levin, S. A. (1997). Mathematical and computational challenges in population biology and ecosystems science. *Science, 275,* 334–343. doi:10.1126/science.275.5298.334

Libralato, S., Christensen, V., & Pauly, D. (2006). A method for identifying keystone species in food web models. *Ecological Modelling, 195,* 153–171. doi:10.1016/j.ecolmodel.2005.11.029

Livi, C. M. (2009). *Modelling and simulating ecological networks with BlenX. The food web of Prince William Sound: a case study.* Unpublished doctoral dissertation, Universita di Bologna, Bologna, Italy.

Livi, C. M., Jordán, F., Lecca, P., & Okey, T. A. (in press). Identifying key species in ecosystems with stochastic sensitivity analysis. *Ecological Modelling.*

Luczkovich, J. J., Borgatti, S. P., Johnson, J. C., & Everett, M. G. (2003). Defining and measuring trophic role similarity in food webs using regular equivalence. *Journal of Theoretical Biology, 220,* 303–321. doi:10.1006/jtbi.2003.3147

Margalef, R. (1991). Networks in ecology. In Higashi, M., & Burns, T. P. (Eds.), *Theoretical Studies of Ecosystems - the Network Perspective* (pp. 288–351). Cambridge: Cambridge University Press.

Martinez, N. D. (1991). Artifacts or attributes? Effects of resolution on the Little Rock Lake food web. *Ecological Monographs, 61,* 367–392. doi:10.2307/2937047

May, R. M., Beddington, J. R., Clark, C. W., Holt, S. J., & Laws, R. M. (1979). Management of multispecies fisheries. *Science, 205,* 267–277. doi:10.1126/science.205.4403.267

McCaig, C. (2009). From individuals to populations: a symbolic process algebra approach to epidemiology. *Mathematics in Computer Science, 2,* 535–556. doi:10.1007/s11786-008-0066-2

Mills, L. S., Soulé, M. L., & Doak, D. F. (1993). The keystone-species concept in ecology and conservation. *Bioscience, 43,* 219–224. doi:10.2307/1312122

Montoya, J. M., Woodward, G., Emmerson, M. C., & Solé, R. V. (2009). Press perturbations and indirect effects in real food webs. *Ecology, 90,* 2426–2433. doi:10.1890/08-0657.1

Norman, R., & Shankland, C. (2004). Developing the use of process algebra in the derivation and analysis of mathematical models of infectious disease. *Lecture Notes in Computer Science, 280,* 404–414.

Okey, T. A. (2004). *Shifted community states in four marine ecosystems: some potential mechanisms.* Unpublished doctoral dissertation, University of British Columbia, Vancouver.

Okey, T. A., & Pauly, D. (Eds.). (1999). *A trophic mass-balance model of Alaska's Prince William Sound ecosystem, for the post-spill period 1994-1996*. 2nd edition, Vol. Fisheries Centre Research Report 7(4), Vancouver, BC: University of British Columbia.

Okey, T. A., & Wright, B. A. (2004). Toward ecosystem-based extraction policies for Prince William Sound, Alaska: Integrating conflicting objectives and rebuilding pinnipeds. *Bulletin of Marine Science, 74*, 727–747.

Okuyama, T. (2009). Local interactions between predators and prey call into question commonly used functional responses. *Ecological Modelling, 220*, 1182–1188. doi:10.1016/j.ecolmodel.2009.02.010

Olff, H., et al. (2009). Parallel ecological networks in ecosystems. *Philosophical Transactions of the Royal Society, London, series B, 364*, 1755-1779.

Paine, R. T. (1966). Food web complexity and species diversity. *American Naturalist, 100*, 65–75. doi:10.1086/282400

Pascual, M. (2005). Computational ecology: from the complex to the simple and back. *PLoS Computational Biology, 1*, e18. doi:10.1371/journal.pcbi.0010018

Pascual, M., & Dunne, J. A. (Eds.). (2006). *Ecological Networks: Linking Structure to Dynamics in Food Webs*. Oxford: Oxford University Press.

Patten, B. C. (1981). Environs: the superniches of ecosystems. *American Zoologist, 21*, 845–852.

Patten, B. C. (1991). Concluding remarks. Network ecology: indirect determination of the life-environment relationship in ecosystems. In Higashi, M., & Burns, T. P. (Eds.), *Theoretical Studies of Ecosystems - the Network Perspective* (pp. 288–351). Cambridge: Cambridge University Press.

Pimm, S. L. (1991). *The Balance of Nature?* Chicago, IL: University of Chicago Press.

Powell, C. R., & Boland, R. P. (2009). The effects of stochastic population dynamics on food web structure. *Journal of Theoretical Biology, 257*, 170–180. doi:10.1016/j.jtbi.2008.11.006

Power, M. E. (1996). Challenges in the quest for keystones. *Bioscience, 46*, 609–620. doi:10.2307/1312990

Priami, C. (2009). Algorithmic systems biology. *Communications of the ACM, 52*, 80–89. doi:10.1145/1506409.1506427

Purcell, J. E. (2000). Aggregations of the jellyfish Aurelia labiata: abundance, distribution, association with age-0 walleye pollock, and behaviors promoting aggregation in Prince William Sound, Alaska, USA. *Marine Ecology Progress Series, 195*, 145–158. doi:10.3354/meps195145

Roff, D. A. (1997). *Evolutionary Quantitative Genetics*. New York, NY: Chapman and Hall. doi:10.1007/978-1-4615-4080-9

Sagarin, R. D., & Taylor, T. (2008). *Natural Security: a Darwinian Approach to a Dangerous World*. Berkeley: University of California Press.

Scheffer, M. (1995). Super-individuals a simple solution for modelling large populations on an individual basis. *Ecological Modelling, 80*, 161–170. doi:10.1016/0304-3800(94)00055-M

Seth, A. K. (2007). The ecology of action selection: insights from artificial life. *Philosophical Transactions of the Royal Society, London, series B, 362*, 1545-1558.

Simberloff, D. (1980). A succession of paradigms in ecology: essentialism to materialism and probabilism. *Synthese, 43*, 3–39. doi:10.1007/BF00413854

Simberloff, D. (2003). Community and ecosystem impacts of single-species extinctions. In Kareiva, P., & Levin, S. A. (Eds.), *The Importance of Species* (pp. 221–233). Princeton, NJ: Princeton University Press.

Solé, R. V., & Montoya, J. M. (2001). Complexity and fragility in ecological networks. *Proceedings. Biological Sciences, 268*, 2039–2045. doi:10.1098/rspb.2001.1767

Stevens, J. D. (2000). The effects of fishing on sharks, rays, and chimaeras (chondrichthyans), and the implications for marine ecosystems. *Journal of Marine Science, 57*, 476–494.

Stibor, H. (2004). Copepods act as a switch between alternative trophic cascades in marine pelagic food webs. *Ecology Letters, 7*, 321–325. doi:10.1111/j.1461-0248.2004.00580.x

Thompson, J. N. (1982). *Interaction and Coevolution*. New York, NY: Wiley and Sons.

Thompson, J. N. (1988). Variation in interspecific interactions. *Annual Review of Ecology and Systematics, 19*, 65–87. doi:10.1146/annurev.es.19.110188.000433

Tofts, C. (1993). Algorithms for task allocation in ants (A study on temporal polyethism: Theory). *Bulletin of Mathematical Biology, 55*, 891–918.

Ulanowicz, R. E. (1986). *Growth and Development -ecosystems phenomenology*. Berlin: Springer Verlag.

Valentini, R., & Jordán, F. (2010). CoSBiLab Graph: the network analysis module of CoSBiLab. *Environmental Modelling & Software, 25*, 886–888. doi:10.1016/j.envsoft.2010.02.001

Williams, T. M. (2008). Killer appetites: assessing the role of predators in ecological communities. *Ecology, 85*, 3373–3384. doi:10.1890/03-0696

Yodzis, P. (2000). Diffuse effects in food webs. *Ecology, 81*, 261–266. doi:10.1890/0012-9658(2000)081[0261:DEIFW]2.0.CO;2

Yodzis, P. (2001). Must top predators be culled for the sake of fisheries? *Trends in Ecology & Evolution, 16*, 78–84. doi:10.1016/S0169-5347(00)02062-0

Yodzis, P., & Winemiller, K. O. (1999). In search of operational trophospecies in a tropical aquatic food web. *Oikos, 87*, 327–340. doi:10.2307/3546748

Chapter 8
The Role of Stochastic Simulations to Extend Food Web Analyses

Marco Scotti
The Microsoft Research - University of Trento, Centre for Computational and Systems Biology, Italy

ABSTRACT

Food webs are schematic representations of who eats whom in ecosystems. They are widely used in linking process to pattern (e.g., degree distribution and vulnerability) and investigating the roles played by particular species within the interaction web (e.g., centrality indices and trophic position). First, I present the dominator tree, a topological structure reducing food web complexity into linear pathways that are essential for energy delivery. Then, I describe how the dominance relations based on dominator trees extracted from binary food webs may be modified by including interaction strength. Consequences related to the skewed distribution of weak links towards the trophic chain are discussed to explain higher risks of secondary extinction that characterize top predators dominated by basal species. Finally, stochastic simulations are introduced to suggest an alternative approach to static analyses based on food web topology. Ranking species importance using stochastic-based simulations partially contradicts the predictions based on network analyses.

INTRODUCTION

Within ecosystems, species interact in various ways (*e.g.*, predator-prey, plant-seed disperser, host parasite, plant-pollinator, and plant-ant). Types and strengths of interaction change through

time and space, varying between individuals that are subject to the rules of natural selection and genetic drift (Case & Taper, 2000; Fussmann *et al.*, 2007; Bascompte & Jordano, 2007).

In community ecology, food relations are certainly the most investigated. Dealing with the whole set of trophic interactions is possible by

DOI: 10.4018/978-1-61350-435-2.ch008

Copyright © 2012, IGI Global. Copying or distributing in print or electronic forms without written permission of IGI Global is prohibited.

graph theory, and ecosystems can be represented as sets of nodes (species or trophospecies) connected by edges (trophic relations). From this idea, two types of tools have come about: food webs (Yodzis, 1989; Cohen *et al.*, 1990; Polis & Winemiller, 1995) and ecological networks (Ulanowicz, 2004; Fath & Patten, 2004). The former describes feeding relations among species in a qualitative way (presence/absence); the latter includes also the magnitude of the interactions, in terms of amount of matter (or energy) that is exchanged in a given time period, over a reference area (*e.g.*, kcal m^{-2} year^{-1}; gC cm^{-2} month^{-1}). Food webs and ecological networks are widely used in linking process to pattern (*e.g.*, degree distribution and vulnerability) and investigating the roles played by particular species within the interaction web (*e.g.*, centrality indices and trophic position).

A central issue in ecology is understanding the processes that shape food webs. This is of key importance as the topology (*i.e.*, static graph configuration associated to trophic links between species) of these networks is one of the major determinants of ecosystem dynamics and is ultimately responsible for response to human impact. For this reason, discovering patterns in food web topology has long been a prominent topic in ecology (Cohen, 1978). To unveil mechanisms lying behind community structure we are asked to identify general rules governing such architectures. Progress towards this knowledge would help advances on applied issues such as understanding the potentially catastrophic consequences of species loss on cascades of further extinctions (Pimm, 1980; Allesina & Bodini, 2004), and predicting the direct and indirect impact of invasive species (Woodward & Hildrew, 2001).

The existence of empirical patterns has stimulated analyses to identify which mechanisms are responsible for shaping the structure of food webs. It has been shown unambiguously that real food webs are topologically distinct from randomly connected networks (Solow & Beet, 1998) and several simple models predict in detail many regularities of food web topology (Cohen & Newman, 1985; Williams & Martinez, 2000; Cattin *et al.*, 2004; Stouffer *et al.*, 2006; Allesina *et al.*, 2008).

Newly developed algorithms aim to identify the role of species by quantifying the effect of their loss on ecosystem structure. Key species are those possessing the greatest strategic value and, from a network perspective, their conservation promotes the persistence of other species (Jordán & Scheuring, 2002; Jordán *et al.*, 2006; Jordán, 2009). A promising issue concerns the forecasting of secondary extinctions (*i.e.*, the possibility that species loss may lead to cascades of further extinctions) based on food web structure. In particular, studies on simulated food web models have focused on the relation between connectance and secondary extinctions, showing how the loss of random species is likely to result only in a few extinctions, whereas there are structurally dominant taxa whose loss is responsible for stronger impact (Dunne *et al.*, 2002a,b, 2004). Other works have shown the potential of the dominator tree (a structure describing the dominance relationship between nodes in a hierarchical digraph) to assess secondary losses caused by species exclusion, and to identify which nodes are likely to cause the greatest impact if removed (Allesina & Bodini, 2004; Bodini *et al.*, 2009).

Models capturing the non-random topology of food webs, and the majority of techniques estimating the robustness of networks, are based on binary (*i.e.*, unweighted) data. Food webs are often considered to have rigid architectures, with links connecting prey to predators summarizing the observed diet. This inflexible structure represents a limit, since it does not describe what really happens in nature. Although binary food webs have been deeply analyzed in recent years, many ecologists claimed the need of using weighted trophic links to unveil important dynamics, such as the role of skewed interaction strength distribution (*e.g.*, many weak and few strong links; Paine, 1992; McCann *et al.*, 1998), or effects of species with few but extremely strong trophic links on secondary extinction (Dunne *et al.*, 2002b).

Despite the observation that link strength varies considerably (Berlow *et al.*, 2004), food web analyses of real networks are still limited by data availability and new efforts and investments should be devoted to solve this inconsistency (Cohen *et al.*, 1993). When qualitative descriptors are analyzed, most of these indices are extremely sensitive to different levels of sampling effort (Goldwasser & Roughgarden, 1997; Martinez *et al.*, 1999). As previously observed, distribution of link strength is likely to be uneven (Paine, 1992; McCann *et al.*, 1998) and the same weight assigned to each link in qualitative food webs distorts the true picture of their structure (Kenny & Loehle, 1991). These aspects emphasize the need of weighting to achieve a more sensible description of food web structure (May, 1983; Kenny & Loehle, 1991; Pimm *et al.*, 1991; Cohen *et al.*, 1993; Bersier *et al.*, 1999). A fascinating question is to find how link strength (*i.e.*, using weighted data) may provide further insight on ecosystem function. Adopting weighted data allows for the extension of the static perspective based on network topology, and represents a partial shift towards dynamics.

In this chapter I show results on the analysis of 14 weighted food webs for which the link density (*i.e.*, the number of links, weighted by their magnitude - see Solé & Montoya, 2001; Dunne *et al.*, 2002b) of each species is estimated. First, a prevalence of weak links in comparison to strong trophic connections is observed (*i.e.*, there exist few main routes through which energy flows in ecosystems). Second, the skewed link magnitude is characterized by a regular distribution, with fewer stronger links dispersed in many weak links at the top of the trophic chain (*i.e.*, herbivores display a generalist trophic behavior, while top predators tend to be strongly specialized). Third, including interaction strengths contradicts the patterns of link distribution computed with binary food webs (*i.e.*, with unweighted data, a generalist

trophic behavior is found when moving towards top predators).

I describe the dominator tree algorithm (Allesina & Bodini, 2004) to forecast secondary extinctions, using both unweighted and weighted data. The apparent robustness observed in binary food webs is strongly attenuated when filtering the whole architecture of trophic links. In fact, after the removal of the weakest links, only the trophic relationships responsible for the larger amount of energy supply are preserved. These latter are considered to be essential for species survival, and they represent a small fraction of the total links in food webs. Using weighted data may substantially improve our understanding of food web organization, and possibly contradict results based on the analysis of binary webs.

Topological analyses are commonly used to extract static features of real food webs. Their logical extension is represented by dynamic models. Progress towards this knowledge would help the development of techniques estimating the vulnerability of biological communities to species extirpations, a central challenge of conservation biology.

After introducing classical topological analyses, and illustrating their refined version by using weighted data, I present a stochastic dynamic framework for food web analysis. I introduce individual-based, stochastic simulations to show the potential of this approach for inferring the importance of species within food webs. In particular, stochastic simulations are performed for studying the dynamics of Prince William Sound (Alaska) food web (Okey, 2004; Okey & Wright, 2004) by applying a programming language called BlenX (Dematté *et al.*, 2008, 2010; Romanel, 2010). BlenX has been developed within the framework of algorithmic systems biology (Priami, 2009). It enhances current modeling capabilities (*i.e.*, easiness, composability and reusability of models) and is explicitly designed to describe interactions of (biological) entities (*i.e.*, quantitative information about speed and probability of actions is provided with systems specification). Individual animals are represented as boxes, composed by a set of interfaces and internal programs that are executed simultaneously. The exchange of a message between the programs of two boxes is equivalent to an interaction involving two biological entities (Regev & Shapiro, 2002). These features allow the user to construct models that are based on simple statements, without dealing with a critical issue of the mathematical approach: the combinatorial explosion of variables needed to characterize the whole set of states through which a single component can pass. The evolution of complex systems can emerge from local interactions between simple components (*e.g.*, boxes representing individuals of different species for which basic rules describing their trophic activities are codified), by setting their elementary behavior (*e.g.*, predator-prey preferences). I use this tool to present new metrics based on the functional importance of species. I also emphasize how the stochastic approach can be of key importance for studying ecological interactions, particularly in models with small population size. In fact, stochastic simulations bypass one of the major drawbacks associated to the application of deterministic dynamic models. These latter are feasible when the population size is sufficiently large to minimize noise in the overall system. In models with small population size, stochasticity can be modeled explicitly. I describe a new perspective for the study of ecological networks. This is based on the idea that stochastic processes and noise are fundamental features of biological systems. I discuss the process algebra-based approach as a promising modeling perspective in the study of complex and heterogeneous biological systems. Actions of conservation biology often aim to protect rare species. These species are characterized by small population size, with individuals showing a highly heterogeneous behavior. For these reasons, stochastic modeling can represent a step ahead in the domain of ecological research.

BACKGROUND

The ever increasing interest in ecosystem status and performance, and the need to approach complex environmental problems, stimulate the application of tools for whole-system assessment (NSF, 1999). The most common method for quantifying system level events is simulation modeling, which implies five main steps: (1) identifying relevant species; (2) defining the significant interactions among those species; (3) modeling such interactions; (4) calibrating and validating the model; (5) making predictions. Despite successful models describing the dynamics of one or a few subjects, mathematical modeling appears complicated when their number increases (Platt *et al.*, 1981). As a consequence, to bypass the above mentioned inconsistencies in applications to system ecology, MacArthur (1955) and Platt *et al.* (1981) suggested an alternative approach, paying more attention to processes (flows) than focusing on what can be inferred from identification and analysis of single objects (stocks). In this conceptual framework, a prominent collection of quantitative methods consists of food web (Yodzis, 1989; Cohen *et al.*, 1990; Polis & Winemiller, 1995) and ecosystem network analyses (ENA; Ulanowicz, 1986; Wulff & Ulanowicz, 1989; Ulanowicz, 2004). The basic assumption behind these approaches is that topology (static graph configuration associated to trophic links between species) reveals much about history, current status and functioning of ecosystems.

In ecology, there have been several independent lines of research using networks (Fath & Patten, 1999). Hannon (1973) first used input-output analysis to investigate the interdependence of organisms in an ecosystem, and to determine the total energy flows that directly and indirectly link the component to its ecosystem. He introduced dynamic analysis as a way to identify control in an ecosystem (Hannon, 1986). Finn (1976) developed standard methods to calculate the total system throughflow, average path length, and a cycling index that is widely used in ecology. Thanks to network models we may know how energy circulates throughout ecosystems. Ulanowicz (1986) emphasized a combination of transactive flows and information theory called ascendancy. In recent years, unweighted food webs (*i.e.*, ecological networks portraying presence/absence of trophic interactions between species, by means of adjacency matrix) have been widely used. Analyzing binary data on feeding relationships helped to understand the structure of food webs from a variety of ecosystems, providing details on properties as characteristic path lengths, clustering coefficients, and degree distributions (Camacho *et al.*, 2002; Dunne *et al.*, 2002a; Montoya & Solé, 2002). By investigating food webs as transportation networks (Banavar *et al.*, 1999, Garlaschelli *et al.*, 2003) it was possible to derive an allometric relation between the amount of energy to any single species and the overall community energy budget, which may improve our knowledge on

the efficiency of energy delivery in ecosystems (Allesina & Bodini, 2005).

All the analyses performed on unweighted and weighted food webs make use of a static representation, which is based on the binary architecture of the trophic interactions between species.

This inflexible structure could be identified as a limitation in this kind of analyses since it does not represent what actually happens in nature. In particular, the static architecture of trophic interactions does not consider a possible shift in species diet (prey switching), that is the ability of species to change or extend their trophic activity, withstanding the cascade effects (Figure 1). In general, diet switching cannot be easily accommodated into food web topology. The binary configuration of food webs lumps together the whole set of trophic interactions displayed by species or trophospecies (*i.e.*, a set of species with similar diet and predators - see Yodzis & Winemiller, 1999), without capturing spatial and temporal variations in the trophic preferences of individuals.

Figure 1. Examples of diet switching: (a) despite the fact that the whole trophic behavior of species A is based on a generalist activity (H, C, D), node H represents a bottleneck to energy flow during the ontogenetic development, being the exclusive food item for juvenile individuals (A_{ju}); (b) in presence of low concentration of suspended organic carbon and high rates of photosynthesis, both of the copepods (C_1 and C_2) feed on the abundant source of phytoplankton (P), while turbulent water (which increases turbidity) stimulates the shift of C_2 to zooplankton (Z), an alternative source of energy for buffering the decrease in primary production; (c) the primary extinction of I_1 does not trigger any secondary extinction, since species T switches its diet to I_2.

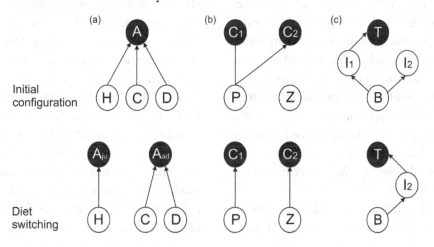

Allesina and Bodini (2004) introduced a simple and elegant algorithm to extract the dominator tree, a structure used to unfold complex food webs into a topologically simpler scheme. Dominator tree allows forecasting indirect effects of a species removal according with topological criteria only (*i.e.*, without focusing on secondary extinctions occurring in case of dynamic instabilities caused by both direct and indirect interactions), and Bodini *et al.* (2009) tested this model in cases where secondary extinction has been observed in nature. By applying the dominator tree model they were able to successfully identify a real secondary extinction observed in the Barents Sea, while two additional extinction events were overestimated. This partial failure was likely caused by difficulties in capturing the diet shift in species trophic activities, since the dominator tree was built starting from the static topology of the food web.

Systems analysis in ecology has a very long tradition, and indeed, systems ecology is older than what is currently called systems biology. It was born well before the application of computers in life sciences and flourished as a major field (Margalef, 1968; Odum, 1969; Ulanowicz, 1986). While systems ecology was focused more on macroscopic properties (*e.g.*, the percentage of material and energy that is recycled by an ecosystem; the transfer efficiency throughout the trophic chain), population biology aimed at describing lower-level details that developed more or less independently. Although network theory principles were introduced in ecology many years ago, recent analytical advances coupled with the enhanced potential of high-speed computation, and the growing number of investigators interested in studying well-resolved networks (*i.e.*, with a higher number of compartments - see Heymans *et al.*, 2002), have opened up new vistas and presented new challenges (Walters *et al.*, 1997; Levin *et al.*, 1997).

Although the debate concerning the use of deterministic or stochastic methods started to per-

meate ecology many years ago (Nisbet & Gurney, 1982; Renshaw, 1993), only recent studies have focused on dynamic simulation of large food webs. Ideas about complex network dynamics are being tested with large datasets adopting a deterministic approach (Christensen & Walters, 2004; Okey, 2004; Okey *et al.*, 2004). Food web and ecological network analyses represent almost unexplored areas for stochastic simulation. In ecology, there exist individual-based approaches and some mixed studies (deterministic models with some stochastic components), but stochastic modeling should still be improved (Ebenman & Jonsson, 2005). Novel conceptual and computational tools (*e.g.*, stochastic programming languages) can help in modeling the link between local and global processes, simulating density dependence (Björnstad *et al.*, 1999) and dealing with several other challenges of ecology, but most likely the explicit modeling of hierarchical organization will be one of the key contributions to ecological research (Levin, 1998; Kolasa, 2005). Other ecologists focused on the demographic and environmental stochasticity in metapopulation dynamics (Bonsall & Hastings), investigated fluctuations affecting the densities of populations in communities and food webs as a consequence of environmental variability (Ripa & Ives), and analyzed the effects of random perturbations on cyclic population dynamics (Kaitala *et al.*, 1996). In practice, these tools may aid in planning systems-based conservation strategies (Berkes, 2004), defining optimum programs for managing multispecies fisheries (May *et al.*, 1979; Yodzis, 2001), creating sustainable agro-ecosystems (Rasmussen *et al.*, 1998), investigating the functioning of bio-geochemical cycles (Botter *et al.*, 2006), predicting risks of secondary extinctions (Ebenman & Jonsson, 2005), and ranking of conservation priorities (Lande *et al.*, 2003).

Linking these organizational levels is still a challenge: the increasing need for hierarchical thinking is present in ecological stoichiometry (community-level patterns of the ratios of certain elements; Elser *et al.*, 2000), and community genetics (how genetic variance influences ecosystem functioning; Huges *et al.*, 2008). Traditional modeling methods, focusing on macroscopic patterns and searching for general laws, seem to be weak in several respects. Primarily, they need to be improved in terms of predictability and accuracy. Also, the inherent stochasticity and variability, as well as the large-scale patterns produced by local rules, are important features that should be more thoroughly investigated. Moreover, even if the importance of these aspects is recognized, modeling approaches have not been developed to form new conceptual frameworks (for example, stochastic processes are modeled by deterministic equations with added random noise).

Then, I suggest how adopting BlenX, a process algebra-based language, is ecologically reasonable, as it can capture the inherent variability of biological systems, as opposed to ODE-based simulations that are based on a homogeneous set of components. While the latter represents a view based on equations to provide general laws with some (mostly external) noise, the former describes a situation where variability is inherent and influential. I argue that, independently of simulation results, the process algebra-based approach is logically more biological in nature.

The broadest goal of this contribution is extending the current methods, based on topological analyses of unweighted food webs, to provide effective tools for policy makers working in the field of environmental management. New tools should be developed for estimating the optimal options to preserve highly endangered species, and for planning actions of biodiversity conservation in complex ecological communities. To achieve these objectives, I present revised versions of some classical structural analyses on unweighted data. This is consistent with the fact that a quantitative approach has been called for by numerous authors (Bersier *et al.* 1999, Dunne *et al.* 2002a, 2002b, Montoya & Solé 2002, Allesina & Bodini 2004, Tylianakis *et al.* 2007) to better understand food web organization and dynamics.

First, the additional information displayed by weighted food webs is used to extract novel patterns in the distribution of weak and strong trophic interactions towards the trophic chain. Then, I emphasize how knowing the distribution of weak links in food webs can help in defining trajectories of environmental sustainability and formulating policies for halting the loss of biodiversity. Finally, by applying a process-algebra based method, I illustrate an alternative approach that makes use of stochastic dynamics within the framework of food web analysis. Simulations represent a step ahead for characterizing the relative importance of species in food webs (Proulx *et al.*, 2005; Quince *et al.*, 2005; Eklöf & Ebenman, 2006; Berlow *et al.*, 2008).

STRUCTURE AND DYNAMICS IN FOOD WEB MODELS

How to Forecast Secondary Extinctions in Binary Food Webs

In any study of evolutionary ecology, food relations seem to be among the most important aspects of the system of animate nature. In this section I deal with the problem of forecasting risks of secondary extinction using unweighted food web data. The dominator tree model represents a network topological structure used for disentangling the architecture of complex networks, reducing food webs to linear pathways that are essential for energy delivery (Allesina & Bodini, 2004). Each species along this rooted and directed tree is responsible for transferring energy to the nodes that follow it, and, as such, it is a dominator essential for their survival. The higher the number of species a node dominates the greater the impact resulting from its removal. Here I compute the dominator trees for 14 food webs, obtaining, for each of them, the number of nodes dominated by a single species and the number of nodes that dominate each species. Table 1 provides name of

Table 1. List of the ecological networks considered in the analysis. Total number of nodes (S) and number of non-living compartments (nl) are given. Flow intensities are measured as carbon (i.e., g C m^{-2} year^{-1} or mg C m^{-2} summer^{-1}), ash free dry weight (g AFDW m^{-2} year^{-1}) and wet weight (t WW km^{-2} year^{-1}). The last column summarizes the references to networks analyzed.

Food web	S	nl	Flow units	References
Chesapeake Mesohaline Network	36	3	mg C m^{-2} summer^{-1}	Baird & Ulanowicz, 1989
Crystal River Creek (control)	21	1	mg C m^{-2} day^{-1}	Homer, M., & Kemp, W.M., unpublished manuscript. See also, Ulanowicz, 1986
St. Marks River (Florida) Flow Network	51	3	mg C m^{-2} day^{-1}	Baird *et al.*, 1998
Lake Michigan Control Network	36	1	g C m^{-2} year^{-1}	Krause, A.E., & Mason, D.M., unpublished manuscript
Mondego Estuary	43	1	g AFDW m^{-2} year^{-1}	Patrício *et al.*, 2004
Final Narraganasett Bay Model	32	1	mg C m^{-2} year^{-1}	Monaco & Ulanowicz, 1997
Cypress Wetlands (dry season)	68	3	g C m^{-2} year^{-1}	Ulanowicz *et al.*, 1997
Marshes and Sloughs (dry season)	66	3	g C m^{-2} year^{-1}	Ulanowicz *et al.*, 2000
Florida Bay (dry season)	125	3	g C m^{-2} year^{-1}	Ulanowicz *et al.*, 1998
Mangroves (dry season)	94	3	g C m^{-2} year^{-1}	Ulanowicz *et al.*, 1999
Lake Santo (Spring 1991)	27	3	g C m^{-2} year^{-1}	Bondavalli et. al, 2006
Huizache-Caimanero	26	1	mg C m^{-2} day^{-1}	Zetina-Rejòn *et al.*, 2004
Gulf of California	26	1	g C m^{-2} year^{-1}	Arreguin-Sanchez *et al.*, 2002
Prince William Sound (Alaska)	51	3	t WW km^{-2} year^{-1}	Okey, 2004

the networks, number of nodes, currency used for weighting, and original reference.

As a static picture of "who eats whom", food webs describe how species feed on each other for their energy requirements. Extinction may have different cascading effects as a consequence of the relative position of species with respect to the flow of energy from producers to consumers. In linear food chains, the loss of a species causes all the others following it to go extinct. However, food webs are characterized by a multiplicity of trophic connections that create complex patterns of reciprocal dependence. Because of this intricacy, the spread of indirect effects is difficult to unveil and, consequently, secondary extinctions very complicated to predict (Yodzis & Winemiller, 1999).

The algorithm for extracting the dominator tree allows association of every food web to another topological structure in which species are sequentially connected, as a consequence of their dominance relations in energy delivery. Ecosystems are sustained by energy input from outside the system (*i.e.*, solar radiation), and every primary producer (*i.e.*, plants) can be connected with this "root" node. Mapping the extent of secondary extinctions is equivalent to measuring how many nodes will be disconnected from the "root" when a primary extinction occurs. Then, the complexity of trophic flows displayed by a food web with S species can be unfolded using another graph, containing S-1 links, called the dominator tree: the removal of a node in the original food web will extinguish all the nodes that belong to its branch in the dominator tree. In Figure 2 I illustrate a hypothetical food web (Figure 2a) and the dominator tree associated to its topological structure (Figure 2b).

With reference to the binary food web of Figure 2a, node C is the dominator of F (C = dom(F)).

Figure 2. The black node represents the external environment (i.e., sunlight energy intended as the ultimate source of energy for all the species), while grey nodes are primary producers (i.e., plants). Energy flows are depicted as arrowhead edges leading from prey to predator nodes. Link strength is quantified by numbers next to arrows, and describes relative prey importance in with respect to the total predator energy demand. The depicted graphs correspond to: (a) a simple rooted food web; (b) the dominator tree extracted for the unweighted food web architecture (i.e., with uniform distribution of interaction strength); (c) the alternative dominator tree computed when a threshold is imposed (i.e., links are selected on the basis of their magnitude and, in this case, only trophic flows providing more than 10% of the predator needs are preserved). The dominator tree in (c) is therefore constructed when links B → D and D → G are removed from the hypothetical food web in (a), as they represent less than 10% of the energy input to predators (D and G).

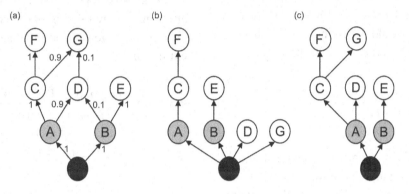

Every path from the "root" (*i.e.*, the external source of solar energy, in the case of food webs) to F contains C (in this specific example, it corresponds to the only route that is available): that is to say, energy (or matter) supply to F cannot be carried out without passing through C. From this definition it follows that every node dominates itself (C = dom(C)). In addition, C can be defined as the "proper dominator" of F because C = dom(F) and C ≠ F. Finally, as C = dom(F) and the other proper dominator of F (A = dom(F), A ≠ C ≠ F) is also dominator of C (A = dom(C)), C is the "immediate dominator" of F. All the energy available to C passes trough the "root" and the species A, so that both are dominators of this node and A is its immediate dominator. Species G receives energy along the pathways (1) "root" → A → C → G, (2) "root" → A → D → G, and (3) "root" → B → D → G. Figure 2b shows that only the "root" dominates G because it is the only node in common between the three paths. When either A or B become extinct, species G may survive be-

cause at least one pathway remains at its disposal. With the removal of the "root" the entire system would vanish.

In summary, (1) a general node i dominates j if and only if every path going from the "root" to j contains i; (2) i is the immediate dominator of j if i dominates j, and every dominator of i is a dominator of j as well; (3) the removal of a node will extinguish all the nodes it dominates; (4) connecting every node to its immediate dominator generates the so-called dominator tree. One of the fundamental theorems of dominator trees (Lengauer & Tarjan, 1979) states that *"every node of a graph except root has a unique immediate dominator"*. Accordingly, in the dominator tree a link connecting i and j exists if and only if i is the immediate dominator of j.

I extracted the dominator tree from the unweighted configuration of the 14 food webs listed in Table 1 (S = number of species; N = S + 1 = number of species + "root" node = total number of nodes in the dominator tree). For each node i, the subset of proper dominators is computed as |dom(i)|-1. Every node dominates itself, and the "root" is excluded from this analysis as no ecosystems can survive without sunlight energy. The probability that the i-th node would go extinct from an ecosystem with S species (and N = S + 1 nodes, since also the "root" is considered), in case of random node removal (excluding the "root" collapse), is calculated by the probability (|dom(i)|-1)/(N-1). The index of error sensitivity (ES) is computed by averaging this probability among all nodes. It quantifies the average fraction of species that would go extinct after a random node removal (Albert *et al.*, 2000):

$$ES = \sum_{i \neq root} \frac{|dom(i)|-1}{(N-1)^2} \qquad (1)$$

Error sensitivity ranges between 1/2 and 1/(N-1). The first value is computed when the dominator tree is a linear chain, while the latter corresponds to a star-like structure. Linear chain and star-like structures are extreme dominator tree configurations that define the range of variation for ES (see Figure 3).

Figure 3. Extreme configurations for the dominator tree: (a) linear chain and (b) star-like architecture. The black node is the "root" (sunlight energy sustaining food webs).

(a)

(b)

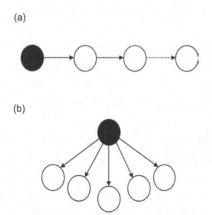

On average, in a linear structure a single node removal is expected to cause half of the nodes to disappear (with N → ∞):

$$ES = \sum_{i \neq root} \frac{|dom(i)|-1}{(N-1)^2} = \frac{1}{(N-1)^2} + \frac{2}{(N-1)^2}$$
$$+ \cdots + \frac{N-1}{(N-1)^2} = \frac{N(N-1)}{2(N-1)^2} = \frac{N}{2(N-1)} \simeq \frac{1}{2} \qquad (2)$$

In a star-like topology, no secondary extinctions are triggered by random node removals, and the average damage is a consequence of the primary extinction only:

$$ES = \sum_{i \neq root} \frac{|dom(i)|-1}{(N-1)^2} = \frac{1}{(N-1)^2} + \frac{1}{(N-1)^2}$$
$$+ \cdots + \frac{1}{(N-1)^2} = \frac{N-1}{(N-1)^2} = \frac{1}{N-1} \qquad (3)$$

In addition to error sensitivity, another index called attack sensitivity (AS) can be measured (Albert *et al.*, 2000). It quantifies the effects of a targeted removal, intended as the extinction of the species that creates as much damage as possible in terms of secondary extinctions:

$$AS = \max \left\{ \frac{|dom(i)|-1}{N-1} \right\}, \forall i \neq root \qquad (4)$$

AS ranges between 1/(N-1) and 1. In a linear dominator tree the percentage of extinction when the basal species (*i.e.*, primary producer) is removed is 100% (all species disappear; AS = 1). The star-like dominator tree is the most resistant structure to attacks: no extinctions are observed as a consequence of targeted species removals (except for the primary extinction; AS = 1/(N-1)). Low ES and low AS values pertain to error-tolerant and attack-tolerant systems, respectively. Error and attack sensitivity obtained with unweighted data, for the studied food webs, are summarized by "FW" columns in Table 2.

All of the food webs in Table 2 show the possibility of multiple secondary extinctions, except for the case of Lake Michigan Network and Lake Santo. The most fragile ecosystem is Gulf of California, with the risk of collapse for the 84% of species predicted as the effect of a single primary extinction (AS = 0.840). The highest level of pathway multiplicity is observed for Lake Michigan Network and Lake Santo, where no secondary extinctions are triggered by primary extinctions (AS=0). Mean and standard deviation for this index are $\mu = 0.114$ and $\sigma = 0.215$. As described by standard deviation, the average

value is strongly biased by three ecosystems, with 11 food webs out of 14 (excluding Gulf of California, Chesapeake Mesohaline Network and Mondego Estuary) that are extremely less sensitive to targeted species removal (*i.e.*, they are characterized by mean and standard deviation well below 10%; $\mu_{11}AS = 0.041$; $\sigma_{11}AS = 0.030$). ES ranges between 0.009 (Florida Bay) and 0.074 (Gulf of California), with average $\mu = 0.032$ and standard deviation $\sigma = 0.019$. ES appears inversely related to food web size, while this relationship is attenuated for AS. I examined log(ES) and log(AS) as linear functions of food web size (S). In the first case I found a strong negative relationship ($\rho = 0.929$; $p \ll 0.001$), while for

Table 2. Error (ES) and attack sensitivity (AS) of the 14 food webs analyzed in this study. Columns under the label "FW" refer to these indices in case of dominator trees extracted from the binary food web configuration. The following values are measured when, in each reference food web, thresholds are imposed to select links on the base of their magnitude: the weaker trophic relationships are removed (i.e., connections representing less than 1%, 5%, 10%, 15% and 20% of the predators' energy supply, respectively). Contrary to all expectations, some ecosystems decrease AS when trophic links are removed (e.g., California: $AS_{FW} = 0.840$; $AS_{20\%} = 0.280$). This is due to network fragmentation after the removal of a few links, with the index estimated for sub-networks of the reference food web, rather than corresponding to the whole ecosystem. When the dominator tree structure displays a star-like configuration (the system is dominated by the "root" node only) AS is 0 (see Michigan & Santo).

Ecosystem	FW		1%		5%		10%		15%		20%	
	AS	ES	AS	ES	AS	ES	AS	ES	AS	ES	AS	ES
Chesapeake	0.182	0.040	0.182	0.040	0.212	0.044	0.242	0.050	0.242	0.051	0.212	0.052
Crystal	0.100	0.060	0.100	0.060	0.100	0.060	0.100	0.062	0.150	0.068	0.150	0.072
Marks	0.042	0.022	0.042	0.022	0.042	0.024	0.062	0.026	0.062	0.028	0.062	0.029
Michigan	0.000	0.029	0.000	0.029	0.000	0.029	0.029	0.029	0.057	0.031	0.171	0.038
Mondego	0.119	0.028	0.119	0.028	0.119	0.030	0.095	0.031	0.190	0.035	0.167	0.032
Narra	0.032	0.034	0.032	0.034	0.032	0.034	0.613	0.055	0.548	0.056	0.387	0.057
Cypress	0.046	0.017	0.077	0.017	0.077	0.017	0.092	0.018	0.092	0.018	0.108	0.019
Marshes	0.032	0.017	0.048	0.017	0.063	0.018	0.063	0.019	0.270	0.024	0.270	0.026
Florida	0.025	0.009	0.025	0.009	0.016	0.009	0.025	0.009	0.049	0.011	0.057	0.011
Mangroves	0.033	0.011	0.022	0.011	0.033	0.012	0.110	0.013	0.154	0.014	0.176	0.016
Santo	0.000	0.042	0.000	0.042	0.042	0.043	0.000	0.042	0.542	0.064	0.000	0.042
Huizache	0.080	0.045	0.080	0.045	0.080	0.046	0.280	0.056	0.280	0.066	0.240	0.067
California	0.840	0.074	0.760	0.083	0.240	0.056	0.520	0.069	0.240	0.072	0.280	0.075
Alaska	0.061	0.022	0.143	0.025	0.163	0.027	0.163	0.027	0.184	0.031	0.204	0.034

the latter this trend is mitigated ($\rho = 0.613$; $p < 0.05$). This means that sensitivity to random removals exponentially diminishes with food web size and, on average, single random extinctions result in 2-3% of species loss. This effect is mostly determined by self-domination. In contrast, a less evident relationship is the link between attack sensitivity (AS) to the number of species in a given ecosystem. In certain food webs, secondary extinctions due to removal of highly dominant species is very similar to patterns shown by random removals (*e.g.*, St. Marks River Flow Network, Final Narraganasett Bay Model, and Prince William Sound food web), with food webs highly resistant to cascade effects regardless of what species is removed. Gulf of California, Chesapeake Mesohaline Network and Mondego Estuary are three ecosystems characterized by AS values beyond 0.1, meaning that a single species extinction can cause enormous damage (California: 84.0% of species loss; Chesapeake: 18.2%; Mondego: 11.9%). The negative exponential correlation linking ES and AS to species richness contradicts results obtained using demographic models, which pointed out that the probability of secondary extinction increases with species richness (Lundberg *et al.*, 2000).

As a final remark, I emphasize that by applying the dominator tree algorithm a bottom-up perspective is adopted to identify bottlenecks in energy delivery (*i.e.*, which species are likely to be responsible for higher risks of secondary extinctions once removed from the ecosystem). Cascading extinctions certainly occur also in a top-down direction, and this scenario cannot be captured using the dominator tree algorithm. This method underestimates secondary extinctions, and it is conceived for predicting events triggered when species are disconnected from their unique source of energy. As suggested by Jordán *et al.* (1999), a reliable approach for dealing with this question from a top-down perspective must include dynamical features of species interaction.

Bottlenecks to Energy Delivery: Dominator Trees in Weighted Food Webs

Forecasting the consequences of a single extinction event was possible according to the idea that whenever a node is removed, all of the species that rely on it for energy supply would go extinct as well. However, only links that are strong enough (*i.e.*, that transport enough currency) can satisfy the energy supply that is essential for the predator's survival. This feature suggests the opportunity of investigating patterns of dominance as a function of link magnitude. In a purely qualitative dominator tree (*i.e.*, the directed tree extracted from the binary architecture of a food web), this distinction is not taken into account, and it is sufficient that a species remains somehow connected to the "root" for preventing its extinction, no matter how much energy is passing through such connection. However, once flow intensity is taken into account, dominance patterns are likely to change. This can be intuitively described with reference to Figure 2. The simple food web depicted in Figure 2a can be considered in terms of a crude binary architecture (presence/absence of links between species), or studied by discriminating the importance of trophic relationships. Numbers next to arrows quantify the relative importance of links in terms of energy supply to predators (*e.g.*, species D is receiving 90% of energy preying upon A, while the remaining 10% comes from feeding on B). As illustrated by Figure 2a, seven trophic links out of nine are fundamental for transporting more than the 90% of the requisite medium consumed by each predator (*i.e.*, all except links B → D and D → G). Once the binary structure is filtered with the notion of interaction strength (*e.g.*, removing links contributing to less than the 10% of the consumer's energy supply), a new dominator tree is extracted (see Figure 2c). Updating the crude binary approach with this more functional analysis identifies species that are responsible for transporting the bulk of energy to predators (bottom-up perspective). In Figure 2a, the species D receives 90% of its food intake from A and the other 10% from B; the extinction of A would likely cause D to vanish, as too little energy would reach D through B. As a consequence, species A is essential for the survival of D, and it appears to be its dominator (Figure 2c). In the qualitative case the node D was directly dominated by the "root" (Figure 2b), as its energy intake was transported by two alternative corridors passing through A and B.

Also with this approach, which considers trophic connections that are fundamental for satisfying the larger amount of predators' energy intake, ecological flow networks provide a means for investigating secondary extinctions from a bottom-up perspective. Variation in the top-down regulatory effects cannot be unveiled, as the mechanism of competitive exclusion triggered by primary extinction of a common predator shared between two prey.

As observed by Borrvall *et al.* (2000), the risk of secondary extinctions increases when the distribution of link strength is skewed. They described how food webs characterized by few strong links and many weak interactions are more exposed to secondary extinction. In this section, the definition of weak and strong trophic relationship is inferred by studying energy flow networks, instead of the dynamics of species interactions, and it represents a different perspective for testing the Borrvall *et al.* (2000) findings. First, I explored how the spectrum of link strength is distributed in the 14 food webs, from a bottom-up perspective (*e.g.*, is species feeding activity evenly distributed between prey? Do weak links prevail in comparison to the whole set of trophic interactions in a food web?). In the 14 food webs analyzed in this study, a strong preponderance of weak links is found (around 80% of the total feeding relationships represent less than 20% of species' food intake - see Figure 4).

Qualitative food webs represent networks with uniform distribution of interaction strength. When thresholds are imposed to select links on the base

of their magnitude, I observed that most links are removed for rather low values of the filter. In these 14 food webs, the distribution of link strength is clearly skewed, an outcome that corroborates previous findings of Ulanowicz and Wolff (1991) and supports the idea that in real food webs there is a prevalence of weak interactions between species (Berlow, 1999; Kokkoris *et al.*, 1999; Montoya & Solé, 2003).

Analyzing food web fragility with the notion of interaction strength can affect the dominator tree construction, with consequences on the prediction of secondary extinction risks. In Table 2, error and attack sensitivity are summarized for the food web structures obtained when removing the weakest links. In some cases, AS and ES indices were decreasing when filtering the binary architecture because after removing a few links the graphs became disconnected, and the main dominator was computed for a subset of the whole network (*e.g.*, Florida Bay, Gulf of California). At one extreme lies the Gulf of California ecosystem for which disconnection occurs when removal involves links whose magnitude is much lower than 20% of each species' diet. At the opposite extreme, the Marshes and Sloughs food web remains connected up to when links representing the 25% of each species' diet are removed. In the former case, relatively weak links are essential to maintain all nodes connected to the root, whereas in the latter this function is performed only by strong links.

Until network fragmentation is not observed, error and attack sensitivity increase as the weak links are progressively removed from the graphs. Some ecosystems are extremely resistant to targeted node deletion (*e.g.*, St. Marks River ecosystem: $AS_{FW} = 0.042$; $AS_{20\%} = 0.062$). In other cases, with the removal of the weakest links a single primary extinction can be responsible for the 28% of system collapse (*e.g.*, Huizache-Caimanero food web), despite the relative network robustness displayed by the binary architecture ($AS_{FW} = 8\%$). Ecosystems that possess the greater threshold for disconnection are also those for which the

Figure 4. Prevalence of weak links in the 14 food webs. On the x-axis, the interaction strength of food links is normalized by the whole energy input entering the predator (relative link strength). Consider, as an example, a predator feeding on five species and receiving 16 kcal m⁻² year⁻¹ from its preferential prey and the remaining 4 kcal m⁻² year⁻¹ evenly distributed between the other four prey. This predator has a total energy input of 20 kcal m⁻² year⁻¹ (16 kcal m⁻² year⁻¹ + 1 kcal m⁻² year⁻¹ + 1 kcal m⁻² year⁻¹ + 1 kcal m⁻² year⁻¹ + 1 kcal m⁻² year⁻¹) that is distributed between one strong link representing the 80% of the energy intake (16 kcal m⁻² year⁻¹/20 kcal m⁻² year⁻¹ = 0.8) and four weak interactions responsible for the remaining 20% of predator's intake (each one transporting the 5% of its needs). On the y-axis the cumulative number of links (l) in comparison to the total trophic interactions of the 14 food webs (M) is summarized. The majority of the links in the selected food webs are weak, and strong interactions (consisting of more than 80% of predators' intake) represent 20% of the total linkage patrimony of these ecosystems. The relationship between l/M (y) and relative link strength (x) can be approximated by the following function (with constant values: $a = 0.737$; $b = 6.238$; $c = 0.032$): $y = a * e^{-bx} + c$.

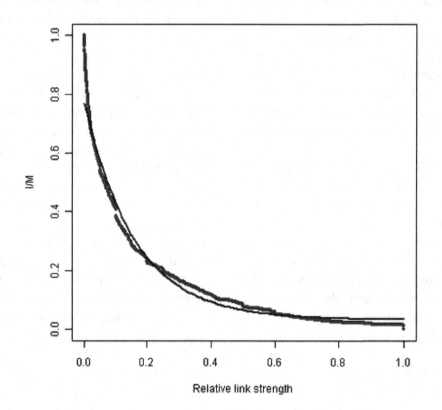

difference between AS and ES is the highest and can reach one order of magnitude (Marshes and Sloughs ecological network: $AS_{20\%} = 0.270$, $ES_{20\%} = 0.026$; Mangroves food web: $AS_{20\%} = 0.176$, $ES_{20\%} = 0.016$). For all of the food webs, when the weakest trophic relationships are filtered, the AS index tends to score close to its maximum (1, extinction of 100% of the species), while ES remains quite far from its upper threshold (0.5). This means that after the majority of weak links are removed these networks are characterized by dominator trees closer to star-like structures than linear chains.

One of the targets of ecosystem network analysis is focusing on the consequences that food web structure can have on ecosystem stability.

Knowledge of how weak links are distributed in food webs can help policy makers identify which species are more prone to extinctions. This feature could be taken into account when planning strategies of ecosystem management, or formulating best practices for biodiversity conservation. The aim of the next section is to investigate whether peculiar patterns exist to explain weak link distribution in ecosystems (*i.e.*, are weak links evenly dispersed or are they mainly restricted to a well defined subset of species?).

This approach based on the removal of all of the weaker links that enter a predator (*i.e.*, those accounting for less than a threshold of the consumer's energy supply) may have some difficulties in capturing the positive consequences of a generalist diet. Indeed, a species feeding on a lot of different prey, each contributing to a small fraction of the total predator's intake, could appear extremely endangered, while it should be described as very well buffered against fluctuations. Such a kind of extreme situation was never realized in the empirical food webs studied in this work. However, future studies should deal with this inconsistency, by analyzing the threshold of a cumulative energy supply provided by multiple links, rather than considering them as separate entities. With this amended version, species that depend mainly on a single resource would be defined as more fragile and prone to risks of secondary extinction. A more comprehensive analysis of the flow structure in food webs is described in the next session, where the effective redundancy of prey links entering each predator is quantified by the average mutual information (AMI, henceforth; Ulanowicz, 2004). This index measures the heterogeneity of predator-prey relationships: the fewer links one node has, and/or the more skewed the distribution of their magnitude, the higher the AMI is for that node. In the next session I investigate whether the food web structure of the links entering each predator (estimated with AMI) is organized in a gradient of trophic positions from producers to consumers.

The Skewed Distribution of Weak Links towards the Trophic Chain

Trophic links trace who eats whom in ecosystems and consequently the species' feeding habits represents a major determinant of food web structure. Sorting species' feeding activity gives rise to the trophic structure of the community. Given these premises, one interesting question is investigating the relationship between trophic structure and link arrangement in food webs (*i.e.*, understanding whether link disposition forms patterns that are characteristically associated to the trophic structure, and whether these patterns hold across ecosystems).

I reconstructed the trophic structure of the 14 food webs by calculating every species' trophic position (TP, henceforth; Kercher & Shugart 1975; Cousins, 1987; Polis & Strong 1996), which gives a view of the average number of steps that energy travels from producers to consumers, without describing the way links are associated to the nodes. Then, I analyzed link arrangement using the average mutual information, which depends on the number of links targeted to each node weighted by their magnitude. AMI measures the contribution that each compartment, through its trophic connections and their strength, gives to the organization of the food web.

Ranking communities through the trophic position of their species yields a continuous trophic spectrum that defines a hierarchy from producers to consumers (van der Zanden *et al.*, 1997; Bondavalli & Ulanowicz, 1999). Conceptually, TP comes out from apportioning each species' feeding activity to a series of discrete trophic levels (Lindeman, 1942) and summing up these fractions. Its computation is made possible by a suite of different techniques that are essentially based on matrix manipulations; in this chapter I used the following three methods: (1) the canonical trophic aggregation (CTA, Ulanowicz & Kemp, 1979; Scotti *et al.*, 2006); (2) the network unfolding approach (Higashi *et al.*, 1989) and

(3) the path-based network unfolding algorithm (Whipple, 1998). The main difference between the three methods concerns the way they treat diet partitioning in ecosystems containing cycles, non-living matter storages (*i.e.*, detrital components) and their accompanying non-trophic flows (*i.e.*, decay, egestion, excretion). For the sake of simplicity I labeled the three indices of trophic position as C (canonical trophic aggregation), H (original matrix-based network unfolding) and W (path-based network unfolding).

TP is computed as the weighted average length of all the pathways from the primary source of energy to any species. Consider a species that bases 20% of its diet on primary producers, being thus a herbivore for this fraction, and the remaining 80% on herbivores, acting here as a primary carnivore; its TP would be $2 \times 0.2 + 3 \times 0.8 = 2.8$. The integer numbers that appear in this calculation label trophic levels and count exactly the number of steps energy travels before arriving at the species (primary producers have TP = 1, because they rely on solar energy and energy travels a pathway of length one: outside → primary producer; herbivores are at level 2 because energy travels a pathway of length two: outside → primary producer → herbivore to reach them, and so forth). So diet fractions are apportioned to the corresponding trophic levels.

AMI estimates the average amount of constraints exerted upon an arbitrary unit of currency when passing from any one species to the next (Rutledge *et al.*, 1976; Ulanowicz, 1986). Both the number of links and their magnitude determine this measure, and AMI is adopted, in the present study, as an index for measuring linkage density. For a single component AMI is similar to the Ulanowicz's effective connectance (m in Ulanowicz & Wolff, 1991) and Bersier's link density (LD, in Bersier *et al.*, 2002). Suffice here to say that effective connectance and link density are computed by averaging the diversity of inputs and outputs for every node, whereas in this study I kept the two contributions separate. In practice for each node I

calculated its AMI based on incoming links first, thus considering it as a predator, and then using outgoing links, viewing the node as a prey. This approach was more appropriate than computing AMI as the average contribution of incoming and outgoing links, because TP classifies each species according to its feeding behavior (*i.e.*, it considers it in its role of consumer). I framed the analysis into two schemes. One, called "AMI-living", in which computation of AMI was done using trophic links (predator-prey) only; the second, called "AMI-whole", in which this index included also the contribution of non-trophic transfers. The two schemes provide a means for comparison of the outcomes when TPs are computed with (original matrix-based network unfolding, and path-based network unfolding algorithms) and without non-trophic links (canonical trophic aggregation).

For each ecosystem I estimated Spearman's correlation coefficients (ρ) between TP and AMI, using both unweighted and weighted data. The way I calculated TP and AMI emphasized different scenarios for the analysis. I considered the nodes in their role of prey (AMI based on outgoing links, OUTPUT scenario) and predator (AMI based on incoming links, INPUT scenario). For each scheme I compared "AMI-living" and "AMI-whole" with TP. In particular, I conceived the following combinations for these indices: C vs. "AMI-living" only, and both H and W with "AMI-whole", as they reflect the coherence in the way indices are computed. So, it seemed reasonable to couple CTA, which calculates species' trophic position on the basis of trophic links only, with "AMI-living" that also makes use of trophic links. On the other hand, both W and H compute trophic positions by including also non-trophic links; accordingly they have been associated with the "AMI-whole" in the correlation analysis.

Overall, weak correlations were observed between AMI and TP when using unweighted data (Figure 5a-b). In two cases the positive association between trophic position and linkage density was clear enough (*i.e.*, those reported under the INPUT scenario for H - $\mu = 0.501$, $\sigma = 0.205$; W - $\mu = 0.619$, $\sigma = 0.166$; see Figure 5a). These coefficients, however, were lower than the corresponding values estimated with weighted data (Figure 5c; H - $\mu = 0.617$, $\sigma = 0.308$ and W - $\mu = 0.723$, $\sigma = 0.289$). In the other cases, average coefficients, either positive (under the INPUT scenario: C - $\mu = 0.067$, $\sigma = 0.236$) or negative (under the OUTPUT scenario: C - $\mu = -0.215$, $\sigma = 0.197$; H - $\mu = -0.071$, $\sigma = 0.223$; W - $\mu = -0.089$, $\sigma = 0.216$), were close to zero, and no correlation emerged between trophic position and linkage density.

TP and AMI in weighted food webs correlated differently in comparison with their unweighted counterparts (Figure 5c-d). Very high correlations were observed between AMI based on incoming links and TP, no matter which form was used for computing the two metrics (Figure 5c). Most of the positive correlations were significant, although there were differences between the single scenarios. When TP was estimated using CTA, and AMI computed without the contribution of non-trophic links, the positive correlation was extremely clear (C - $\mu = 0.857$, $\sigma = 0.092$). The other two indices of trophic position (H and W) did not perform as well as CTA when compared to their AMI counterpart, and the intensity of the association was less pronounced. The same analysis performed with AMI based on outgoing links produced irregularly scattered points, which resulted in absence of any correlation (C - $\mu = 0.144$, $\sigma = 0.236$; H - $\mu = -0.078$, $\sigma = 0.262$; W - $\mu = -0.051$, $\sigma = 0.245$; see Figure 5d).

In summary, when the species are considered in their role as predators, a strong positive association between linkage density (AMI) and trophic position emerges. This association vanishes when

Figure 5. Box plots of correlation coefficients (Spearman's rho) for TP (C = canonical trophic aggregation; H = original matrix-based network unfolding method; W = path-based trophic unfolding method) vs. AMI (on inflows left diagrams, on outflows right plots). Box plots in (a) and (b) refer to unweighted food webs, while weighted data are used for constructing charts in (c) and (d).

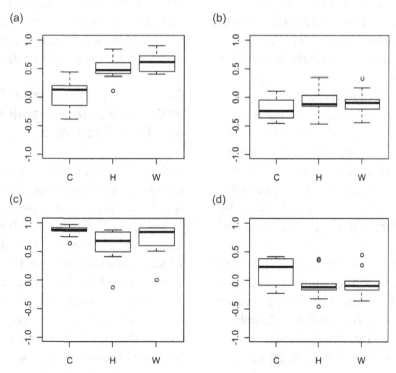

AMI is computed using outgoing links (*i.e.*, when species are seen in their role as prey).

The fewer links one node has, and/or the more skewed the distribution of their magnitude, the higher the AMI is for that node. Thus, the positive correlation observed between AMI and TP in the weighted food webs under the INPUT scenario indicates that links entering a node are fewer and/or total inflow more unevenly distributed among links for species that feed higher in the food chain. According to this, species that occupy higher trophic position tend towards diet specialization whereas a more generalist alimentary behavior would be common at the bottom of the trophic spectrum. This pattern holds across ecosystems and is irrespective of the way one calculates the trophic position. It is possible that diet specialization may prevent top species from competition, but this cannot be inferred from our results.

The absence of correlation between AMI and TP when the effect of link strength is removed would indicate that trophic links are not distributed according to a specific pattern and would be equally distributed between basal and top species. On the other hand, the negative correlation found in certain ecosystems indicates that predators would establish more connections than basal species.

Overall, by combining the results obtained for weighted and non-weighted webs one can infer that top species would possess the same or greater number of trophic links than species feeding lower in the food chain, but most of these connections are weak in magnitude and the skewed link magnitude would be responsible for lower link density of top species in weighted food webs. Moving towards the top of the trophic hierarchy we would encounter fewer stronger links dispersed in many weak links.

Evidences accumulated in the literature about link distribution and interaction strength are mostly in favor of a strong skew towards weaker interactions (McCann *et al.*, 1998, Sala & Graham 2002; Emmerson & Yearsley 2004). The results presented here provide further insight because

such skewness seems to be in relation with the gradient of trophic positions and more pronounced at the top of the trophic hierarchy.

This evidence on the skewed distribution of weak links towards the trophic chain can be associated to the modeling perspective introduced with the dominator tree algorithm. Food web fragility seems to be more pronounced at the upper limit of the trophic hierarchy, and the multiplicity of weak links in the top-predators' diets poses serious concerns on the stability of their energy intake.

Although these results could be biased by the strict bottom-up perspective characterizing the dominator tree algorithm, they clearly describe structural features that are common to the majority of food webs analyzed. These findings are also in agreement with studies conducted on dynamics-based models that revealed how the loss of species from lower trophic levels would cause greater risk of losing additional species (Borrvall *et al.*, 2000): primary extinctions of species with lower trophic levels are expected to increase the risks of halting energy delivery to top predators. In the next section I describe the case study of the Prince William Sound food web. I rank species importance using the dominator tree algorithm and compare these topological outcomes with results inferred from stochastic simulations.

Case Study: Dominator Trees and Stochastic Dynamics of a Real Food Web

In this section I illustrate the potential of dominator tree and stochastic simulations for identifying species that play a major role in energy delivery. The case study is performed for the Prince William Sound ecosystem, a weighted food web for which interaction strength is assigned to each trophic link (Okey, 2004; Okey & Wright, 2004). The network model contains 48 living components. The non-living components (Nekton falls, Inshore Detritus, Offshore Detritus) as well as the self-loops ("cannibalistic" trophic flows) have been omitted from the model. I have included flows between living nodes as they pertain to ingestion-assimilation events (trophic flows), showing a different dynamic in comparison to transfers between living and non-living compartments (Whipple, 1998). Since the focus is on predator-prey interactions, I excluded egestive transfers (*i.e.*, flows from biotic compartments to non-living nodes or flows between non-living compartments). Also self-loops were removed as their presence does not strongly affect food web dynamics, but poses serious constraints when extracting the dominator-tree.

Figure 6 shows that the number of bottlenecks increases if the minimum and viable amount of energy that has to be transported by each single link is set to higher values. Bottlenecks are nodes upon which other species depend for their energy requirements. The higher the number of bottlenecks the greater the risk of secondary extinction. If species survival is guaranteed when they receive energy transported by strong links (those representing >20% of each species' food intake), this bulk of energy is concentrated in 56 out of the 355 original links. This energy is channeled through fundamental nodes that are not visible when all links (and pathways) are considered equivalent. In particular, these nodes are #38 (omnivorous zooplankton), #42 (shallow small epibenthos), #46 (nearshore phytoplankton) and #47 (offshore phytoplankton); their extinction would produce a cascade of secondary extinctions and they can be considered as key species in the Prince William Sound ecosystem. Among the species that are likely to cause greater damage in terms of secondary extinctions, two are primary producers (nearshore phytoplankton and offshore phytoplankton), while the other two nodes (omnivorous zooplankton and shallow small epibenthos) feed at trophic positions 2.3 and 2.1, in a food web that counts up to five trophic levels (Okey & Wright, 2004).

In the last part of this section I describe the stochastic simulations performed for the Prince William Sound food web. Many stochastic programming languages have been developed to explicitly model interactions of biological entities (*e.g.*, WSCCS and BlenX; see Tofts, 1993; Dematté *et al.*, 2008; Romanel, 2010). Here I adopted BlenX, a language implementing the Beta-binders calculus. In BlenX, biological entities are represented as boxes, which are composed of an internal program and a set of interfaces. The interaction sites on boxes are called binders; as for biological entities, a box has an interface (its set of binders) and an internal structure that drives its behavior. Internal structures of the process influence interactions of each box with other boxes, modify the interface of the process, and can also be changed by interactions through the binders. For example, when a box is used to model an individual organism, binders are characterized by different levels of affinity to interact with other species (*e.g.*, predator-prey or plant-pollinator relationships). In case of food webs, the interaction behavior is defined on the basis of relative interaction strength (*i.e.*, prey preference extracted from weighted food webs). The internal structure codifies the mechanism that transforms an input signal into demographic (*e.g.*, reproduction, death) or behavioral (*e.g.*, changed prey preference) change of individuals. Signals are represented as messages exchanged over communication channels. Once internal processes within boxes and interactions involving several boxes are represented, the system behavior emerges out of lower-level dynamics. Since the hierarchical view is implicit, it is suitable for modeling the links between different organizational levels and among interconnected, multiple, parallel processes. The propensity of communication between processes is quantified by the affinity (rate) between the different types of binders: it is a real number that measures how strong an interaction between two processes can be.

Important features of BlenX are composability, propensity to describe parallel events and the opportunity of including multiple interactions.

Figure 6. Prince William Sound ecosystem: the food web structure (a), dominator trees extracted from the binary architecture (b), and computed for the more fragile topologies that were obtained by filtering the topological configuration. Links with fractionary importance smaller than 10% (c) and 20% (d) of the predators' intake are eliminated for computing the last dominator trees. Consequently, when increasing the threshold magnitude, dominator trees possess more branches and their fragility is increased ($AS_{FW} = 0.061$; $ES_{FW} = 0.022$; $AS_{20\%} = 0.204$; $ES_{20\%} = 0.034$). Correspondence between numbers and species is as follows: 0 - "root"; 1 - Transient orca; 2 - Salmon sharks; 3 - Resident orca; 4 - Sleeper sharks; 5 - Halibut; 6 - Pinnipeds; 7 - Porpoise; 8 - Lingcod; 9 - Adult arrowtooth; 10 - Adult salmon; 11 - Pacific cod; 12 - Sablefish; 13 - Juvenile arrowtooth.; 14 - Spiny dogfish; 15 - Avian predators; 16 - Octopods; 17 - Seabirds; 18 - Deep demersals; 19 - Pollock 1+; 20 - Rockfish; 21 - Baleen whales; 22 - Salmon fry 0-12; 23 - Nearshore demersal; 24 - Squid; 25 - Eulachon; 26 - Sea otters; 27 - Deep epibenthos; 28 - Capelin; 29 - Adult herring; 30 - Pollock 0; 31 - Invertebrate-eating bird; 32 - Sandlance; 33 - Shallow large epibenthos; 34 - Juvenile herring; 35 - Jellies; 36 - Deep small infauna; 37 - Nearshore omnivorous-zooplankton; 38 - Omnivorous zooplankton; 39 - Shallow small infauna; 40 - Meiofauna; 41 - Deep large infauna; 42 - Shallow small epibenthos; 43 - Shallow large infauna; 44 - Nearshore herbivorous-zooplankton; 45 - Herbivorous-zooplankton; 46 - Nearshore phytoplankton; 47 - Offshore phytoplankton; 48 - Macroalgae/gras.

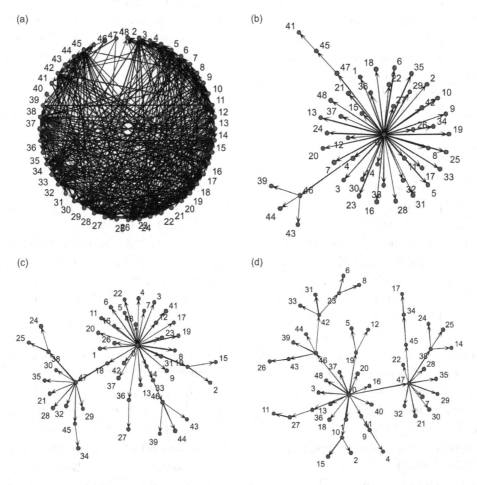

Composability refers to model construction and development. It allows the user to extend models by adding simple and modular elements instead of complete rewriting of the code. Biological events are concurrent as they often occur simultaneously. In ecology, predation and facilitation shape animal communities, but their concurrent interactions are difficult to integrate. BlenX offers an environment for modeling these parallel (*i.e.*, concurrent) events. Simulating concurrent interactions also corresponds to investigating predator-prey, plant-pollinator and host-parasite relationships under a single framework (*i.e.*, stochastic simulations). In a classical study of network analysis, these interactions should be measured by means of different currencies, reducing the opportunity of a direct comparison. All of these properties (*i.e.*, composability, concurrency and multiplicity of interactions) are relevant for modeling ecological systems.

In this case study I considered predator-prey connections only. Trophic flows extracted from the weighted food web were directly translated into interaction rates. Death rates were chosen from a realistic range (from 0.001 to 0.1, typically 0.01). Equations describing the predator-prey interaction between couples of species are:

$$A + B \xrightarrow{k1} A \tag{5}$$

$$A + B \xrightarrow{k2} 2A \tag{6}$$

In (5), the rate $k1$ defines the propensity of species A to feed on B, while in (6), the species A is preying upon B with rate $k2$, and this event is also associated to its reproduction. Once the initial scenario based on weighted food web data was set, 20 simulations on a time scale of 30 years were performed.

To test the relative importance of each species, pulse perturbations were simulated by reducing the number individuals by half, one by one, in different runs. The response function adopted

is based on a metric inspired by the Hurlbert response index (Hurlbert, 1997). In this case the comparison is done between the reference value (average population size in absence of any disturbance) and the average population density after perturbations. The absolute value of the difference is normalized by the undisturbed population size, and finally averaged by the total number of species. The importance of species i is measured as,

$$I_{H(i)}(\mu) = \sum_{j=1}^{S} \frac{\mid P_{ij}(\mu) - P_j(\mu) \mid}{P_j(\mu)} \cdot \frac{1}{S} \tag{7}$$

where S is the number of living nodes in the Prince William Sound food web ($S = 48$), $P_j(\mu)$ is the average number of individuals of species j at time t in the undisturbed scenario, and $P_{ij}(\mu)$ is the mean number of individuals of j during time t (averaged over 20 simulations) when species i was perturbed. This index is used to quantify the impact on the system emerging from a perturbation involving the target species i. Another version of the previous index is used to assess the overall response of species i to perturbations of any other species in the ecosystem:

$$I^*_{H(i)}(\mu) = \sum_{j=1}^{S} \frac{\mid P_{ji}(\mu) - P_i(\mu) \mid}{P_i(\mu)} \cdot \frac{1}{S} \tag{8}$$

with $P_i(\mu)$ as the average number of individuals of species i at time t in the reference simulation, and $P_{ji}(\mu)$ standing for the mean number of individuals of the species i (averaged over 20 simulations) when, in turn, all the other species j were perturbed.

Then, I calculated an alternative version of the same index that is based on standard deviation rather than mean values. Population standard deviation of each species, in the 20 runs of each simulation, was normalized with the mean to compute the response in terms of coefficient of variation (CV).

First, I focused on the spread of impacts that were triggered by disturbing the target species i:

$$I_{H(i)}(CV) = \sum_{j=1}^{S} \frac{|P_{ij}(CV) - P_j(CV)|}{P_j(CV)} \cdot \frac{1}{S} \tag{9}$$

where $P_j(CV)$ is the coefficient of variation for the number of individuals of species j after time t in the undisturbed scenario (ratio between the standard deviation of the population j and the absolute value of its average population; $P_j(CV) = P_j(\sigma)/|P_j(\mu)|$), while $P_{ij}(CV)$ indicates the coefficient of variation for the density of species j once the population size of i is halved.

The following equation is used for analyzing the effects of global impacts on a target species i:

$$I^*_{H(i)}(CV) = \sum_{j=1}^{S} \frac{|P_{ji}(CV) - P_i(CV)|}{P_i(CV)} \cdot \frac{1}{S} \tag{10}$$

with $P_i(CV)$ standing for the coefficient of variation computed for the population density of species i in the reference scenario (no perturbation), after time t; the coefficient of variation for the same species i is $P_{ji}(CV)$, once the population size of j has been halved.

The first index ($I_H(CV)$) estimates the global response to local changes, while the second ($I_H^*(CV)$) summarizes the local response to global changes (Table 3).

Based on the sensitivity analysis of mean values ($I_H(\mu)$, Table 3), the higher rank of importance in terms of global effects is led by shallow large infauna (#43), followed by herbivorous zooplankton (#45) and nearshore demersals (#23). These species occupy the lower levels of the trophic chain. Shallow large infauna and herbivorous zooplankton are herbivorous nodes, while the compartment called nearshore demersals is feeding at trophic positions 3.3 (Okey & Wright, 2004). The higher levels of fragility, intended as

how much species are influenced by disturbing other members of the community ($I_H^*(\mu)$, Table 3), are displayed by shallow large infauna (#43), seabirds (#17) and halibut (#5). The trophic group ranking highest with both the indices is shallow large infauna (#43). Estimating global impacts from variance-based dynamics ($I_H(CV)$) suggests shallow large infauna in the first rank. Capelin is characterized by higher fluctuations in his population density ($I_H^*(CV) = 0.599$), despite the fact that it was affected by intermediate levels of average disturbance ($I_H^*(\mu) = 0.101$). Note that halibut (#5) is one of the worst species in the I_H rankings, but it occupies leading positions in the I_H^* rankings.

Both I_H and I_H^* are higher in the middle of the trophic scale (TP of living species are extracted from Okey & Wright, 2004). All importance indices extracted using deterministic dynamics suggest either top-predators or producers to be of highest importance (Okey, 2004; Libralato *et al.*, 2006). Using the dominator tree algorithm, the removal of species feeding at lower trophic levels would result in greater risk of secondary extinction, a finding that partially matches the outcomes of dynamic analysis (*e.g.*, nearshore phytoplankton and offshore phytoplankton are ranked at higher levels when their ecosystem level impacts are obtained with stochastic simulations and measured with the coefficient of variation).

I performed the Kruskal-Wallis test to measure the differences between species rankings that are obtained with the dominator tree and using the impacts determined by local changes (simulated with the stochastic approach). Species importance estimated by the dominator tree is significantly different from the species rankings computed in terms of average global impacts ($I_H(\mu)$; $p < 0.001$) or variance ($I_H(CV)$; $p < 0.001$). Also a significant difference is found between species rankings extracted from mean values of impacts and their variance ($p < 0.001$). I repeated the same analysis to understand whether measuring the impacts affecting each species may change according to the

Table 3. For each living species of the Prince William Sound food web I summarized code number and the corresponding species (or trophic group) in the network. The third column ($D_{20\%}$) shows the number of species dominated by each node when links transporting less than 20% of the predators' food intake are removed. The last four columns illustrate results of the stochastic simulations. Effects emerging from the perturbation of target species (i.e., global responses to local impacts) are estimated using mean values ($I_H(\mu)$) and coefficients of variation ($I_H(CV)$). An alternative version makes use of mean values ($I_H^*(\mu)$) and coefficients of variation ($I_H^*(CV)$) for estimating the local responses to global impacts (i.e., consequences of perturbations involving all the species, except the target one, on the studied trophic group).

code	name	$D_{20\%}$	$I_H(\mu)$	$I_H^*(\mu)$	$I_H(CV)$	$I_H^*(CV)$
1	Transient orca	0	0.657	0.071	2.756	0.233
2	Salmon sharks	0	0.189	0.075	1.166	0.384
3	Resident orca	0	0.164	0.057	1.104	0.243
4	Sleeper sharks	0	0.107	0.049	0.870	0.243
5	Halibut	0	0.014	0.250	0.006	0.396
6	Pinnipeds	0	0.060	0.078	0.438	0.272
7	Porpoise	0	0.258	0.031	2.281	0.268
8	Lingcod	0	0.067	0.053	0.379	0.344
9	Adult arrowtooth	4	0.233	0.091	0.649	0.158
10	Adult salmon	2	0.053	0.179	0.277	0.153
11	Pacific cod	0	0.058	0.066	0.420	0.271
12	Sablefish	0	0.066	0.106	0.465	0.216
13	Juvenile arrowtooth	0	0.140	0.054	0.545	0.170
14	Spiny dogfish	0	0.168	0.209	0.262	0.178
15	Avian predators	0	0.059	0.051	0.416	0.214
16	Octopods	0	0.152	0.162	0.404	0.168
17	Seabirds	0	1.161	0.527	0.246	0.352
18	Deep demersals	0	0.000	0.000	0.000	0.000
19	Pollock 1+	2	0.132	0.125	0.405	0.287
20	Rockfish	0	0.399	0.123	0.667	0.201
21	Baleen whales	0	0.125	0.058	0.717	0.193
22	Salmon fry 0-12	0	0.055	0.038	0.802	0.270
23	Nearshore demersal	2	1.368	0.191	2.597	0.211
24	Squid	0	0.351	0.060	1.708	0.152
25	Eulachon	0	0.164	0.141	0.732	0.170
26	Sea otters	0	0.155	0.146	0.526	0.253
27	Deep epibenthos	1	0.097	0.138	0.163	0.247
28	Capelin	0	0.110	0.101	0.410	0.599
29	Adult herring	0	0.077	0.025	1.182	0.288
30	Pollock 0	0	0.520	0.070	2.341	0.196
31	Invertebrate-eating bird	0	0.038	0.064	0.418	0.300
32	Sandlance	0	0.000	0.000	0.000	0.000
33	Shallow large epibenthos	0	0.020	0.070	0.090	0.233

continues on following page

Table 3. Continued

code	name	$D_{20\%}$	$I_H(\mu)$	$I_H*(\mu)$	$I_H(CV)$	$I_H*(CV)$
34	Juvenile herring	1	0.040	0.102	0.070	0.131
35	Jellies	0	0.061	0.056	0.143	0.245
36	Deep small infauna	1	0.047	0.036	0.637	0.319
37	Near Omnivorous-zooplankton	0	0.040	0.037	0.582	0.333
38	Omnivorous-zooplankton	3	0.048	0.081	0.473	0.233
39	Shallow small infauna	0	0.783	0.199	1.368	0.165
40	Meiofauna	0	0.677	0.246	1.333	0.219
41	Deep large infauna	3	0.100	0.068	0.455	0.146
42	Shallow small epibenthos	0	0.079	0.058	0.352	0.187
43	Shallow large infauna	1	13.271	0.742	5.714	0.350
44	Near Herbivorous-zooplankton	0	0.053	0.047	0.746	0.466
45	Herbivorous-zooplankton	1	1.562	0.207	3.211	0.176
46	Nearshore phytoplankton	4	0.058	0.028	1.765	0.507
47	Offshore phytoplankton	10	0.031	0.042	0.762	0.298
48	Macroalgae/gras	0	0.103	0.074	0.522	0.276

way this indicator is estimated. Kruskal-Wallis test revealed a significant difference ($p < 0.001$) between measuring the local response to global impacts in terms of average values ($I_H*(\mu)$) or coefficient of variation ($I_H*(CV)$).

Adopting all of these approaches (simulations, binary and weighted data), I have found a prevalence of weak interactions. Performing structural analyses I have observed the prevalence of bottom-up effects, while this pattern is challenged and partially contradicted when using stochastic simulations.

CONCLUSION

As human activity threatens the functioning of ecological systems by habitat destruction, fragmentation, and possibly climate change and invasions, we face the problem of how to understand and hopefully manage the consequences of these impacts. If the goal of environmental policy actions is to preserve the food web structure for maintaining a reliable supply of ecosystem outputs, then identifying and protecting important species will be the only viable long term solution for managing biodiversity loss. This "functional" approach is complementary to classical symptomatic treatments which mainly focus on protecting rarest species. There are several kinds of key species in ecology, and a variety of studies have identified endemic, dominant, link, indicator, invasive, introduced, reintroduced and keystone species (Dale & Beyeler, 2001); conservation biologists also consider umbrella, charismatic and flagship species (Simberloff, 1998).

The aim of this chapter is to provide an alternative perspective, based on food web analysis, for identifying species that play a major role in energy delivery and are likely to cause the greatest damage if removed. Risks of secondary extinctions, spread of indirect effects, and persistence and resilience of the community were described using weighted data, making a comparison with classical analyses based on unweighted food webs and introducing a stochastic-based approach for the dynamics. I emphasized how exploring the distribution of weak interactions may provide further insight on food web functioning and processes of community assembly. Food webs are inherently complex, and with the choice of a single algorithm there is the risk to neglect the role played by certain species, or the network fragility. In this framework, the dominator tree model provides an elegant way to understand and predict which species are essential for the survival of others. It does this by unfolding food-web structures into linear pathways that are essential for energy delivery. Binary food webs are special representations of networks with uniform distribution of interaction strength. When thresholds are imposed to select links based on their magnitude, most of the links are removed for relatively low values. Weak links are unevenly distributed towards the trophic chain and this would affect risks of secondary extinctions as predicted by the dominator tree (*i.e.*, top predators seem to be more prone to experiencing energy intake collapse than intermediate species). Applications of stochastic, individual-based modeling are helpful when large differences between individuals are likely to occur. With heterogeneous population dynamics (*e.g.*, size-overfishing; Okey *et al.*, 2004), deterministic models based on the hypothesis of homogeneous population dynamics can be misleading. These scenarios call for novel conceptual and computational tools capturing demographic noise and local interactions in the case of small populations, both of which are accounted for in stochastic simulations.

FUTURE RESEARCH DIRECTIONS

Studying positions of nodes in food webs may be a key to better understand community dynamics, helping to identify structurally important species which should deserve particular attention in conservation practices. For example, epibenthos species may be functionally much more important than rare and charismatic megafauna, and their protection may have tremendous direct and indirect positive effects on ecosystem integrity

(a feature that could also indirectly support rare species). How to set conservation priorities is an enduring question (Mace & Collar, 2002): future conservation biology should probably focus more on *"the little things that run the world"* (Wilson, 1987), if they are in special network position. This static system perspective should be updated with dynamic simulations. In food web analyses, there is the need to improve stochastic modeling for better understanding demographic noise and local interactions, especially in case of small populations. Stochasticity is not a source of unpredictability and randomness; rather, it represents a set of various unknown or unmodeled processes, producing higher-level patterns (Clark, 2009). Ecosystem management would benefit from novel computational tools that allow researchers to extend stochastic-based dynamics towards spatial and temporal simulations. Results extracted from these analyses could serve for suggesting best strategies of environmental sustainability, and planning actions for biodiversity conservation. The BlenX model proposed in this chapter could be further implemented using mathematical functions to set the propensity of communication between species. Currently, constant rates are adopted to define the propensities of trophic relationships between species. I argue that next studies should consider different mathematical formulations, replacing constant rates with Holling's functional responses (Holling, 1965). Other methods could be adopted for refining the simplistic way used to model predator behavior. In the stochastic analysis presented here, two rates are supplied for describing the trophic activities of consumers: the first stands for "eat" (5), while the second refers to "eat and reproduce" (6). A more realistic modification should classify each population in terms of hungry individuals, who are actively involved in feeding, and sated individuals, who are not and can reproduce (Powell & Boland, 2009). Another aspect that should be investigated concerns the effects of using different perturbation techniques to perform sensitivity analysis. Instead of disturbing the species by reducing their population abundance, the consequences of a decline in the reproduction rates could be tested (Okey, 2004).

Novel computational methods do not compete with the more traditional ones but can complement them if particular questions need particular answers. Classical topological analyses may be useful for revealing general principles of ecosystem organization. Using weighted data and introducing stochastic simulations may help considering the rarity and noisy behavior of the smallest populations to protect. I emphasize that both of these perspectives should be taken into account when dealing with complex topics as biodiversity conservation and ecosystem management.

ACKNOWLEDGMENT

I am grateful to Ferenc Jordán, Paola Lecca, Davide Prandi, Federica Ciocchetta, Tommaso Mazza, Alessandro Romanel, Michele Forlin and Bianca Baldacci for their help and cooperation. Melissa J. Morine is acknowledged for checking the language. Three anonymous reviewers are acknowledged for their useful comments.

REFERENCES

Albert, R., Jeong, H., & Barabási, A. L. (2000). Error and attack tolerance of complex networks. *Nature, 406*, 378–381. doi:10.1038/35019019

Allesina, S., Alonso, D., & Pascual, M. (2008). A General Model for Food Web Structure. *Science, 320*(5876), 658–661. doi:10.1126/science.1156269

Allesina, S., & Bodini, A. (2004). Who dominates whom in the ecosystem? Energy flow bottlenecks and cascading extinctions. *Journal of Theoretical Biology, 230*, 351–358. doi:10.1016/j.jtbi.2004.05.009

Allesina, S., & Bodini, A. (2005). Food web networks: Scaling relation revisited. *Ecological Complexity, 2*, 323–338. doi:10.1016/j.ecocom.2005.05.001

Arreguin-Sanchez, F., Arcos, E., & Chavez, E. A. (2002). Flows of biomass and structure in an exploited benthic ecosystem in the gulf of California, Mexico. *Ecological Modelling, 156*, 167–183. doi:10.1016/S0304-3800(02)00159-X

Baird, D., Luczkovich, J. J., & Christian, R. R. (1998). Assessment of spatial and temporal variability in ecosystem attributes of the St Marks National Wildlife Refuge, Apalachee Bay, Florida. *Estuarine, Coastal and Shelf Science, 47*, 329–349. doi:10.1006/ecss.1998.0360

Baird, D., & Ulanowicz, R. E. (1989). The seasonal dynamics of the Chesapeake Bay ecosystem. *Ecological Monographs, 59*, 329–364. doi:10.2307/1943071

Banavar, J. R., Maritan, A., & Rinaldo, A. (1999). Size and form in efficient transportation networks. *Nature, 399*, 130–132. doi:10.1038/20144

Bascompte, J.,[REMOVED HYPERLINK FIELD] & Jordano, P. (2007). Plant-Animal Mutualistic Networks: The Architecture of Biodiversity. *Annual Review of Ecology Evolution and Systematics, 38*, 567–593. doi:10.1146/annurev.ecolsys.38.091206.095818

Berkes, F. (2004). Rethinking community-based conservation. *Conservation Biology, 18*, 621–630. doi:10.1111/j.1523-1739.2004.00077.x

Berlow, E. L. (1999). Strong effects of weak interactions in ecological communities. *Nature, 398*, 330–334. doi:10.1038/18672

Berlow, E. L., Dunne, J. A., Martinez, N. D., Stark, P. B., Williams, R. J., & Brose, U. (2008). Simple prediction of interaction strengths in complex food webs. *Proceedings of the National Academy of Sciences of the United States of America, 106*, 187–191. doi:10.1073/pnas.0806823106

Berlow, E. L., Neutel, A.-M., Cohen, J. E., de Ruiter, P. C., Ebenman, B., & Emmerson, M. (2004). Interaction strengths in food webs: issues and opportunities. *Journal of Animal Ecology, 73,* 585–598. doi:10.1111/j.0021-8790.2004.00833.x

Bersier, L.F., Banašek-Richter, C., & Cattin, M.F. (2002). Quantitative descriptors of food-web matrices. *Ecology, 83,* 2394–2407. doi:10.1890/0012-9658(2002)083[2394:QDOFWM]2.0.CO;2

Bersier, L.-F., Dixon, P., & Sugihara, G. (1999). Scale-invariant or scale-dependent behavior of the link density property in food webs: A matter of sampling effort? *American Naturalist, 153,* 676–682. doi:10.1086/303200

Björnstad, O. N., Fromentin, J. M., Stenseth, N. C., & Gjøsæter, J. (1999). Cycles and trends in cod populations. *Proceedings of the National Academy of Sciences of the United States of America, 96,* 5066–5071. doi:10.1073/pnas.96.9.5066

Bodini, A., Bellingeri, M., Allesina, S., & Bondavalli, C. (2009). Using food web dominator trees to catch secondary extinctions in action. *Philosophical Transactions of the Royal Society of London. Series B, Biological Sciences, 364*(1524), 1725–1731. doi:10.1098/rstb.2008.0278

Bondavalli, C., Bodini, A., Rossetti, G., & Allesina, S. (2006). Detecting stress at a whole ecosystem level. The case of a mountain lake: Lake Santo (Italy). *Ecosystems (New York, N.Y.), 9,* 1–56. doi:10.1007/s10021-005-0065-y

Bondavalli, C., & Ulanowicz, R. E. (1999). Unexpected effects of predators upon their prey: The case of the American alligator. *Ecosystems (New York, N.Y.), 2,* 49–63. doi:10.1007/s100219900057

Bonsall, M. B., & Hastings, A. (2004). Demographic and environmental stochasticity in predator-prey metapopulation dynamics. *Journal of Animal Ecology, 73,* 1043–1055. doi:10.1111/j.0021-8790.2004.00874.x

Borrvall, C., Ebenman, B., & Jonsson, T. (n.d.). (200). Biodiversity lessens the risk of cascading extinction in model food webs. *Ecology Letters, 3,* 131–136. doi:10.1046/j.1461-0248.2000.00130.x

Botter, G., Settin, T., Marani, M., & Rinaldo, A. (2006). A stochastic model of nitrate transport and cycling at basin scale. *Water Resources Research, 42,* W04415. doi:10.1029/2005WR004599

Camacho, J., Guimerà, R., & Amaral, L. A. N. (2002). Robust patterns in food web structure. *Physical Review Letters, 88,* 228102. doi:10.1103/PhysRevLett.88.228102

Case, T. J., & Mark, L. (2000). Taper Interspecific Competition, Environmental Gradients, Gene Flow, and the Coevolution of Species' Borders. *American Naturalist, 155*(5), 583–605. doi:10.1086/303351

Cattin, M. F., & Bersier, L.-F., Banašek-Richter, C., Baltensperger, R., & Gabriel, J.-P. (2004). Phylogenetic constraints and adaptation explain food-web structure. *Nature, 427,* 835–839. doi:10.1038/nature02327

Christensen, V., & Walters, C. J. (2004). Ecopath with Ecosim: methods, capabilities and limitations. *Ecological Modelling, 172,* 109–139. doi:10.1016/j.ecolmodel.2003.09.003

Clark, J. S. (2009). Beyond neutral science. *Trends in Ecology & Evolution, 24,* 8–15. doi:10.1016/j.tree.2008.09.004

Cohen, J. E. (1978). *Food Webs and Niche Space.* Princeton University Press.

Cohen, J. E., Beaver, R. A., Cousins, S. H., DeAngelis, D. L., Goldwasser, L., & Heong, K. L. (1993). Improving food webs. *Ecology, 74,* 252–258. doi:10.2307/1939520

Cohen, J. E., Briand, F., & Newman, C. M. (Eds.). (1990). *Community Food Webs: Data and Theory. (Biomathematics).* Springer-Verlag.

Cohen, J. E., & Newman, C. M. (1985). A stochastic theory of community food webs. I. Models and aggregated data. *Proceedings of the Royal Society of London. Series B. Biological Sciences, 224*, 421–448. doi:10.1098/rspb.1985.0042

Cousins, S. H. (1987). The decline of the trophic level concept. *Trends in Ecology & Evolution, 2*, 312–316. doi:10.1016/0169-5347(87)90086-3

Dale, V. H., & Beyeler, S. C. (2001). Challenges in the development and use of ecological indicators. *Ecological Indicators, 1*, 3–10. doi:10.1016/S1470-160X(01)00003-6

Dematté, L., Larcher, R., Palmisano, A., Priami, C., & Romanel, A. (2010). Programming Biology in BlenX. In Choi, S. (Ed.), *Systems Biology for Signaling Networks 1* (pp. 777–820). New York: Springer. doi:10.1007/978-1-4419-5797-9_31

Dematté, L., Priami, C., & Romanel, A. (2008). The Beta Workbench: a computational tool to study the dynamics of biological systems. *Briefings in Bioinformatics, 9*(5), 437–449. doi:10.1093/bib/bbn023

Dunne, J. A., Williams, R. J., & Martinez, N. D. (2002a). Food-web structure and network theory: the role of connectance and size. *Proceedings of the National Academy of Sciences of the United States of America, 99*, 12917–12922. doi:10.1073/pnas.192407699

Dunne, J. A., Williams, R. J., & Martinez, N. D. (2002b). Network structure and biodiversity loss in food webs: Robustness increases with connectance. *Ecology Letters, 5*, 558–567. doi:10.1046/j.1461-0248.2002.00354.x

Dunne, J. A., Williams, R. J., & Martinez, N. D. (2004). Network structure and robustness of marine food webs. *Marine Ecology Progress Series, 273*, 291–302. doi:10.3354/meps273291

Ebenman, B., & Jonsson, T. (2005). Using community viability analysis to identify fragile systems and keystone species. *Trends in Ecology & Evolution, 20*, 568–575. doi:10.1016/j.tree.2005.06.011

Eklöf, A. & Ebenman, B. (2006). Species loss and secondary extinctions in simple and complex model

Elser, J. J., Sterner, R. W., Gorokhova, E., Fagan, W. F., Markow, T. A., & Cotner, J. B. (2000). Biological stoichiometry from genes to ecosystems. *Ecology Letters, 3*, 540–550. doi:10.1046/j.1461-0248.2000.00185.x

Emmerson, M., & Yearsley, J. M. (2004). Weak interactions, omnivory and emergent food-web properties. *Proceedings. Biological Sciences, 271*, 397–405. doi:10.1098/rspb.2003.2592

Fath, B. D., & Patten, B. C. (1999). Review of the foundations of network environ analysis. *Ecosystems (New York, N.Y.), 2*, 167–179. doi:10.1007/s100219900067

Finn, J. T. (1976). Measures of ecosystem structure and function derived from analysis of flows. *Journal of Theoretical Biology, 56*, 363–380. doi:10.1016/S0022-5193(76)80080-X

Fussmann, G. F., Loreau, M., & Abrams, P. A. (2007). Eco-evolutionary dynamics of communities and ecosystems. *Functional Ecology, 21*(3), 465.477.

Garlaschelli, D., Caldarelli, G., & Pietronero, L. (2003). Universal scaling relations in food webs. *Nature, 423*, 165–168. doi:10.1038/nature01604

Goldwasser, L., & Roughgarden, J. (1997). Sampling effects and estimation of food-web properties. *Ecology, 78*, 41–54. doi:10.1890/0012-9658(1997)078[0041:SEATEO]2.0.CO;2

Hannon, B. (1973). The structure of ecosystems. *Journal of Theoretical Biology, 41*, 535–546. doi:10.1016/0022-5193(73)90060-X

Hannon, B. (1986). Ecosystem control theory. *Journal of Theoretical Biology, 121,* 417–437. doi:10.1016/S0022-5193(86)80100-X

Heymans, J. J., Ulanowicz, R. E., & Bondavalli, C. (2002). Network analysis of the South Florida Everglades Gramminoid Marshes and comparison with nearby Cypress ecosystems. *Ecological Modelling, 149,* 5–23. doi:10.1016/S0304-3800(01)00511-7

Higashi, M., Burns, T. P., & Patten, B. C. (1989). Food network unfolding - an extension of trophic dynamics for application to natural ecosystems. *Journal of Theoretical Biology, 140,* 243–261. doi:10.1016/S0022-5193(89)80132-8

Holling, C. S. (1965). The functional response of predator to prey density and its role in mimicry and population regulation. *Memoirs of the Entomological Society of Canada, 45,* 1–60. doi:10.4039/entm9745fv

Hughes, A. R., Inouye, B. D., Johnson, M. T. J., Underwood, N., & Vellend, M. (2008). Ecological consequences of genetic diversity. *Ecology Letters, 11,* 609–623. doi:10.1111/j.1461-0248.2008.01179.x

Hurlbert, S. H. (1997). Functional importance vs. keystoneness: reformulating some questions in theoretical biocenology. *Australian Journal of Ecology, 22,* 369–382. doi:10.1111/j.1442-9993.1997.tb00687.x

Jordán, F. (2009). Keystone species and food webs. *Philosophical Transactions of the Royal Society of London. Series B, Biological Sciences, 364*(1524), 1733–1741. doi:10.1098/rstb.2008.0335

Jordán, F., Liu, W., & Davis, A. J. (2006). Topological keystone species: measures of positional importance in food webs. *Oikos, 112,* 535–546. doi:10.1111/j.0030-1299.2006.13724.x

Jordán, F., & Scheuring, I. (2002). Searching for keystones in ecological networks. *Oikos, 99,* 607–612. doi:10.1034/j.1600-0706.2002.11889.x

Jordán, F., Takács-Sánta, A., & Molnár, I. (1999). A reliability theoretical quest for keystones. *Oikos, 86,* 453–462. doi:10.2307/3546650

Kaitala, V., Ranta, E., & Lindstroem, J. (1996). Cyclic population dynamics and random perturbations. *Journal of Animal Ecology, 65,* 249–251. doi:10.2307/5728

Kenny, D., & Loehle, C. (1991). Are food webs randomly connected? *Ecology, 72,* 1794–1799. doi:10.2307/1940978

Kercher, J. R., & Shugart, H. H. (1975). Trophic structure, effective trophic position, and connectivity in food webs. *American Naturalist, 109,* 191–206. doi:10.1086/282986

Kokkoris, G. D., Troumbis, A. Y., & Lawton, J. H. (1999). Patterns of species interaction strength in assembled theoretical competition communities. *Ecology Letters, 2,* 70–74. doi:10.1046/j.1461-0248.1999.22058.x

Kolasa, J. (2005). Complexity, system integration, and susceptibility to change: biodiversity connection. *Ecological Complexity, 2,* 431–442. doi:10.1016/j.ecocom.2005.05.002

Lande, R., Engen, S., & Swether, B.-E. (2003). *Stochastic population dynamics in ecology and conservation.* Oxford, UK: Oxford University Press. doi:10.1093/acprof:oso/9780198525257.001.0001

Lengauer, T., & Tarjan, R. E. (1979). A fast algorithm for finding dominators in a flowgraph. *ACM Transactions on Programming Languages Systems, 1,* 121–141. doi:10.1145/357062.357071

Levin, S. A. (1998). Ecosystems and the biosphere as complex adaptive systems. *Ecosystems (New York, N.Y.), 1,* 431–436. doi:10.1007/s100219900037

Levin, S. A., Grenfell, B., Hastings, A., & Perelson, A. S. (1997). Mathematical and computational challenges in population biology and ecosystems science. *Science*, *275*, 334–343. doi:10.1126/science.275.5298.334

Libralato, S., Christensen, V., & Pauly, D. (2006). A method for identifying keystone species in food web models. *Ecological Modelling*, *195*, 153–171. doi:10.1016/j.ecolmodel.2005.11.029

Lindeman, R. (1942). The trophic-dynamic aspect of ecology. *Ecology*, *23*, 399–418. doi:10.2307/1930126

Lundberg, P., Ranta, E., & Kaitala, V. (2000). Species loss leads to community closure. *Ecology Letters*, *3*, 465–468. doi:10.1046/j.1461-0248.2000.00170.x

MacArthur, R. H. (1955). Fluctuations of animal populations and a measure of community stability. *Ecology*, *36*, 533–536. doi:10.2307/1929601

Mace, G. M., & Collar, N. J. (2002). Priority-setting in species conservation. In Norris, K., & Pain, D. J. (Eds.), *Conserving bird biodiversity* (pp. 61–73). Cambridge, UK: Cambridge University Press. doi:10.1017/CBO9780511606304.005

Margalef, R. (1968). *Perspectives in ecological theory*. University of Chicago Press.

Martinez, N. D., Hawkins, B. A., Dawah, H. A., & Feifarek, B. P. (1999). Effects of sampling effort on characterization of food-web structure. *Ecology*, *80*, 1044–1055. doi:10.1890/0012-9658(1999)080[1044:EOSEOC]2.0.CO;2

May, R. M. (1983). The structure of foodwebs. *Nature*, *301*, 566–568. doi:10.1038/301566a0

May, R. M., Beddington, J. R., Clark, C. W., Holt, S. J., & Laws, R. M. (1979). Management of multispecies fisheries. *Science*, *205*, 267–277. doi:10.1126/science.205.4403.267

McCann, K., Hastings, A., & Huxel, G. R. (1998). Weak trophic interactions and the balance of nature. *Nature*, *395*, 794–798. doi:10.1038/27427

Monaco, M. E., & Ulanowicz, R. E. (1997). Comparative ecosystem trophic structure of three U.S. mid-Atlantic estuaries. *Marine Ecology Progress Series*, *161*, 239–254. doi:10.3354/meps161239

Montoya, J. M., & Solé, R. V. (2002). Small world patterns in food webs. *Journal of Theoretical Biology*, *214*, 405–412. doi:10.1006/jtbi.2001.2460

Montoya, J. M., & Solé, R. V. (2003). Topological properties of food webs: from real data to community assembly models. *Oikos*, *102*, 614–622. doi:10.1034/j.1600-0706.2003.12031.x

Nisbet, R. M., & Gurney, W. S. C. (1982). *Modelling fluctuating populations*. New York: John Wiley & Sons.

NSF. (1999). *Decision-making and Valuation for Environmental Policy. NSF Bulletin 99-14*. Ballston, VA: National Science Foundation.

Odum, E. P. (1969). The strategy of ecosystem development. *Science*, *164*, 262–270. doi:10.1126/science.164.3877.262

Okey, T. A. (2004). *Shifted community states in four marine ecosystems: some potential mechanisms*. Unpublished doctoral dissertation, University of British Columbia, Vancouver, Canada.

Okey, T. A., Banks, S., Born, A. R., Bustamante, R. H., Calvopina, M., & Edgar, G. J. (2004). A trophic model of a Galápagos subtidal rocky reef for evaluating fisheries and conservation strategies. *Ecological Modelling*, *172*, 383–401. doi:10.1016/j.ecolmodel.2003.09.019

Okey, T. A., & Wright, B. A. (2004). Toward ecosystem-based extraction policies for Prince William Sound, Alaska: Integrating conflicting objectives and rebuilding pinnipeds. *Bulletin of Marine Science*, *74*, 727–747.

Paine, R. T. (1992). Food-web analysis through field measurement of per capita interaction strength. *Nature, 355,* 73–75. doi:10.1038/355073a0

Patrício, J., Ulanowicz, R. E., Pardal, M. A., & Marques, J. C. (2004). Ascendency as an ecological indicator: a case study of estuarine pulse eutrophication. *Estuarine, Coastal and Shelf Science, 60,* 23–35. doi:10.1016/j.ecss.2003.11.017

Pimm, S. L. (1980). Food web design and the effect of species deletion. *Oikos, 35,* 139–149. doi:10.2307/3544422

Pimm, S. L., Lawton, J. H., & Cohen, J. E. (1991). Food web patterns and their consequences. *Nature, 350,* 669–674. doi:10.1038/350669a0

Platt, T. C., Mann, K. H., & Ulanowicz, R. E. (1981). *Mathematical Models in Biological Oceanography.* Paris, France: UNESCO Press.

Polis, G., & Winemiller, K. (1995). *Food Webs: Integration of Patterns and Dynamics.* New York: Chapman and Hall.

Polis, G. A., & Strong, D. R. (1996). Food web complexity and community dynamics. *American Naturalist, 147,* 813–846. doi:10.1086/285880

Powell, C. R., & Boland, R. P. (2009). The effects of stochastic population dynamics on food web structure. *Journal of Theoretical Biology, 257,* 170–180. doi:10.1016/j.jtbi.2008.11.006

Priami, C. (2009). Algorithmic systems biology. *CACM, 52,* 80–88.

Proulx, S. R., Promislow, D. E. L., & Phillips, P. C. (2005). Network thinking in ecology and evolution. *Trends in Ecology & Evolution, 20,* 345–353. doi:10.1016/j.tree.2005.04.004

Quince, C., Higgs, P. G., & McKane, A. J. (2005). Deleting species from model food webs. *Oikos, 110,* 283–296. doi:10.1111/j.0030-1299.2005.13493.x

Rasmussen, P. E., Goulding, K. W. T., Brown, J. R., Grace, P. R., Janzen, H. H., & Körschens, M. (1998). Long-term agroecosystem experiments: assessing agricultural sustainability and global change. *Science, 282,* 893–896. doi:10.1126/science.282.5390.893

Regev, A., & Shapiro, E. (2002). Cells as computations. *Nature, 419,* 343. doi:10.1038/419343a

Renshaw, E. (1993). *Modelling biological populations in space and time.* Cambridge, UK: Cambridge University Press.

Ripa, J., & Ives, A. R. (2003). Food web dynamics in correlated and autocorrelated environments. *Theoretical Population Biology, 64,* 369–384. doi:10.1016/S0040-5809(03)00089-3

Romanel, A. (2010). *Dynamic Biological Modelling: a language-based approach.* Unpublished doctoral dissertation, University of Trento, Italy.

Rutledge, R. W., Basorre, B. L., & Mulholland, R. J. (1976). Ecological stability: an information theory viewpoint. *Journal of Theoretical Biology, 57,* 355–371. doi:10.1016/0022-5193(76)90007-2

Sala, E., & Graham, M. H. (2002). Community-wide distribution of predator-prey interaction strength in kelp forests. *Proceedings of the National Academy of Sciences of the United States of America, 99,* 3678–3683. doi:10.1073/pnas.052028499

Scotti, M., Allesina, S., Bondavalli, C., Bodini, A., & Abarca-Arenas, L. G. (2006). Effective trophic positions in ecological acyclic networks. *Ecological Modelling, 198,* 495–505. doi:10.1016/j.ecolmodel.2006.06.005

Simberloff, D. (1998). Flagships, umbrellas, and keystones: is single-species management passé in the landscape area? *Biological Conservation, 83,* 247–257. doi:10.1016/S0006-3207(97)00081-5

Solé, R. V., & Montoya, J. M. (2001). Complexity and fragility in ecological networks. *Proceedings. Biological Sciences*, *268*, 2039–2045. doi:10.1098/rspb.2001.1767

Solow, A. R., & Beet, A. R. (1998). On lumping species in food webs. *Ecology*, *79*, 2013–2018. doi:10.1890/0012-9658(1998)079[2013:OLSIFW]2.0.CO;2

Stouffer, D. B., Camacho, J., & Amaral, L. A. N. (2006). A robust measure of food web intervality. *Proceedings of the National Academy of Sciences of the United States of America*, *103*, 19015–19020. doi:10.1073/pnas.0603844103

Tofts, C. (1993). Describing social insect behavior using process algebra. *Transactions on Social Computing Simulation*, *10*, 227–283.

Tylianakis, J. M., Tscharntke, T., & Lewis, O. T. (2007). Habitat modification alters the structure of tropical host-parasitoid food webs. *Nature*, *455*, 202–205. doi:10.1038/nature05429

Ulanowicz, R. E. (1986). *Growth & Development: Ecosystems Phenomenology*. New York: Springer Verlag.

Ulanowicz, R. E. (2004). Quantitative methods for ecological network analysis. *Computational Biology and Chemistry*, *28*(5-6), 321–339. doi:10.1016/j.compbiolchem.2004.09.001

Ulanowicz, R.E., Bondavalli, C., & Egnotovich, M.S. (1997). *Network Analysis of Trophic Dynamics in South Florida Ecosystems, FY 96: The Cypress Wetland Ecosystem*. - Tech. Rep. [UMCES] CBL 97-075, Chesapeake Biological Laboratory, Solomons.

Ulanowicz, R.E., Bondavalli, C., & Egnotovich, M.S. (1998). *Network Analysis of Trophic Dynamics in South Florida Ecosystems, FY 97: The Florida Bay Ecosystem*. - Tech. Rep. [UMCES] CBL 98-123, Chesapeake Biological Laboratory, Solomons.

Ulanowicz, R.E., Bondavalli, C., Heymans, J.J., & Egnotovich, M.S. (1999). *Network Analysis of Trophic Dynamics in South Florida Ecosystem, FY 98: The Mangrove Ecosystem*. - Tech. Rep. [UMCES] CBL 99-0073, Chesapeake Biological Laboratory, Solomons.

Ulanowicz, R.E., Heymans, J.J., & Egnotovich, M.S. (2000). *Network Analysis of Trophic Dynamics in South Florida Ecosystems FY 99: The Graminoid Ecosystem*. - Tech. Rep. [UMCES] CBL 00-0176, Chesapeake Biological Laboratory, Solomons.

Ulanowicz, R. E., & Kemp, W. M. (1979). Toward canonical trophic aggregations. *American Naturalist*, *114*, 871–883. doi:10.1086/283534

Ulanowicz, R. E., & Wolff, W. F. (1991). Ecosystem flow networks: loaded dice? *Mathematical Biosciences*, *103*, 45–68. doi:10.1016/0025-5564(91)90090-6

van der Zanden, M. J., Cabana, G., & Rasmussen, J. B. (1997). Comparing trophic position of freshwater littoral fish species using stable nitrogen isotopes (d15N) and literature dietary data. *Canadian Journal of Fisheries and Aquatic Sciences*, *54*, 1142–1158. doi:10.1139/f97-016

Walters, C., Christensen, V., & Pauly, D. (1997). Structuring dynamic models of exploited ecosystems from trophic mass-balance assessments. *Reviews in Fish Biology and Fisheries*, *7*, 139–172. doi:10.1023/A:1018479526149

Whipple, S. J. (1998). Path-based network unfolding: A solution for the problem of mixed trophic and non-trophic processes in trophic dynamic analysis. *Journal of Theoretical Biology*, *190*, 263–276. doi:10.1006/jtbi.1997.0551

Williams, R. J., & Martinez, N. D. (2000). Simple rules yield complex food webs. *Nature*, *404*, 180–183. doi:10.1038/35004572

Wilson, E. O. (1987). The little things that run the world. *Conservation Biology, 1*, 344–346. doi:10.1111/j.1523-1739.1987.tb00055.x

Woodward, G., & Hildrew, A. G. (2001). Invasion of a stream food web by a new top predator. *Journal of Animal Ecology, 70*, 273–288. doi:10.1046/j.1365-2656.2001.00497.x

Wulff, F., & Ulanowicz, R. E. (1989). A comparative anatomy of the Baltic Sea and Chesapeake Bay ecosystems. In Wulff, F., Field, J., & Mann, K. (Eds.), *Network analysis in marine ecology - methods and applications. Vol. 32 of Coastal and Estuarine Studies.* Springer-Verlag, New York.

Yodzis, P. (1989). Patterns in food webs. *Trends in Ecology & Evolution, 4*(2), 49–50. doi:10.1016/0169-5347(89)90140-7

Yodzis, P. (2001). Must top predators be culled for the sake of fisheries? *Trends in Ecology & Evolution, 16*, 78–84. doi:10.1016/S0169-5347(00)02062-0

Yodzis, P., & Winemiller, K. O. (1999). In search of operational trophospecies in a tropical aquatic food web. *Oikos, 87*, 327–340. doi:10.2307/3546748

Zetina-Rejon, M. J., Arreguin-Sanchez, F., & Chavez, E. A. (2004). Exploration of harvesting strategies for the management of a Mexican coastal lagoon fishery. *Ecological Modelling, 172*, 361–372. doi:10.1016/j.ecolmodel.2003.09.017

ADDITIONAL READING

Bertness, M. D., & Callaway, R. (1994). Positive interaction in communities. *Trends in Ecology & Evolution, 9*, 191–193. doi:10.1016/0169-5347(94)90088-4

Caswell, J., & John, A. M. (1992). From the individual to the population in demographic models. In DeAngelis, D. L., & Gross, L. J. (Eds.), *Individual-based models and approaches in ecology: populations, communities and ecosystems* (pp. 33–61). London, UK: Chapman & Hall.

DeAngelis, D. L., & Gross, L. J. (1992). *Individual-based Models and Approaches in Ecology.* New York: Chapman and Hall.

DeAngelis, D. L., & Mooij, W. M. (2005). Individual-based modeling of ecological and evolutionary processes. *Annual Review of Ecology Evolution and Systematics, 36*, 147–168. doi:10.1146/annurev.ecolsys.36.102003.152644

Gillespie, D. T. (1977). Exact stochastic simulation of coupled chemical reactions. *Journal of Physical Chemistry, 81*, 2340–2361. doi:10.1021/j100540a008

Greenman, J. V., & Benton, T. G. (2003). The amplification of environmental noise in population models: Causes and consequences. *American Naturalist, 161*, 225–239. doi:10.1086/345784

Grimm, V., & Railsback, S. F. (2005). *Individual-based modeling and ecology.* Princeton University Press.

Grimm, V., Revilla, E., Berger, U., Jeltsch, F., Mooij, W. M., & Railsback, S. F. (2005). Pattern-oriented modeling of agent-based complex systems: lessons from ecology. *Science, 310*, 987–991. doi:10.1126/science.1116681

Holland, J. N., & DeAngelis, D. L. (2009). Consumer-resource theory predicts dynamic transitions between outcomes of interspecific interactions. *Ecology Letters, 12*, 1357–1366. doi:10.1111/j.1461-0248.2009.01390.x

Holling, C. S. (2001). Understanding the complexity of economic, ecological and social systems. *Ecosystems (New York, N.Y.), 4*, 390–405. doi:10.1007/s10021-001-0101-5

Johnson, M. T. J., & Stinchcombe, J. R. (2007). An emerging synthesis between community ecology and evolutionary biology. *Trends in Ecology & Evolution*, *22*, 250–257. doi:10.1016/j.tree.2007.01.014

Judson, O. P. (1994). The rise of the individual-based model in ecology. *Trends in Ecology & Evolution*, *9*, 9–14. doi:10.1016/0169-5347(94)90225-9

Klipp, E., Herwig, R., Kowald, A., Wierling, C., & Lehrach, H. (2009). *Systems Biology in Practice: Concepts, Implementation and Application*. Weinheim: Wiley.

Loreau, M. (2010). Linking biodiversity and ecosystems: towards a unifying ecological theory. *Philosophical Transactions of the Royal Society B*, *365*, 49–60. doi:10.1098/rstb.2009.0155

McKane, A. J., & Drossel, B. (2006). Models of food-web evolution. In Pascual, M., & Dunne, J. A. (Eds.), *Ecological Networks: Linking Structure to Dynamics in Food Webs* (pp. 223–243). Oxford: Oxford University Press.

McNamara, J. M., & Houston, A. I. (2009). Integrating function and mechanism. *Trends in Ecology & Evolution*, *24*, 670–675. doi:10.1016/j.tree.2009.05.011

Memmott, J., Craze, P. G., Waser, N. M., & Price, M. V. (2007). Global warming and the disruption of plant-pollinator interactions. *Ecology Letters*, *10*, 710–717. doi:10.1111/j.1461-0248.2007.01061.x

Mills, L. S., Soulé, M. E., & Doak, D. F. (1993). The keystone-species concept in ecology and conservation. *Bioscience*, *43*, 219–224. doi:10.2307/1312122

Olff, H., Alonso, D., Berg, M. P., Eriksson, B. K., Loreau, M., Piersma, T., & Rooney, N. (2009). Parallel ecological networks in ecosystems. *Philosophical Transactions of the Royal Society B*, *364*, 1755–1779. doi:10.1098/rstb.2008.0222

Pascual, M. (2005). Computational ecology: from the complex to the simple and back. *PLoS Computational Biology*, *1*, e18. doi:10.1371/journal.pcbi.0010018

Priami, C. (2009). Algorithmic systems biology. *Communications of the ACM*, *52*, 80–89. doi:10.1145/1506409.1506427

Ruokolainen, L., Lindén, A., Kaitala, V., & Fowler, M. S. (2009). Ecological and evolutionary dynamics under coloured environmental variation. *Trends in Ecology & Evolution*, *24*, 555–563. doi:10.1016/j.tree.2009.04.009

Scheller, R. M., Sturtevant, B. R., Gustafson, E. J., Ward, B. C., & Mladenoff, D. J. (2010). Increasing the reliability of ecological models using modern software engineering techniques. *Frontiers in Ecology and the Environment*, *8*, 253–260. doi:10.1890/080141

Schwager, M., Johst, K., & Jeltsch, F. (2006). Does red noise increase or decrease extinction risk? Single extreme events versus series of unfavorable conditions. *American Naturalist*, *167*, 879–888. doi:10.1086/503609

Williams, T. M., Estes, J. A., Doak, D. F., & Springer, A. M. (2008). Killer appetites: assessing the role of predators in ecological communities. *Ecology*, *85*, 3373–3384. doi:10.1890/03-0696

Chapter 9
Process Algebra Models in Biology:
The Case of Phagocytosis

Ozan Kahramanoğulları
The Microsoft Research – University of Trento Centre for Computational and Systems Biology, Italy

ABSTRACT

Process algebras are formal languages, which were originally designed to study the properties of complex reactive computer systems. Due to highly parallelized interactions and stochasticity inherit in biological systems, programming languages that implement stochastic extensions of processes algebras are gaining increasing attention as modeling and simulation tools in systems biology. The author discusses stochastic process algebras from the point of view of their broader potential as unifying instruments in systems biology. They argue that process algebras can help to complement conventional more established approaches to systems biology with new insights that emerge from computer science and software engineering. Along these lines, the author illustrates on examples their capability of addressing a spectrum of otherwise challenging biological phenomena, and their capacity to provide novel techniques and tools for modeling and analysis of biological systems. For the example models, they resort to phagocytosis, an evolutionarily conserved process by which cells engulf larger particles.

INTRODUCTION

Systems biology is a relatively recent term, which is often used to describe the general interdisciplinary effort in using techniques from biology, mathematics, physics and computing to provide

DOI: 10.4018/978-1-61350-435-2.ch009

insight into the workings of biological systems (Boogerd et al., 2007). Thus, the paradigm of systems biology covers a broad range of approaches, including those for obtaining massive amounts of information about whole biology systems. Another line of research in systems biology aims at building, with such a data, a science of principles

Copyright © 2012, IGI Global. Copying or distributing in print or electronic forms without written permission of IGI Global is prohibited.

of operation that is based on the interactions between components of biological systems. In this chapter, we discuss this latter consideration from the point of view of computer science (Cardelli, 2005; Fisher & Henzinger, 2007), in particular, of process algebras (Priami et al., 2001; Regev & Shapiro, 2002; Priami, 2009).

Biological systems are evolutionarily engineered, highly structured systems (Oltvai & Barabási, 2002). The underlying mechanisms enjoy an immense complexity, which is necessary for their functioning and survival, but difficult to reverse engineer. One of the reasons for this difficulty lies in obtaining 'complete' and 'accurate' data on these systems or their components for conceptualizing the acquired knowledge in (formal or informal) models. Another difficulty is that, in the presence of such data, the principles and analysis techniques imported from other disciplines are often not directly applicable to cover their complexity in an obvious way, and require an adjustment to the characteristics of the particular biological system being studied.

One of the main stream approaches for modeling and simulating the dynamics of biological systems is using differential equations, which can be traced back to the sixties (Noble, 1960) and earlier (Lotka, 1927; Volterra, 1926), and has its roots in Newton's physics. Being equipped with well understood analysis techniques, differential equations provide the 'deterministic' approach (as opposed to the stochastic approach) for modeling and simulating biological systems. In comparison to stochastic simulations, simulations with differential equation models are advantageous in terms of computational cost. However, differential equation models are inherently difficult to change, extend and upgrade, when modification to the model structure is required. For example, as new data about the modeled system is acquired, local changes in the structure of a model need to be carried over to all the equations that describe the structure of the model. Moreover, differential equations have limitations in expressivity when,

for example, complexations of unbounded number of (diverse) entities are being modeled. Because of these reasons, differential equation models are better suited for models with a smaller size and fewer number of species (Danos et al., 2007). In addition, within the last few years, a general consensus has emerged that noise and stochastic effects, which are not directly captured by ordinary differential equations, are essential attributes of biological systems, especially when molecule numbers of certain species are smaller (Blossey et al, 2008; Shahrezaei & Swain, 2008).

Biological systems are massively parallel, highly complex systems, in which system components interact with each other in various ways. Similarly, complex reactive systems, as they are studied in computer science, maintain ongoing interactions with their environment rather than producing some final value upon termination. This observation points to an analogy, which provides means to study biological systems as complex reactive systems. The basic idea here is to describe the interactions of biological system components and the consequences of these interactions by means of computer language constructs in models and run simulations on these models. Such an algorithmic treatment (Priami, 2009) results in a mechanistic, systems-level consideration of the modeled biological system. In such a setting, the computer simulations can be seen as in silico experiments that are performed prior to in vitro wet-lab experiments to make predictions and guide the wet-lab experiments. Then, the newly obtained biological knowledge serves as feedback to improve the models for new predictions. In return, this approach provides feedback to develop and adapt the computer science technologies with respect to the needs of the modeled systems.

In recent years, pioneered by Regev and Shapiro's (2002) seminal work, there has been a considerable amount of research on applying computer science technologies to modeling biological systems. Various languages with stochastic simulation capabilities based on, for example, process algebras, term rewriting (Danos et al., 2007; Curien et al., 2008; Danos et al., 2008; Hlavacek et al., 2006) and Petri nets (Heiner et al, 2008; Talcott, 2008) have been proposed. The focus of this chapter is on process algebras. Process algebras (Baeten, 2005) are formal languages, which were originally introduced as a means to study the properties of complex reactive systems. In these systems, concurrency, that is, the view of systems in which interacting and synchronizing computational processes are executing in parallel, is a central aspect. As it was proposed by Regev and Shapiro (2002), the capability to describe such complex behavior qualifies the process algebra languages as appropriate tools to describe the dynamics of biological systems (Priami et al., 2001), which employ concurrency immensely in their functioning.

Having emerged as an area of theoretical computer science, process algebras profit from a mathematical foundation that provides a rich arsenal of formal techniques and tools as well as a broadly expending culture of software engineering. Such a positioning gives rise to two fundamental aspects that qualify these languages as promising instruments for systems biology: (1) Due to their algebraic origin, process algebras are compositional languages. That is, the meaning of a system component is given in terms of its components and the meaning of the algebraic operator that composes them. This way, each component of a biological system can be modeled independently, rather than, for example, modeling the reactions that the components participate. This allows large models to be constructed by composition of simple components. Furthermore, because one can work on individual components, modifications to the dynamics of a model can be made locally on the appropriate component of the model without modifying the rest of the model. (2) Availability of techniques from language design makes it possible to tailor the process algebra languages with respect to the domain specific needs while remaining on formal grounds. In this respect, on one hand, the

theoretical notion of Turing-completeness can be exploited in the process algebra setting as an indicator of expressive power (Cardelli & Zavattaro, 2008; 2010) in the sense that a biological system, which can be described as computation in any other language, can also be expressed as a process model. On the other hand, the process algebra languages can be re-designed to capture the structure of the systems that they model with their syntax, instead of providing a complex encoding that captures the desired behavior.

Phagocytosis, which we introduce below, is a biological process whereby cells engulf large particles. *In the next sections, we provide evidence for the arguments above by using certain sub-systems of phagocytosis as examples for illustrating the following facts.*

1. For the models of biological systems as chemical reactions, the relationship between their ordinary differential equation (ODE) and process algebra representations are well understood from a syntactic point of view: there are now a number of algorithms for translating given sets of chemical reactions into sets of ODEs or programs in process algebra languages, see for example (Cardelli, 2008). In this respect, supported by computer science technologies, process algebra based languages provide compositional means for studying models consisting of sets of chemical reactions.

2. Although many biological systems such as signaling pathways can be modeled as sets of chemical reactions, there are other biological systems, which require models with richer structures and dynamics that exceed the expressivity limits of chemical reactions (Cardelli & Zavattaro, 2010). Models of filament formation, such as actin polymerization, and models describing the dynamics of proteins on a membrane, which are typically modeled in biophysics on dynamic grids, are examples to such biological systems.

3. Techniques from various areas of computer science can be imported to the process algebra languages and developed into modeling aids for constructing models, and also for analyzing these models and simulations with them.

In the following, we use a stochastic extension of the pi calculus (Milner, 1999), which is a broadly studied process algebra. Because of its compactness and generality, the pi calculus is well suited for the above mentioned purpose of this chapter. We use the Stochastic Pi Calculus Machine (SPiM) (Phillips & Cardelli, 2007) for the implementation of the models, thus use the SPiM syntax for the presentation of the models. However, it is possible to carry the ideas presented in this chapter to various other process algebra based languages (Dematté et al., 2008; Ciocchetta & Hillston, 2008).

The chapter is organized as follows. We first introduce process algebra modeling with respect to the stochastic pi calculus, and give an overview of the Fcγ receptor mediated phagocytosis, which serves as an example biological system for the concepts presented here. Following this, we discuss different levels of representation in models of biological systems within the process algebra framework. We first consider the class of models that are given as sets of chemical reactions, and then others that involve more complicated structures that exceed the expressivity limits of chemical reactions. We then review how techniques and tools from other disciplines of computer science and software engineering can be imported to enhance the process algebra models. We conclude the chapter with a discussion of future research directions.

BACKGROUND

In this section, we give an overview to the stochastic pi calculus and Fcγ receptor medi-

ated phagocytosis, which we use in the example models below.

The Stochastic Pi Calculus Machine

In the stochastic pi calculus, we build models by composing processes by using the algebraic composition operators. A model, obtained this way, provides a precise description of the actions that each component of the modeled system can undertake with what rate. Once a system is expressed in this manner, we can use a simulation engine, for example, one which implements the Gillespie (1977) algorithm, to run simulations, and observe how the system evolves over time.

The Stochastic Pi Calculus Machine (SPiM) is an implementation language for a stochastic extension of the process algebra pi calculus. In SPiM, stochasticity is implemented by means of the Gillespie algorithm. For the rest of this chapter, we use the SPiM syntax and semantics, as defined in (Cardelli et al, 2009). For an in depth exposure to the pi calculus and the stochastic pi calculus, we refer the reader to (Milner, 1999) and (Priami, 1995), respectively.

Before going into the syntax and semantics of the SPiM language, let us first illustrate some of the ideas on an example: while modeling biological systems with the pi calculus, we often follow the abstraction of species as stateful entities with connectivity interfaces to other species as in, for example, (Danos et al., 2007; Danos et al., 2008; Dematté et al., 2008). A biochemical species can have a number of sites, through which it interacts with other species, and changes its state as a result of these interactions. Examples to this include binding of two proteins in order to form a complex, and phosphorylation of a site on a protein. In both of these examples, the resulting biochemical species have different functionalities from their components, hence they change state. We can implement this idea in the pi calculus by resorting to private names between species that represent their connectivity. For example, consider the species A and B, each with a binding site that allows one to bind to the other, in SPiM syntax:

```
let A() = (new e@r:chan()!bind(e); Ab(e))
let B() = ?bind(e); Bb(e)
```

When process expressions A and B interact over the channel bind by performing complementary output(!) and input(?) actions, A sends the private name e to B. Then Ab(e) and Bb(e) are bound forms of A and B, and the private name e then becomes the bond between them. The evolution of this scenario is depicted in an interacting au-tomata representation (Cardelli, 2009) in Figure 1 together with the plot of a simulation with this model. In modeling with the stochastic pi calculus, we exploit this idea to model biological phenomena that vary from chemical reactions to diffusion of proteins on membranes, and the representation of other more complex structures.

Now, let us bring these ideas to formal grounds by introducing the syntax and the semantics of the stochastic pi calculus.

The syntax and the semantics of the stochastic pi calculus, implemented in SPiM, is shown in Definition 1, Definition 2 and Definition 3. The

Figure 1. Interacting automata representation of the evolution of the model for a reaction, where species A and species B form a complex and the time series resulting from a simulation with this model. Species A sends to species B the private name e on channel bind. At the next state, species Ab and species Bb share the private name e. On the right-hand-side, we have the simulation plot with this model with 1000 A and 1000 B at time zero. The rate of channel bind is set to 1.0.

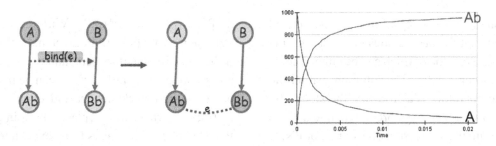

Definition 1. Syntax of SPi. Each channel x is associated with a rate ρ(x).

P,Q ::=	M	Choice
	X(n)	Instance
	P | Q	Parallel
	new x P	Restriction

M ::=	()	Null
	π; P	Action
	do π1;P1 or … or πN;PN	Actions

E ::= {}	Empty
	E, X(m) = P	Definition
	fn(P) ⊆ m	

π ::=	?x(m)*r	Input
	!x(n)*r	Output
	delay@r	Delay

Definition 2. Reduction in SPi.

$$(1) \quad \texttt{do delay@r; P or ...} \xrightarrow{\ r\ } \texttt{P}$$

$$(2) \quad \texttt{(do !x(n)*r1;P1 or ...)} \mid \texttt{(do ?x(m)*r2;P2 or ...)} \xrightarrow{\ \rho(x).r1.r2\ } \texttt{P1|P2 \{m:=n\}}$$

$$(3) \quad \texttt{P} \xrightarrow{\ r\ } \texttt{P}' \quad\Longrightarrow\quad \texttt{new x P} \xrightarrow{\ r\ } \texttt{new x P}'$$

$$(4) \quad \texttt{P} \xrightarrow{\ r\ } \texttt{P}' \quad\Longrightarrow\quad \texttt{P} \mid \texttt{Q} \xrightarrow{\ r\ } \texttt{P}' \mid \texttt{Q}$$

$$(5) \quad \texttt{Q} \equiv \texttt{P} \xrightarrow{\ r\ } \texttt{P}' \equiv \texttt{Q}' \quad\Longrightarrow\quad \texttt{Q} \xrightarrow{\ r\ } \texttt{Q}'$$

Definition 3. Structural Congruence Axioms in SPi. Structural congruence is defined as the least congruence that satisfies the axioms below. Processes in SPi are assumed to be equal up to renaming of bound names and reordering of terms in a choice.

$$\texttt{P} \mid \texttt{()} \equiv \texttt{P}$$
$$\texttt{P} \mid \texttt{Q} \equiv \texttt{Q} \mid \texttt{P}$$
$$\texttt{P} \mid \texttt{(Q} \mid \texttt{R)} \equiv \texttt{(P} \mid \texttt{Q)} \mid \texttt{R}$$
$$\texttt{X(n)} \equiv \texttt{P\{m:=n\}}$$
$$\texttt{new x ()} \equiv \texttt{()}$$
$$\texttt{new x new y P} \equiv \texttt{new y new x P}$$
$$x \notin fn(P) \quad \texttt{new x (P} \mid \texttt{Q)} \equiv \texttt{P} \mid \texttt{new x Q}$$

reduction rules, given in Definition 2, are labeled with rates that denote the rates of the single corresponding reactions, which can be either a communication or a delay. The intuition behind the algebraic operators is as follows: the stochastic choice between zero or more alternative actions is given with the expression do P1 or ... or PN. If there is only one alternative then we write P1 and we denote the empty choice with (). The parallel composition, which denotes the co-existence of processes is written as P1 | ... | PN. A process P can also be given a name X with parameter m, written as let X(m) = P.

The atomic actions that a process can perform consist of delay actions, and input and output actions. A process can perform a delay at rate *r* and then do P, written delay@r;P. The rate *r* is a real number value denoting the rate of an exponential distribution such that the average duration of the delay is *1/r*. A process can also send (output) a value n on channel x with weight r1 and then do P1, written !x(n)*r1;P1, or it can receive a value (input) m on channel x with weight r2 and then

do P2, written ?x(m)*r2;P2. With respect to the reduction semantics of SPi given in Definition 2, if these complementary send and receive actions are running in parallel, they can synchronize on the common channel x and evolve to P1 | P2{m:=n}, where m is replaced by n in process P2. This allows messages to be exchanged from one process to another. The operator new x@r:t P creates a fresh channel x of rate r to be used in the process P. In SPiM, each channel has a type, denoted with t in this expression. As an example, consider the type chan(chan,chan). This expression denotes a channel that can transmit the names of two channels. When a process is prefixed with the declaration of a fresh channel, that channel remains private to the process and does not conflict with any other channel.

Fc Receptor-Mediated Phagocytosis

Phagocytosis is the process, by which cells engulf particles that are usually larger than 0.5μm. Phagocytosis is evolutionarily conserved from amoeba, which obtain food this way, to mammals, and it is performed by a large variety of cells. For example, in multi-cellular organisms, 'professional' phagocytic (white blood) cells such as macrophages, neutrophils and dendritic cells can recognize bacteria, viruses or cancerous body cells with their surface receptors and protect the organism by internalizing and digesting them. Phagocytic mechanisms that are involved in the recognition and uptake of the pathogens by professional phagocytes is paramount for the induction of protective immunity. Phagocytosis plays also an important role in clearance of cell corpses generated by apoptosis (programmed cell death).

Phagocytosis is a triggered process, often initiated by the interaction of particle-bound ligands (opsonins) with specific receptors on the cell membrane of the phagocytes. Although the mechanisms underlying phagocytosis have been being studied extensively, a complete understanding is far from being established. Among dozens of receptors that can mediate phagocytic uptake, probably the best understood experimental model is the internalization of IgG-coated particles by Fcγ receptors (Swanson & Hoppe, 2004).

Fcγ receptor mediated phagocytosis is initiated by the antibodies called immunoglobulin G (IgG), which bind to the surface of the particle, to be internalized, to form a coat. This process is called opsonization. When a particle is opsonized, the tail region of each IgG molecule, called the Fc region, is exposed on the exterior on the particle surface. Fcγ receptors are trans-membrane proteins with a cytoplasmic tail. The recognition of the IgGs by the phagocyic cell is performed by the ligands of the Fcγ receptor, which bind to the Fc regions of the IgG molecules. This binding activates a signaling cascade that drives the remodeling of the cytoskeleton close to the membrane. The cell then extends pseudopods to form a phagosome while proceeding with binding its ligands in a zipper-like fashion around the internalized particle, and eventually closes the plasma membrane-derived phagosome (Garcia-Garcia & Rosales, 2002).

Fcγ receptor contains within its cytoplasmic tail an immune-receptor tyrosine-based activation motif (ITAM), which has two tyrosine residues. The signaling cascade proceeding the Fcγ-Fc interaction on the exterior surface of the cell membrane propagates as a result of the phosphorylation of these tyrosine residues by a protein tyrosine kinase of the Src family: another protein tyrosine kinase (Syk) binds to the phosphorylated ITAMs. This results in auto-phosphorylation and activation of Syk. Among other tasks, activated Syk is responsible for the activation of the protein Vav (Hall et al. 2006), which activates the Rho GTP-binding protein Rac (Etienne-Manneville & Hall, 2002; Patel et al., 2002). In a parallel independent pathway, another Rho GTP binding protein Cdc42 gets activated. Cdc42 and Rac act at distinct stages to regulate actin filament polymerization and organization: Cdc42 and Rac control actin filament polymerization through proteins WASP (Wiskott Aldrich Syndrome Protein) and WAVE, respectively, that stimulate the activity of the Arp2/3 complex. Activation of Arp2/3 results in actin polymerization and the extrusion of actin-based protrusions around the particle. While Rac is generally responsible for the branching structure of actin filaments, Cdc42 causes the actin to polymerize in a linear structure (Hoppe & Swanson, 2004; Chimini & Chavrier, 2000).

PROCESS ALGEBRA MODELS IN BIOLOGY

In this section, we illustrate on examples that process algebras are equipped with a rich arsenal of theoretical and practical means to provide complementary strengths to other broadly used techniques in systems biology. By using process algebras, we can model biological phenomena varying from chemical reactions to others, which can be challenging to model faithfully, for example, with differential equations. Moreover, within the process algebra framework, we can import and use techniques and tools from computer science and software engineering without sacrificing from formal coherence. In the following, we provide evidence for this by resorting to stochastic pi calculus models of certain stages of Fcγ receptor mediated phagocytosis.

From Chemical Reactions to Process Algebra Models

Chemical reactions are commonly used in systems biology as a convenient, intuitive and scalable notation. By using existing algorithms and tools, models consisting of sets of chemical reactions can be easily translated into models in ordinary differential equations, Petri nets, and process algebras (Cardelli, 2008).

In the stochastic pi calculus, we can model chemical reactions, in particular, complexations by using private names as illustrated by the introductory example of the previous section, where we model the reaction $A + B \rightarrow AB$. In this encoding, Ab and Bb are distinct syntactic objects, representing the bond states of the species A and B. The private name e represents the bond between these two species. During simulation, the complex of A and B takes the form 'new e (Ab(e) | Bb(e))'. The advantage of modeling with private names is the capability of being able to trace A and B individually during a simulation in their unbound states as well as in their bound states in complexes. An alternative to this is modeling the complex consisting of A and B as a single syntactic object as we demonstrate with the following SPiM code.

```
let A() =    (!bind; AB())
let B() =    (?bind; ())
```

Here, as a result of the interaction between the species A and B on channel bind, species A becomes the complex AB and B disappears. In fact, these two programs model the same reaction, and they can be interchanged for different purposes: the first alternative has more informa-

tion, whereas the latter provides a simpler model. Reactions with more than two reactants can also be encoded by using this schema, for example, by using transactions (Ciocchetta & Priami, 2007). Reactions with a single reactant are modeled with the delay action as illustrated in the following example that models the reaction $C \rightarrow P1 + P2 + P3$. This code also provides a schema for modeling reactions with multiple products.

```
let C() =   delay@r; (P1() | P2() | P3())
```

Returning to phagocytosis, the proteins Cdc42 and Rac, which participate in the phagocytic signaling pathway, belong to the Rho GTP-binding protein family (Bustelo et al., 2007). These proteins serve as molecular switches in various cellular activities. They regulate the transmission of an incoming signal further to effectors in a molecular module by cycling between inactive and active states, depending on being GDP or GTP bound, respectively. As depicted in Figure 2, GDP/ GTP cycling is regulated by guanine nucleotide exchange factors (GEFs) that stimulate the GDP dissociation and GTP binding, whereas GTPase-activating proteins (GAPs) have the opposite effect and stimulate the hydrolysis of Rho-GTP into Rho-GDP. In the active GTP-bound state, Rho proteins interact with and activate downstream effectors, for example, to control actin polymerization in the context of Fcγ receptor mediated phagocytosis (Jaffe & Hall, 2005).

Goryachev and Pokhilko (2006) give an ordinary differential equations (ODE) model of the Rho GTP-binding proteins, based on a set of chemical reactions. These reactions are depicted on the left-hand-side of Figure 3: the three forms of the Rho protein (GDP-bound RD, GTP-bound RT, and nucleotide free R) in the middle layer form complexes with GEF (E) in the bottom layer and with GAP (A) in the top layer. All the reactions, except those for GTP hydrolysis, are reversible. In their model, Goryachev and Pokhilko use the quantitative biochemical data on the

Figure 2. Mechanisms underlying Fcγ receptor mediated phagocytosis: (Left) upon the binding of the Fcγ receptor with the IgG on the opsonized particle, the two tyrosine residues on the ITAM domain get phosphorylated (Garcia-Garcia & Rosales, 2002). (Middle) This triggers a signaling cascade where Rho GTP-binding proteins Rac and CdC42 get activated and propagate the signal to downstream effectors (Etienne-Manneville & Hall, 2002). (Right) Actin polymerization results in protrusions around the internalized particle (Weeds & Sharon, 2001).

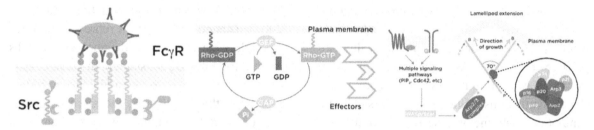

Cdc42p member of the Rho family proteins. This results in an explanation of the experimentally observed rapid cycling of the Rho GTP-binding proteins between their GDP-bound off states and GTP-bound on states while displaying high activity. The activity of the system is measured by the relative concentration of the GTP-bound Rho proteins (RT in Figure 3).

Cardelli et al (2009) give a stochastic pi calculus model of the Rho GTP-binding proteins that implements the set of chemical reactions of Goryachev and Pokhilko. The stochastic simulations with this model display an excellent agreement with the simulations with the deterministic

ODE model of Goryachev & Pokhilko (2006). The plots in Figure 3 provide a comparison of both models with respect to the RT activity on simulations with varying regimes of initial concentrations.

As this example model illustrates, the stochastic pi calculus is well suited for modeling sets of chemical reactions. In this respect, compositionality of the process algebra operators brings about an added value: compositionality becomes instrumental, for example, in combining models consisting of sets of chemical reactions with the models of entities that require more involved constructs that cannot be expressed as chemical

Figure 3. The model of Rho GTP-binding proteins in (Goryachev & Pokhilko, 2006). (Left:) the structure of the model where the Rho GTP-binding protein (R) forms a complex with either GEF (E) or GAP (A). (Middle:) The simulation results with the ordinary differential equations model with respect to the RT activity with varying regimes of initial concentrations. (Adapted from (Goryachev & Pokhilko, 2006).) (Right:) The simulation results with the stochastic pi calculus model with respect to the RT activity with the same initial conditions as the ODE model.

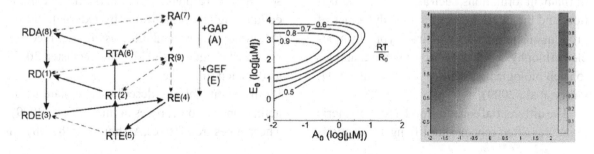

reactions (such as those that we illustrate in the next section). However, it is important to observe that in order to compare the process algebra models with the ODE models, a conversion and factoring of the initial concentrations into quantities of individual species is necessary (Wolkenhauer et al., 2004). This is because in process algebra models, we work with quantities of individuals whereas in ODE models concentration values are positive real values. As it can be seen on these examples, when the numbers of individuals in stochastic simulations are high enough, the stochastic simulations with the process algebra models are in agreement with the simulations with the ODE models. However, when the number of certain species are low, stochastic simulations and ODE simulations can demonstrate different behaviors. For example, in the stochastic simulations with Lotka-Volterra (Lotka, 1927; Volterra, 1926) predator-prey interaction models, certain species can go extinct, whereas they can demonstrate an oscillatory behavior with the ODE simulations. In this respect, the stochastic simulation capabilities that the process algebra languages employ is an advantage for example in ecosystem models (Powell & Boland, 2009), where species extinctions are of central importance.

Modeling Polymers and Grids

Although many biological systems such as signaling pathways can be modeled as sets of chemical reactions, there are other biological systems that require models with richer structures and dynamics and exceed the expressivity limits of chemical reactions (Cardelli & Zavattaro, 2010). Models of filament formations, such as actin polymerization, and the models describing the dynamics of proteins on membranes, which are typically modeled in biophysics on dynamic grids, are examples to such biological systems (Alberts et al., 2004; Gurry et al., 2009).

The differential equation models of polymeric structures often rely on simplifying assumptions on the structure of the polymers. Because differential equation models describe the concentration changes of species in a system at infinitesimal time intervals, they require the polymers of different lengths to be defined as distinct species. They thus require each polymer of different length to be modeled with a distinct equation (Hu et al., 2007). This poses barriers in representation, for example, when filaments with unbounded lengths or rich structures are considered. In the stochastic pi calculus, because we can model the individual monomers that polymerize, polymeric structures can be modeled without any restriction: in a model we describe the actions each monomer can undertake, and the polymerization occurs as the emergent behavior in the form of self-assembly during simulation with respect to the modeled capabilities of the monomers. Moreover, it is also possible to assign different states to each monomer, which are independent of the states of the other free and bound monomers in the system. In particular, this capability is challenging to achieve in differential equation models.

As an example for the stochastic pi calculus models of polymerization, in the following we discuss models of actin dynamics with respect to the models presented in (Cardelli, 2009; Cardelli et al., 2009b). Actin is the monomeric subunit of actin filaments, which form one of the three major cytoskeleton networks in eukaryotic cells. Actin dynamics plays a key role in phagocytosis as well as other cellular activities that involve cell shape modifications. In cells, actin polymerization is highly regulated, firstly through the interaction of actin monomers and polymers with a variety of actin-binding proteins (Pollard, 2007); and secondly in response to the activation of intracellular signaling pathways by external stimuli (Mogilner & Oster, 2008), as in Fcγ receptor mediated phagocytosis (Mogilner & Oster, 2003) as depicted in Figure 2.

In our model, we describe each state of an actin monomer by a process as in (Cardelli, 2009). These states are Af (free), Al (bound on the left), Ar (bound on the right), and Ab (bound on both sides). Each monomer can move between these states by interacting with another monomer. Actin filaments are polarized with a barbed end and a pointed end. In this setting, Al represents a monomer at the barbed end of the filament and Ar represents a monomer at the pointed end. Actin monomers can in fact polymerize and depolymerize at both ends. However, depolymerization at the barbed end and polymerization at the pointed end are very slow. We can reflect this in the model with rate constants, however here in this first model

we simplify further by allowing the polymers to grow only at the barbed end and shrink only at the pointed end.

In Figure 4, there are the graphical representations of the processes for two monomers. Their possible interactions are depicted as dashed arrows: the arrows 1 and 2 are the association interactions whereas the arrows 3 and 4 are the disassociation interactions. The SPiM code for this model is shown in Exhibit 1.

By building on this idea, we can incrementally add information to the model about the

Figure 4.(Left) Interacting automata representation of the actin monomer model. (1) a process Af can interact with another process Af, and as a result of this, one of them evolves to process Al and the other one evolves to process Ar. This describes the association of two monomers forming a dimer. (2) A process Af can also interact with a process Al, and as a result of this Af evolves to process Al whereas Al evolves to process Ab. This describes the association of monomers at the barbed end of the actin filament. (3) A process Ar can dissociate from Ab by interacting on a name, private to both processes, and as a result of this, Ar evolves to process Af whereas Ab evolves to process Ar. This describes the disassociation of a monomer from the pointed end of the actin filament. (4) A process Al can dissociate from a process Ar, and as a result of this, both of them evolve to process Af. This describes the disassociation of a dimer to two monomers. (Right) A SPiM simulation with this model.

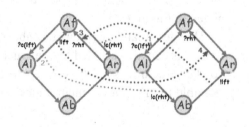 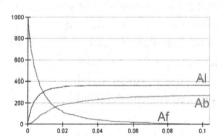

Exhibit 1.

```
new c@0.116:chan(chan)
let Af() = (new rht@0.0027:chan              (* Arrows in Figure 4: *)
              do ?c(lft); Al(lft)            (* 1 and 2 *)
              or !c(rht); Ar(rht))           (* 1 *)
and Al(lft:chan) = (new rht@0.0027:chan
              do !lft; Af()                  (* 4 *)
              or !c(rht); Ab(lft,rht))       (* 2 *)
and Ar(rht:chan) = ?rht; Af()                (* 3 and 4 *)
and Ab(lft:chan, rht:chan) = !lft; Ar(rht)   (* 3 *)
```

system being studied (Cardelli et al., 2009b). For example, actin filaments can have a branching structure (Weeds & Sharon, 2001). This branching is induced by the binding of an Arp2/3 molecule to the side of a pre-existing actin filament. In order to model the branching in the filaments, we extend the model above with an additional binding site that we call mid. We then introduce a process R that models the Arp2/3 molecule with the capability to bind to the actin monomer. During branching, processes representing actin monomers bind to R processes to form daughter filaments that are attached to the mother filaments. However, the introduction of a new binding site in the model depicted in Figure 5 results in eight states for each monomer. This is because each of the previously available four states of the monomer are extended with a capability of binding to process R. In order to simplify this model, we can introduce an alternative model by restricting the binding of each process R only to a monomer in bound state (Ab), and this way reduce the number of states of each monomer to five as depicted in Figure 5.

By exploiting the compositionality feature of the process algebra operators, we can work locally on the model above to extend it with further aspects of actin filaments. For example, we can include their capability to grow and shrink at both barbed and pointed ends as depicted in Figure 6

(although shrinking at the barbed end and growth at the pointed end are much slower). Similarly, we can include the mechanisms related to their regulation into this model. For example, capping of the barbed ends by capping proteins is a mechanism, which reduces the rate of drawdown on the pool of monomeric actin (Iwasa & Mullins, 2007; Jaffe & Hall, 2005). The free end of the new filament elongates until a capping protein becomes available, and binds to the barbed end and terminates the growth. As a result of this, each filament grows only transiently. We model capping proteins as a process, which can bind to the barbed end of filaments by interacting with process Al as depicted in Figure 6. We can then include the mechanisms that involve the role of ATP/ADP. The biochemical mechanism for this can be summarized as follows: filamental or monomeric actin are bound to ATP molecules, which can hydrolyze to ADP-Pi-actin, which can then evolve to ADP-actin by dissociating the phosphate unit (Fujivara et al., 2007). In order to model this, we use a three-layered monomer model where the layers describe the dynamics of the monomer in its ATP, ADP-Pi and ADP bound forms as depicted in Figure 6.

The ideas that we demonstrate above on actin filaments can also be used to construct more involved structures such as grids, which are for example used to model membranes. In order to

Figure 5. An interacting automata representation of the model that extends the model of Figure 4 with the branching capability. (Left) Adding the branching capability to this model increases the number of states from four to eight. We simplify this model by omitting the states where the branching structure can occur on free monomers, or on monomers at the either end of the filaments. (Right) Interactions of the monomers with each other and with the Arp2/3 molecule.

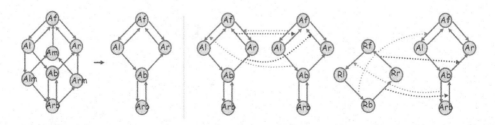

Figure 6. Models that incrementally extend the model in Figure 5. (Left) Interacting automata representation of the actin model where filaments can grow and shrink at both ends, they can branch, and they can be prevented from growing further by the association of capping proteins at the barbed ends. Here, Cf and Cb denote free and bound capping proteins. (Right) The model combines the previous models with the effect of ATP/ADP exchange. AfT, AlT, ArT, AbT denote the ATP-actin in its free and bound forms. AfPi and AfD denote the free ADP-Pi-actin and ADP-actin, respectively. We denote their bound forms as in the previous models. Similarly, ATC, APC, and ADC denote the monomers that are bound to a capping protein process. In this model, ADP-actin can hydrolyze to ADP-Pi-actin and ADP-Pi-actin can dissociate its phosphate to become ADP-actin. We assume that the exchange to ATP actin is quick in the free monomer and we reflect this assumption also in the structure of the model by not allowing the hydrolysis of free ATP-actin.

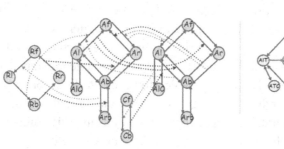

illustrate this, let us consider a square grid, where neighbors can interact with each other and as a result of their interactions they change state. This idea can be seen, for example, as a model of epidemic spread of a disease or spread of information on a membrane-like structure. The following SPiM code illustrates this example.

```
let S(x:chan, y:chan) = do ?x; I(x,y)
                        or ?y; I(x,y)
and I(x:chan, y:chan) = do !x; I(x,y)
                        or !y; I(x,y)
new c1@1.0:chan new c2@1.0:chan
new c3@1.0:chan new c4@1.0:chan
run (I(c1,c2)  | S(c1,c3)
    | S(c2,c4)  | S(c4,c3))
```

When an infected individual (I) interacts with one of its susceptible (S) neighbors, the neighbor becomes infected as well. Here, individuals can only interact with their connected neighbors, where neighborhood is implemented by private names.

Getting Help

As the examples above illustrate, process algebras are well equipped with the technical means for modeling and simulating biological systems with various structures. However, it is often desirable to combine the expressive power and the technical capabilities that the process algebras provide with techniques and tools from other disciplines of computer science and software engineering to bring ease to the *modeling* and *analysis* of various biological phenomena.

Modeling: Process algebras, such as the pi calculus, enjoy the theoretical result of Turing-completeness. This indicates that a biological system, which can be described as computation in any other language, can also be expressed as a process model. Moreover, due to the compositional algebraic operators such as 'choice' and 'parallel composition', the process algebra languages capture the mechanistic structure of the systems that they model with their syntax. For example, the syntax of the pi calculus directly captures the notions such as association and dissociation of biochemical species as illustrated above. In this respect, compositionality makes it possible to define the behavior of a model component in terms of its actions and process algebra operators that compose these actions. This capability allows the modelers to move easily between different levels of abstraction, and work locally on the system component, for example, for refinement, or to undo a refinement. This is an advantage in contrast to other programming languages and differential equation models, that can provide complex encodings of the desired behavior or the biological phenomena. However, mathematical syntax of these languages, due to their algebraic origin, makes them difficult to use for the non-specialist. It is, however, crucial for the biologists to work with 'easy-to-use' languages with which they can communicate their expert knowledge and convert it into models.

Along these lines, one of the central objectives of computational systems biology is the development of modeling languages that are accessible to users who are not specialists of formal languages. There are ongoing efforts for this within the process algebra framework. Examples to this include graphical and natural-language-like-narrative-language interfaces to process algebra languages (Phillips et al., 2006; Priami et al., 2007; Priami et al., 2009; Kahramanoğulları et al., 2009; Kahramanoğulları et al., 2011). The idea here is that the domain expert writes the model in a way with which she is comfortable, and then an automated translation algorithm translates the model into a process algebra language for simulation and analysis.

As an example for this, in the context of phagocytsis consider a model which describes the initial phosphorylation of the Fcγ receptor, as depicted in Figure 2, with the following English sentences.

```
site f on FcR associates site I on IgG
site x on FcR gets phosphorylated if
site f on f FcR is bound
site y on FcR gets phosphorylated if
site f on f FcR is bound
```

These sentences can be automatically translated into a process algebra language as it is done in (Kahramanoğulları et al., 2009; Kahramanoğulları et al., 2011) for the stochastic pi calculus. By using such interface languages, it becomes easier to bridge biological expertise with the capabilities that the process algebra framework makes available. However, the development of interface languages, that scale through various biological phenomena, requires interdisciplinary effort that brings together knowledge on biological primitives as well as concepts and technologies from language design.

Analysis: The stochastic semantics of process algebra models are given by continuous time Markov chains. In such a setting, the data that is output as a result of simulations with the stochastic process algebra models are often given in the form of time-series that are generated by the Gillespie algorithm. This data is then usually analyzed by statistical tools to draw conclusions on the simulated system. An alternative to this approach is processing the simulation output by means of techniques that are borrowed from various fields of theoretical computer science. This way, the simulation output can be observed from a different point of view prior to statistical analysis.

A simple and effective application of this idea is designing and processing the simulation output delivered by the Gillespie algorithm to interpret and plot the simulations graphically as in (Cardelli et al., 2009b). This approach, on SPiM models, is based on decorating each process expression in the model with a coordinate parameter and a vector parameter. In this setting, the coordinate parameter denotes a position and the vector denotes its direction in the coordinate space. Then by using affine transformations, these two parameters are updated at each state transition during the simulation. This way, a dynamic behavior is captured in the encoded geometry of the processes without hampering the stochastic semantics of the models. This is because the encoded geometry information does not interfere with the dynamics of the model, and serves only as a data-register on the location and movement of the processes. This allows the modeler to interpret the simulation data graphically. The visualization is performed by means of a plotting algorithm, which then reads the reaction trace together with the time steps of the reactions. For each reaction, at each time step, the algorithm displays the reaction by erasing the reactants of the reaction from the screen and plotting the products. This results in a movie that is obtained from the simulation and visualizes how the system graphically evolves in time with respect to the encoded geometry.

To illustrate these ideas, let us return to the actin filament model in (Cardelli et al., 2009b). In this model, each bound monomer process is equipped with parameters for its location in space and for its growth direction. When a filament grows along its axis, its direction vector remains unaltered. The model is designed to reflect the experimentally measured 70 degrees angle be-

tween the mother actin filament and the daughter filament (Weeds & Yeoh, 2001). This is done by updating the direction vector of the daughter filament with respect to a rotation matrix for 70 degrees in case of branching. The SPiM code in Exhibit 2 implements this idea.

In this code, when an actin monomer (Arb) and an Arp2/3 (Rf) molecule interact to form a complex, the direction vector of the actin monomer is modified with an affine transformation and communicated to the Arp2/3 molecule: upon interaction over the channel r, the process Arb sends its coordinates to the process Rf together with its direction vector, rotated with a 70 degrees rotation matrix. Because actin filaments take a rotating helical shape, the model stochastically chooses between 70 or -70 degrees with equal probability in order to be able to mimic the growth of a tree-shaped filament in 2D. This new direction vector determines the direction of the daughter filament.

Screenshots of graphical plots with this model are depicted in Figure 7. In these simulations, the monomers are assumed to be freely diffusing until they become bound to polymers. In this setting, geometric models remain consistent with the hypotheses of the Gillespie algorithm. However, it is also possible to use the geometric information to constrain the simulation dynamics. For example, in a model of the phagocytic cup formation, we model the internalized particle with a circle (in

Exhibit 2.

```
...
and Arb(x:float, y:float, x1:float, y1:float, lft:chan, rht:chan) =
(new e@lam:chan
   do !r(x,y,(x1*0.34)+(y1*0.94),(x1*(-0.94))+(y1*0.34),e);
Arbb(x,y,x1,y1,e,lft,rht)
   or !r(x,y,(x1*0.34)-(y1*0.94),(x1*0.94)+(y1*0.34),e);
Arbb(x,y,x1,y1,e,lft,rht))
...
let Rf() = ?r(x,y,x1,y1,er); Rl(x,y,x1,y1,er)
...
```

Figure 7. Screenshots of the graphical visualizations with simulations. (a)An actin filament that branches as it grows due to polymerization, and (b) its visualization with a smaller resolution at a later time in the simulation. (c) We use a meshwork of such filaments to model and visualize the formation of the phagocytic cup. (d)The visualization of a 4×4 grid where neighbors change state by interacting with each other.

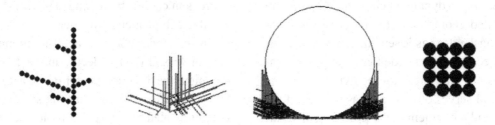

2D) and do not allow the monomers to polymerize in a way such that they would enter in this circle as depicted in Figure 7c.

The geometric parameterization of the processes can also be used to visualize the grid models that we have discussed above. In Figure 7d, we illustrate such a visualization of a 4×4 grid, where neighbors change state by interacting with each other. The two different states are depicted by different colors.

FUTURE RESEARCH DIRECTIONS

There is now consensus within the systems biology community on the perception of biological systems as complex reactive systems such as those studied in computer science where systems maintain ongoing interactions with their environment. Based on this perspective, various modeling languages have been developed together with their simulation engines. In this regard, the recently emerging algorithmic consideration of biological systems, with respect to the stochastic interactions between processes, is prone to provide perspectives that are complementary to those provided by other well established approaches such as differential equations. However, the process algebra based approach to systems biology is currently in its infancy when it is compared to these other approaches with a longer history of development.

Thus, there is a pressing need for development to bring the process algebra based languages to a further level, where they can be employed by a broader community.

Along these lines, an important discussion around the process algebra languages is on appropriate modeling language constructs, which scale through different levels of abstraction and various biological phenomena. Another related topic of investigation is the accessibility of the modeling languages to a broader audience of non-programming-specialist, domain-focused modelers. In this respect, an important and necessary topic of investigation is singling out the biological phenomena with respect to their process algebra representations as primitives. This would also make it possible to equip process algebra languages with intuitive, domain-specific modeling interfaces, since these primitives can be used as building blocks of such languages. Moreover, technologies for automated mapping of data between different modeling languages and also for transferring data from databases to models are other essential topics of further development.

As we have demonstrated above, the data that is output by process algebra models is often given in the form of time-series resulting from simulations that are generated by the Gillespie algorithm. These simulations are often analyzed by statistical means with respect to the time series data to draw conclusions on the emerging model behavior. An alternative to this approach is processing the simulation output by means of techniques that are borrowed from other fields of computer science. This way, the simulation output can be observed from a different point of view prior to statistical analysis. In fact, concurrency theory provides an expending variety of results on the analysis techniques and tools that are tailored for the computer systems. For example, availability of a notion of behavioral equivalence is a desirable feature for biology models, since this would make it possible to formally compare models and simulations with them. In fact, when process algebra models are considered from a concurrency theory point of view, there are various results for observing the behavioral equivalence between two given systems, for example, bisimulation. However, these techniques and tools are meaningful for the typical nondeterministic systems studied in computer science, and are not directly applicable for drawing conclusions on the quantitative behavior of the biological systems. In this respect, the analysis techniques on the process algebra models, that achieve the maturity of the traditional deterministic techniques, are yet to be developed. Thus, re-interpreting, developing and adapting the techniques from concurrency theory in the quantitative setting of biology models is a promising direction of further investigation. A desired feature of these techniques to be achieved is efficient reasoning capabilities. This way, it would be possible to deduce and infer properties of larger biological systems that are not obvious from the topological structure of these systems or from the quantitative data on their components.

CONCLUSION

Process algebras enjoy the availability of notions such as compositionality and stochasticity that are meaningful from the point of view of biological system models. In particular, for the models of systems where the number of species are smaller,

stochasticity becomes an essential feature. Moreover, compositionality allows the modelers to describe the systems in terms of their components. This way, compositionality provides a formal means for modular construction of models. This capability thus has the potential to provide the formal grounds for powerful modeling suites that combine technologies from different disciplines.

Availability of expressive, intuitive (easy-to-use) modeling languages, equipped with analysis tools that are capable of bringing insights into the functioning of modeled systems, would be a valuable asset from the points of view of both scientific and technological development. In this regard, process algebras are promising platforms for the development of instruments that are complementary to those, which are in use in systems biology.

REFERENCES

Alberts, J. B., & Odell, G. M. (2004). In silico reconstitution of listeria propulsion exhibits nanosaltation. *PLoS Biology, 2*, 2054–2066. doi:10.1371/journal.pbio.0020412

Baeten, J. C. M. (2005). A brief history of process algebra. *Theoretical Computer Science, 335*(2–3), 131–146. doi:10.1016/j.tcs.2004.07.036

Blossey, R., Cardelli, L., & Phillips, A. (2008). Compositionality, stochasticity and cooperativity in dynamic models of gene regulation. *HFSP (Human Frontier Science Program Organization). Journal, 2*(1), 17–28.

Boogerd, F., Bruggeman, J. F., Hofmeyr, J.-H. S., & Westerhoff, H. V. (Eds.). (2007). *Systems Biology: Philosophical Foundations*. New York: Elsevier.

Bustelo, X. R., Sauzeau, V., & Berenjeno, I. M. (2007). GTP-binding proteins of the Rho/Rac family: Regulation, effectors and function in vivo. *BioEssays, 29*, 356–370. doi:10.1002/bies.20558

Cardelli, L. (2005). Abstract machines of systems biology. In Priami, C., Merelli, E., Gonzalez, P. P., & Omicini, A. (Eds.), *Transactions on Computational Systems Biology. III, Lecture Notes in Bioinformatics 3737* (pp. 145–168). New York: Springer.

Cardelli, L. (2008). From processes to ODEs by chemistry. In Ausiello, G. & Karhumäki J. & Mauri G. & Ong C.-H. L. (Eds.). *Fifth IFIP International Conference On Theoretical Computer Science - TCS 2008, IFIP 20th World Computer Congress, International Federation for Information Processing 273*, (pp. 261-281). New York: Springer.

Cardelli, L. (2009). Artificial biochemistry. In Condon, A., Harel, D., Kok, J. N., Salomaa, A., & Winfree, E. (Eds.), *Algorithmic Bioprocesses. Natural Computing Series, Part 7* (pp. 429–462). Springer.

Cardelli, L., Caron, E., Gardner, P., Kahramanoğulları, O., & Phillips, A. (2009). A process model of Rho GTP-binding proteins. *Theoretical Computer Science, 410*(33-34), 3166–3185. doi:10.1016/j.tcs.2009.04.029

Cardelli, L., Caron, E., Gardner, P., Kahramanoğulları, O., & Phillips, A. (2009b). A process model of actin polymerization. In Cannata N. & Merelli E. & Ulidowski, I. (Eds.). *From Biology To Concurrency and Back, Sattelite Workshop of ICALP '08*. Electronic Notes in Theoretical Computer Science 229, (pp. 127-144). New York: Elsevier.

Cardelli, L., & Zavattaro, G. (2008). Termination problems in chemical kinetics. In Breugel, F. v. & Chechik, M. (Eds.), *CONCUR 2008 - Concurrency Theory, 19th International Conference,* Proceedings, Lecture Notes in Computer Science 5201, (pp. 477-491), Springer.

Cardelli, L., & Zavattaro, G. (2010). Turing universality of the Biochemical Ground Form. *Mathematical Structures in Computer Science, 20*(1), 45–73. doi:10.1017/S0960129509990259

Chimini, G., & Chavrier, P. (2000). Function of Rho family proteins in actin dynamics during phagocytosis and engulfment. *Nature Cell Biology, 2*, 191–196. doi:10.1038/35036454

Ciocchetta, F., & Hillston, J. (2008). Process Algebras in Systems Biology. Bernardo, M. & Degano, P. & Zavattaro G. (Eds.). *Formal Methods for Computational Systems Biology, 8th International School on Formal Methods for the Design of Computer, Communication, and Software Systems, SFM 2008,* Advanced Lectures. Lecture Notes in Computer Science 5016, (pp. 265-312). New York: Springer.

Ciocchetta, F., & Priami, C. (2007). Biological Transactions for Quantitative Models. Busi, N. & Zandron, C. (Eds.), *Proceedings of the First Workshop on Membrane Computing and Biologically Inspired Process Calculi, MeCBIC 2006,* Electronic Notes in Theoretical Computer Science 171(2), (pp. 55-67), Elsevier.

Curien, P.-L., Danos, V., Krivine, J., & Zhang, M. (2008). Computational self-assembly. *Theoretical Computer Science, 404*(1-2), 61–75. doi:10.1016/j.tcs.2008.04.014

Danos, V., Feret, J., Fontana, W., Harmer, R., & Krivine, J. (2007). Rule-based modelling of cellular signalling. In Caires, L. & Vasconcelos, V. T. (Eds.). *CONCUR 2007 - Concurrency Theory, 18th International Conference,* Proceedings. Lecture Notes in Computer Science 4703, (pp. 17-41). New York: Springer.

Danos, V., Feret, J., Fontana, W., Harmer, R., & Krivine, J. (2008). Rule-based modelling, symmetries, refinements. In Fisher J. (Ed.). *Proceedings of the 1st international workshop on Formal Methods in Systems Biology,* Lecture Notes in Computer Science 5054, (pp 103 – 122). New York: Springer.

Dematté, L., Priami, C., & Romanel, A. (2008). The Beta workbench: A tool to study the dynamics of biological systems. *Briefings in Bioinformatics, 9*(5), 437–449. doi:10.1093/bib/bbn023

Etienne-Manneville, S., & Hall, A. (2002). Rho GTPases in cell biology. *Nature, 420,* 629–635. doi:10.1038/nature01148

Fisher, J., & Henzinger, T. (2007). Executable cell biology. *Nature Biotechnology, 25,* 1239–1249. doi:10.1038/nbt1356

Fujivara, I., Vavylonis, D., & Pollard, T. D. (2007). Polymerization kinetics of ADP- and ADP-Pi actin determined by fluoresence microscopy. *Proceedings of the National Academy of Sciences of the United States of America, 104*(21), 8827–8832. doi:10.1073/pnas.0702510104

Garcia-Garcia, E., & Rosales, C. (2002). Signal transduction during Fc receptor-mediated phagocytosis. *Journal of Leukocyte Biology, 72,* 1092–1108.

Gillespie, D. T. (1977). Exact stochastic simulation of coupled chemical reactions. *Journal of Physical Chemistry, 81*(25), 2340–2361. doi:10.1021/j100540a008

Goryachev, A. B., & Pokhilko, A. V. (2006). *Computational model explains high activity and rapid cycling of Rho GTPases within protein complexes.* PLOS Computational Biology, 2, 151-1521. For the license terms of the figures adapted from this work, see http://creativecommons.org/licenses/by/2.5/.

Gurry, T., Kahramanoğulları, O., & Endres, R. G. (2009). Biophysical mechanism for Ras-nanocluster formation and signaling in plasma membrane. *PLoS ONE, 4*(7). doi:10.1371/journal.pone.0006148

Hall, A. B., Gakidis, M. A., Glogauer, M., Wilsbacher, J. L., Gao, S., Swat, W., & Brugge, J. S. (2006). Requirements for Vav guanine nucleotide exchange factors and Rho GTPases in FcγR- and complement-mediated phagocytosis. *Immunity, 24,* 305–316. doi:10.1016/j.immuni.2006.02.005

Heiner, M., Gilbert, D., & Donaldson, R. (2008). Petri Nets for Systems and Synthetic Biology. Bernardo, M. & Degano, P. & Zavattaro G. (Eds.). *Formal Methods for Computational Systems Biology, 8th International School on Formal Methods for the Design of Computer, Communication, and Software Systems, SFM 2008,* Advanced Lectures. Lecture Notes in Computer Science 5016, (pp. 215-264), Springer.

Hlavacek, W. S. & Faeder, J. R. & Blinov, M. L. & Posner, R. G. & Hucka M. & Fontana W. (2006). Rules for modeling signal-transduction systems. *Science Signaling* (STKE).

Hoppe, A. D., & Swanson, J. A. (2004). Cdc42, Rac1, and Rac2 display distinct patterns of activation during phagocytosis. *Molecular Biology of the Cell, 15*(8), 3509–3519. doi:10.1091/mbc.E03-11-0847

Hu, J., Matzavinos, A., & Othmer, H. G. (2007). A theoretical approach to actin filament dynamics. *Journal of Statistical Physics, 128*(1/2), 111–138. doi:10.1007/s10955-006-9204-x

Iwasa, J. H., & Mullins, R. D. (2007). Spatial and temporal relationships between actin-filament nucleation, capping, and disassembly. *Current Biology, 17,* 395–406. doi:10.1016/j.cub.2007.02.012

Jaffe, A. B., & Hall, A. (2005). Dynamic changes in the length distribution of actin filaments during polymerization can be modulated by barbed end capping proteins. *Cell Motility and the Cytoskeleton, 61,* 1–8. doi:10.1002/cm.20061

Jaffe, A. B., & Hall, A. (2005). Rho GTPases: Biochemistry and biology. *Annual Review of Cell and Developmental Biology, 21,* 247–269. doi:10.1146/annurev.cellbio.21.020604.150721

Kahramanoğulları, O., & Cardelli, L. (2011). (in press). An intuitive modelling interface for systems biology. *International Journal of Software and Informatics.*

Kahramanoğulları, O., Cardelli, L., & Caron, E. (2009). An intuitive automated modelling interface for systems biology. *Electronic Proceedings in Theoretical Computer Science, 9,* 73–86. doi:10.4204/EPTCS.9.9

Lotka, A. J. (1927). Fluctuations in the abundance of a species considered mathematically. *Nature, 119,* 12.

Milner, R. (1999). *Communicating and mobile systems: the pi-calculus.* Cambridge, UK: Cambridge University Press.

Mogilner, A., & Oster, G. (2003). Force generation by actin polymerization II: The elastic ratchet and tethered filaments. *Biophysical Journal, 84,* 1591–1605. doi:10.1016/S0006-3495(03)74969-8

Mogilner, A., & Oster, G. (2008). Cell motility driven by actin polymerization. *Biophysical Journal, 71,* 3030–3045. doi:10.1016/S0006-3495(96)79496-1

Noble, D. (1960). Cardiac action and pacemaker potentials based on the Hodgkin-Huxley equations. *Nature, 188,* 495–497. doi:10.1038/188495b0

Oltvai, Z. N., & Barabási, A.-L. (2002). Life's complexity pyramid. *Science, 298,* 763–764. doi:10.1126/science.1078563

Patel, J. C., Hall, A., & Caron, E. (2002). Vav regulates activation of Rac but not Cdc42 during FcγR -mediated phagocytosis. *Molecular Biology of the Cell, 13,* 1215–1226. doi:10.1091/mbc.02-01-0002

Phillips, A., & Cardelli, L. (2007). Efficient, correct simulation of biological processes in the stochastic pi-calculus. In Calder, M. & Gilmore, S. (Eds.), *Computational Methods in Systems Biology, International Conference, CMSB 2007,* Proceedings. Lecture Notes in Computer Science 4695, (pp. 184-199), Springer.

Phillips, A., Cardelli, L., & Castagna, G. (2006). A graphical representation for biological processes in the stochastic pi-calculus. *Transactions in Computational Systems Biology, 4230,* 123–152.

Pollard, T. D. (2007). Regulation of actin filament assembly by Arp2/3 complex and formins. *Annual Review of Biophysics and Biomolecular Structure, 36,* 451–477. doi:10.1146/annurev.biophys.35.040405.101936

Powell, C. R., & Boland, R. P. (2009). The effects of stochastic population dynamics on food web structure. *Journal of Theoretical Biology, 257,* 170–180. doi:10.1016/j.jtbi.2008.11.006

Priami, C. (1995). Stochastic pi-calculus. *The Computer Journal, 38*(7), 578–589. doi:10.1093/comjnl/38.7.578

Priami, C. (2009). Algorithmic systems biology. *Communications of the ACM, 52*(5), 80–88. doi:10.1145/1506409.1506427

Priami, C., Ballarini, P., & Quaglia, P. (2009). BlenX4Bio - BlenX for Biologists. Degano, P. & Gorrieri, R. (Eds.), *Computational Methods in Systems Biology, 7th International Conference, CMSB 2009,* Proceedings. Lecture Notes in Computer Science, 5688, (pp. 26-51), Springer.

Priami, C., Guerriero, M. L., & Heath, J. K. (2007). An automated translation from a narrative language for biological modelling into process algebra. In Calder, M. & Gilmore S. (Eds.). *Computational Methods in Systems Biology, International Conference, CMSB 2007,* Proceedings. Lecture Notes in Computer Science 4695, (pp 136–151), Springer.

Priami, C., Regev, A., Shapiro, E., & Silverman, W. (2001). Application of a stochastic name-passing calculus to representation and simulation of molecular processes. *Information Processing Letters, 80*(1), 25–31. doi:10.1016/S0020-0190(01)00214-9

Regev, A., & Shapiro, E. (2002). Cellular abstractions: Cells as computation. *Nature, 419,* 343. doi:10.1038/419343a

Shahrezaei, V., & Swain, P. S. (2008). The stochastic nature of biochemical networks. *Current Opinion in Biotechnology, 19*(4), 369–374. doi:10.1016/j.copbio.2008.06.011

Swanson, J. A., & Hoppe, A. D. (2004). The coordination of signaling during Fc receptor-mediated phagocytosis. *Journal of Leukocyte Biology, 76,* 1093–1103. doi:10.1189/jlb.0804439

Talcott, C. L. (2008). Pathway Logic. Bernardo, M. & Degano, P. & Zavattaro G. (Eds.). *Formal Methods for Computational Systems Biology, 8th International School on Formal Methods for the Design of Computer, Communication, and Software Systems, SFM 2008,* Advanced Lectures. Lecture Notes in Computer Science 5016, (pp. 21-53), Springer.

Volterra, V. (1926). Fluctuations in the abundance of species considered mathematically. *Nature, 118,* 558–560. doi:10.1038/118558a0

Weeds, A., & Yeoh, S. (2001). Action at the Y-branch. *Science, 294,* 1660–1661. doi:10.1126/science.1067619

Wolkenhauer, O., Ullah, M., Kolch, W., & Cho, K. H. (2004). Modeling and simulation of intracellular dynamics: Choosing an appropriate framework. *IEEE Transactions on Nanobioscience, 3,* 200–207. doi:10.1109/TNB.2004.833694

ADDITIONAL READING

Alberts, B., Johnson, A., Walter, P., Lewis, J., Raff, M., & Roberts, K. (2008). *Molecular Biology of the Cell* (5th ed.). Garland Science.

Bergstra, J. A., Ponse, A., & Smolka, S. A. (Eds.). (2001). *Handbook of Process Algebra.* Elsevier.

Cardelli, L. (2008b). On process rate semantics. *Theoretical Computer Science, 391*(3), 190–215. doi:10.1016/j.tcs.2007.11.012

Cardelli, L. (2008c). Molecules as Automata. Corradini, A. & Montanari U. (Eds.). *Recent Trends in Algebraic Development Techniques, 19th International Workshop, WADT 2008, Revised Selected Papers.* Lecture Notes in Computer Science 5486, (pp. 18-20). New York, Springer.

Cardelli, L., & Gardner, P. (2010). Processes in Space. Ferreira, F. & Löwe, B. & Mayordomo, E. & Gomes L. M. (Eds.). *Programs, Proofs, Processes, 6th Conference on Computability in Europe, CiE 2010.* Proceedings. Lecture Notes in Computer Science 6158, (pp. 78-87). New York: Springer.

Cardelli, L., & Priami, C. (2009). Visualization in process algebra models of biological systems. In Hey, T. & Tansley, S. & Tolle, K. (Eds.). *The Fourth Paradigm: Data Intensive Scientific Discovery. Creative Commons Attribution Share Alike License,* 99-105.

Dematté, L., Priami, C., & Romanel, A. (2008). The BlenX Language: A Tutorial. In Bernardo, M., Degano, P., & Zavattaro, G. (Eds.), *Formal Methods for Computational Systems Biology, 8th International School on Formal Methods for the Design of Computer, Communication, and Software Systems, SFM 2008. Advanced Lectures. Lecture Notes in Computer Science, 5016* (pp. 313–365). Springer.

Fages, F., & Soliman, S. (2008). From reaction models to influence graphs and back: A theorem. Fisher, J. (Ed.), *Formal Methods in Systems Biology, First International Workshop, FMSB 2008,* Proceedings. Lecture Notes in Computer Science, 5054, (pp 90–102). New York: Springer.

Galpin, V., & Hillston, J. (2009). Equivalence and discretisation in Bio-PEPA. Degano, P. & Gorrieri, R. (Eds.). *Computational Methods in Systems Biology, 7th International Conference, CMSB 2009.* Proceedings. Lecture Notes in Computer Science, 5688, (pp. 189-204). New York: Springer.

Hillston, J. (1996). *A compositional approach to performance modelling.* Distinguished dissertation in Computer Science. Cambridge, UK: Cambridge University Press.

Hinton, A., Kwiatkowska, M., Norman, G., & Parker, D. (2006). PRISM: a tool for automatic verification of probabilistic systems. Hermanns, H. & Palsberg. J. (Eds.). *Tools and Algorithms for the Construction and Analysis of Systems, 12th International Conference, TACAS 2006,* Proceedings. Lecture Notes in Computer Science, 3920, (pp. 441-444). New York: Springer.

Kahramanoğulları, O. (2010). Flux analysis in process models via causality. *Electronic Proceedings in Theoretical Computer Science, 19,* 20–39. doi:10.4204/EPTCS.19.2

Kazanci, C. (2007). EcoNet: a new software for ecological modeling, simulation and network analysis. *Ecological Modelling, 208*(1), 3–8. doi:10.1016/j.ecolmodel.2007.04.031

Kitano, H. (2002a). Systems biology: A brief overview. *Science, 295,* 1662–1664. doi:10.1126/science.1069492

Kitano, H. (2002b). Computational systems biology. *Nature, 420,* 206–210. doi:10.1038/nature01254

Kitano, H., Funahashi, A., Matsuoka, Y., & Oda, K. (2005). Using process diagrams for the graphical representation of biological networks. *Nature Biotechnology, 23,* 961–966. doi:10.1038/nbt1111

Klipp, E., Herwig, R., Kowald, A., Wierling, C., & Lehrach, H. (2005). *Systems Biology in Practice: Concepts, Implementation and Application.* WILEY-VCH Verlag. doi:10.1002/3527603603

Kohn, K. W., Aladjem, M. I., Kim, S., Weinstein, J. N., & Pommier, Y. (2006). Depicting combinatorial complexity with the molecular interaction map notation. *Molecular Systems Biology, 2,* 51. doi:10.1038/msb4100088

Kwiatkowska, M., Normann, G., Segala, R., & Sproston, J. (1999). Automatic verification of real-time systems with discrete probability distributions. *Lecture Notes in Computer Science, 1601,* 79–95. doi:10.1007/3-540-48778-6_5

Larcher, R., Priami, C., & Romanel, A. (2010). Modelling Self-assembly in BlenX. In Priami, C. & Breitling, R. & Gilbert, D. & Heiner, M. & Uhrmacher, A. M. (Eds.), *Transactions on Computational Systems Biology, 12, Special Issue on Modeling Methodologies.* Lecture Notes in Computer Science, 5945, 163-198. New York: Springer.

Mardare, R., & Cardelli, L. (2010). *The measurable space of stochastic processes*. In Proceedings of Seventh International Conference on the Quantitative Evaluation of Systems, QEST 2010, 171-180, Williamsburg, VA, USA, IEEE Publishing.

Milner, R. (1980). *A calculus of communicating systems*. Springer.

Pimm, S. L. (1991). *The Balance of Nature? Ecological Issues in the Conservation of Species and Communities*. The University of Chicago Press.

Prusinkiewicz, P., & Lindenmayer, A. (1990). *The algorithmic beauty of plants*. New York: Springer.

Sangiorgi, D., & Walker, D. (2001). *The pi-calculus: A theory of mobile processes*. Cambridge, UK: Cambridge University Press.

Wilkinson, D. J. (2006). *Stochastic Modelling for Systems Biology*. Chapman & Hall/CRC.

Chapter 10
Intelligent Classifiers Fusion for Enhancing Recognition of Genes and Protein Pattern of Hereditary Diseases

Parthasarathy Subashini
Avinashilingam Deemed University for Women, Thadagam Post, India

Bernadetta Kwintiana Ane
Universität Stuttgart, Germany

Dieter Roller
Universität Stuttgart, Germany

Marimuthu Krishnaveni
Avinashilingam Deemed University for Women, Thadagam Post, India

ABSTRACT

Most the objective of intelligent systems is to create a model, which given a minimum amount of input data or information, is able to produce reliable recognition rates and correct decisions. In the application, when an individual classifier has reached its limit and, at the same time, it is hard to develop a better one, the solution might only be to combine the existing well performing classifiers. Combination of multiple classifier decisions is a powerful method for increasing classification rates in difficult pattern recognition problems. To achieve better recognition rates, it has been found that in many applications, it is better to fuse multiple relatively simple classifiers than to build a single sophisticated classifier. Such classifiers fusion seems to be worth applying in terms of uncertainty reduction. Different individual classifiers performing on different data would produce different errors. Assuming that all individual methods perform well, intelligent combination of multiple experts would reduce overall classification error and as consequence increase correct outputs. To date, content interpretation still remains as a highly complex task which requires many features to be fused. However, the fusion mechanism can be done at different levels of the classification. The fusion process can be carried out on three levels of abstraction closely connected with the flow of the classification process, i.e. data level fusion, feature level fusion, and classifier fusion. The work presented in this chapter focuses on the fusion of classifier outputs for intelligent models.

DOI: 10.4018/978-1-61350-435-2.ch010

Copyright © 2012, IGI Global. Copying or distributing in print or electronic forms without written permission of IGI Global is prohibited.

INTRODUCTION

To date the computational methods and computer-based systems deployed in science, engineering, industry, business and many other aspects of life has become powerful tools for problem solving, particularly when human beings have to cope with such variety of data at such a rate that precludes human analysis. Prime examples are found in medical and bioinformatics sciences. Currently, with the advancement of soft-computing methods and parallel computing systems it is possible to identify some diseases in humans by sequencing and recognition of genes and proteins pattern.

Generally speaking, genetic disorder or hereditary diseases is a result of mutations. There are two primary pathways to genetic defects. First, genetic disorders caused by the abnormal number of chromosomes, e.g., in Down syndrome there are three instead of two "number 21" chromosomes, therefore a total of 47. Second, triplet expansion repeat mutations caused by modification of gene expression or gain of function respectively, e.g., fragile *X*-syndrome and Huntington's diseases (Mehta, 2007). Defective genes are often inherited from the parents. Often, this happens unexpectedly when two healthy carriers of a defective recessive gene reproduce. In other cases, it can also happen when the defective gene is dominant. Currently around 4,000 genetic disorders are known, with more being discovered.

Four types of genetic disorders are known. First, single gene disorder occurs as the result of a single mutated gene due to genomic imprinting and uniparental disomy that might include Mendelian disorders (e.g., Autosomal, X-linked and Y-linked) and non-Mendelian disorders (e.g., mitochondrial inheritance). Second, multi-factorial and polygenic disorders occur likely associated with the effects of multiple genes in combination with lifestyle and environmental factors. Third, disorders with variable modes of transmission, called heredity malformations, are congenital malformations which might be familial and genetic

or might be acquired by exposure to teratogenic agents in the uterus. Fourth, cytogenetic disorder exists due to alterations in the number or structure of the chromosomes and might cause autosomal disorders and sex chromosome disorders. Presently, heart disease, dermatitis, and cancer are known as genetic diseases that likely to occur due to multi-factoral disorders. Although in most cases complex disorders often cluster in families, but they do not have a clear-cut pattern of inheritance. This fact makes it difficult to determine a person's risk of inheriting or passing on these disorders. This chapter would like to describe and further discuss the discovery of heart disease, dermatitis, and cancer through recognition of genes and protein patterns.

Pattern recognition is an integral part of machine vision and image processing (Duda, 2000; Fu, 1982, Gonzales, 1978; Pavlidis, 1977; Perner, 1996). The objective in pattern recognition is to recognize objects in the scene from a set of measurements of physical objects (Acharya, 2005). Each object is a pattern and the measured values are the features of the pattern. A set of similar objects possessing more or less identical features are said to belong to a certain pattern class. Presently, there are many classification techniques can be used for the recognition of patterns. These techniques work in which the classification of an unknown pattern is decided based on some deterministic or statistical or even fuzzy set theoretic principle.

The classification methods are mainly of two categories, i.e., supervised learning and unsupervised learning. Then, the supervised classification algorithms can further be classified into parametric classifiers and non-parametric classifiers. In parametric supervised classification, the classifier is trained with a large set of labeled training pattern samples in order to estimate the statistical parameters of each class of patterns such as arithmetic-mean, standard deviation, variance, etc. The term "labeled pattern samples" means the set of patterns whose class memberships are known in advance. Here the input feature vectors obtained during the training phase of the supervised classification are assumed to be Gaussian in nature. On the other hand, in the non-parametric supervised classification techniques the parameters are not taken into consideration. Meanwhile, in unsupervised classification cases, the machine partitions the entire data set based on some similarity criteria. This partition results in a set of clusters, where each cluster of patterns belongs to a specific class.

Quite often, in safety critical system such as medical diagnosis system or intensive care unit system, the correctness of the decision need to be taken immediately in real-time, is of crucial importance. Most the objective of intelligent systems is to create a model, which given a minimum amount of input data or information, is able to produce correct perception and decisions. Regarding to expert's approach, the development of intelligent systems should be based on continuous progress of existing methods, i.e., the classifiers, as well as discovering new ones. Meanwhile, other expert's approach suggests as the existing individual methods reach its limit and it is hard to develop a better one, then, the solution might be just to combine existing well performing methods (Ruta, 2000).

During the last decade, classifiers fusion has been well-recognized as a powerful technique for increasing classification rates in the complex pattern recognition. Classifiers fusion is an established research area based on both statistical pattern recognition and machine learning. It is also known as committee of learners, mixtures of experts, classifier ensembles, multiple classifier systems, or consensus theory (Haghighi, 2009).

In pattern recognition, each of individual classifiers is potential to produce errors, not mentioning that the input information might be corrupted and incomplete. Hence, classifier fusion seems to be worth applying in terms of uncertainty reduction. In many applications, it is found that combining multiple relative simple classifiers is better than to build a single sophisticated classifier. The application of different classifiers on different data should produce different errors. Assuming all individual classifiers perform well, combination of such multiple classifiers will reduce overall classification error, therefore, increasing correct outputs.

Generally, fusion can be carried out on three levels of abstraction that closely connected with the flow of classification process, i.e., data-level fusion, feature-level fusion, and classifier fusion [10]. For data-level and feature-level fusions, there have been successful attempts to make use of heuristic methods to transform the numerical, interval and linguistic data into a single space of symmetric trapezoidal fuzzy numbers (Pedrycz, 1998),(Ho, 1994). For classifier fusion, a number of methods referring to decision fusion or mixture of experts have been developed.

Essentially, there are two general groups of classifier fusion methods. The first method is subjectively to operate on the classifiers and put an emphasis on the development of classifier structure. They do not do anything with the classifier outputs until the combination process finds a single best classifier, or a selected group of classifiers, and only their outputs are taken as a final decision or for further processing (Jordan, 1994), (Woods, 1997), (Gader, 1996). Another group of methods operate mainly on classifiers outputs, and effectively the combination of classifiers outputs is calculated (Tahani, 1990), (Keller, 1994; Kuncheva, 1998; Cho, 1995; Wang, 1998; Hinton, 1999), (Huang, 1995; Ueda, 2000; Nayer, 2006). The methods operating on classifiers outputs can be further divided according to the type of the output produced by individual classifiers. To date, content interpretation in pattern recognition still remains as highly complex tasks which requires many information need to be considered. Particularly in the area of hereditary diseases, prime features of genes and proteins are needed as proxy to recognize pattern of diseases and produce accurate diagnosis. This chapter aims to describe the mechanism of classifier fusion needed to achieve higher accuracy and higher classification rates. This capability is built through an intelligent classifier fusion, so does by the acting of individual classifiers to normalize each other the overlapping misclassified regions produced by different classifiers. Each of individual classifier design offers complementary information on the pattern being classified, thus, improve overall performance of the combined classifiers.

In the following paragraphs, Section 2 reviews the existing works on classifier fusion, Section 3 describes the state-of-the-art of existing classifiers, Section 4 explains the developed procedure and algorithm of classifier fusion, Section 5 evaluates the fusion model, Section 6 discuss the application of the fusion model for pattern recognition of hereditary diseases and, finally, Section 7 summarizes all findings and brings them to the conclusions, and also discuss future works in the area of intelligent classifier ensembles.

EXISTING WORKS

Classification is the process of assigning unknown input patterns of data to some known classes based on their properties (Haghighi, 2009). During the last decade, prior studies and researches have been devoted in designing classifiers and improving efficiency, accuracy and reliability of classifiers for a wide range of applications. Fusing outputs of base classifiers as an ensemble working in parallel on input feature space is an attractive method to build more reliable classifiers. It is evident in prior studies, combining outputs of several classifiers leads to improved classification results.

Classifier combination has received considerable attention by experts in the last decade and become an established pattern recognition offspring. Recently, the focus has been shifting from practical heuristic solutions of the combination problem toward explaining why combination methods and strategies work so well and in what cases some methods are better than others.

In principle, a set of classifiers can vary in terms of their weights, the time they take to converge, and their architecture, yet constitute the same solution and present the same patterns of error when they are tested (Kuncheva, 2005). Obviously, when designing an ensemble, the aim is to find classifiers which generalize the different diversity (Sharkey, 1999).

Generally, there are two main categories combination of classifiers, i.e., fusion and selection. In classifier fusion, each ensemble member has knowledge of the whole feature space. Meanwhile, in classifier selection each ensemble member knows well only a part of the space. Therefore, different types of fuser are used for each method and problems being solved. Instead of those main categories, there are also combination schemes lying between the two principle strategies. In this regard, the combination of fusion and selection is called competitive/cooperative classifier or ensemble/modular approach or multiple/hybrid topology (Lam, 2000; Xu, 1992).

Classifiers Fusion Taxonomy

In fusion category, the possible ways of combining outputs of classifiers in an ensemble depend on the information obtained from the individual members (Ho, 2002). A general categorization based on types of outputs of classifiers in the ensemble is fused according to labeled outputs together with fusion of continuous valued outputs. A number of methods based on labeled outputs are Majority vote, weighted majority vote, Naive Bayes Combination, Behavior Knowledge Space Method, and Wernecke's Method and SVD2 (Haghighi, 2009). The methods introduced for fusion of continuous valued outputs are divided in two general categories, i.e., class conscious combiners and class indifferent Combiners. Some fusers do not need to be trained after the classifiers in the ensemble have been trained individually, while other fuser need additional training. These two types of fusers are called trainable/non-trainable fusers or data dependent/data independent ensembles. Some of class indifferent combiners are Decision Templates and Dempster Shafer.

The main idea in classifier selection is an "oracle" that can identify the best expert for a particular input x. This expert's decision is accepted as the estimated decision of the ensemble for x. Two general approaches are proposed in selection, i.e., Decision-Independent Estimate or priory approach and Decision-Dependent Estimate or posteriori approach. In Decision-Independent Estimate the competence is determined based only on the location of x, prior to finding out what labels are suggested for x by the classifiers. In Decision-Dependent Estimates, the class predictions for x by all classifiers are known. Some of the algorithms proposed on these approaches are direct k-NN Estimate, Distance-Based k-NN Estimate and Potential Functions Estimate. From another point of view, there are two other methods of gaining optimized fusers. One method is based on choosing and optimizing the fuser for a fixed ensemble of base classifiers, called decision optimization or non generative ensembles. The other method creates an ensemble of diverse base classifiers by assuming a fixed combiner, called coverage optimization or generative ensembles. Combination of these methodologies is also used in applications as decision/coverage optimization or non generative/generative ensembles (Valentini, 2002; Alexandre, 2001).

Classifiers Fusion Methods

Once an ensemble of classifiers has been created, an effective way of combining their outputs should be found. Amongst the methods proposed the majority vote is by far the most simple and popular approach. Other voting schemes include the minimum, maximum, median, average, and product (Tax, 2000; Kuncheva, 2001). The weighted average approach evaluates optimal weights for the individual classifiers and combines them accordingly (Ueda, 2000). The Behavior Knowledge Space (BKS) method selects the best classifier

in some region of the input space, and bases its decision on the best classifier's output. Other approaches include rank-based methods such as the Borda count, Bayes approach, Dempster–Shafer theory, decision template (Huang, 1995), fuzzy integral, fuzzy connectives, fuzzy templates, probabilistic schemes, and combination by neural networks (Kamel, 2003).

The fuser could also be viewed as a scheme to assign data independent or data dependent weights to classifiers (Woods, 1997; Kuncheva, 2004; Freund, 1996). The boosting algorithm of Freund and Schapire (Wolpert, 1992) maintains a weight for each sample in the training set that reflects its importance. Adjusting the weights causes the learner to focus on different examples leading to different classifiers. After training the last classifier, the decisions of all classifiers are aggregated by weighted voting. The weight of each classifier is a function of its accuracy.

A layered architecture named stacked generalization framework, has been proposed by Wolpert (Jia, 2007). The classifiers at Level-0 receive as input the original data, and each classifier outputs a prediction for its own sub problem. Each layer receives as input the predictions immediately preceding layer. A single classifier at the top level produces the final prediction. Stacked generalization is an attempt to minimize the generalization error by making classifiers at higher layers to learn the types of errors made by the classifiers immediately below them.

Another method of designing classifiers fuser based on fuzzy integral and MSVM4 was proposed by Kexin Jia (Cevikalp, 2008). The method employs multi-class support vector machines classifiers and fuzzy integral to improve recognition reliability. In another approach, Hakan, et al. (n.d.) proposed a dynamic method to combine classifiers that have expertise in different regions of input space. The approach uses local classifier accuracy estimate to weight classifier outputs. The problem is formulated as a convex quadratic optimization problem, which returns optimal nonnegative classifier weights with respect to the chosen objective function, and the weights ensure that locally most accurate classifiers are weighted more heavily for labeling the query sample.

REVIEW ON EXISTING CLASSIFIERS

A Classifier system constantly endures two major crisis when it is under supervised learning environment namely performance and efficiency. The first depends upon the training samples and the latter deals with space and time complexity. In practice, intact these two complexity are will inter-related. This section deals with the existing classifiers and the fusion methods which are effective approaches to enhance the performance of weak classifiers.

Weak Classifiers

There are three aspects that determine a weak classifier, i.e., its architecture, potency of individual classifier, and computational efficiency. Initially, the architecture of weak classifiers should be very simple, but it should not be too preliminary without affecting the efficiency of the space constraint. In order for combinations of weak classifiers to acquire an efficient time-complexity, they have to be generated in a computationally easy and less-costly way. In particular, two steps are involved in producing a fuser, i.e., generating individual weak classifiers through a simple randomized algorithm, and combining a collection of weak classifiers through different fusion techniques. Classifier combination can be applied to class labels, class rankings or confidence estimates on class labels.

Fusion of Weak Classifiers

A set of weak classifiers should satisfy the following two conditions, i.e., each weak classifier should do better than random guessing, and the set of classifiers should have enough computational power to learn a problem. The first condition is to ensure that each weak classifier possess a minimum computational power. The second condition suggests that individual weak classifiers should learn different parts of a problem so that a collection of weak classifiers can learn an entire problem. If all the weak classifiers in a collection learned the same part of a problem, their combination would not do better than the individual classifiers.

Methods of Classifier Fusion

Currently, there are three existing approaches can be used for decision fusion:

- Voting. The simplest approach. But, is it the best?
- Weighted Linear Combination. Using generalized voting.
- Stack Generalization, or also called Classifier of Classifiers. The most general approach. But, specific method is not specified.

Basic ideas to perform Stack Generalization is as follow:

- output of each expert (individual decisions) are regarded as a meta-feature for the decision fusion algorithm to make the fused decision,
- fusion and performing mapping from local decisions (meta-feature) to the final decision.

Soft-Output Fusion Methods

Fusion based on soft/fuzzy outputs produce the greatest improvement in classification performance. The range of outputs belongs to real values ranging from 0 to 1. It is therefore referred to as fuzzy measures. This method takes four trials of evidence to reduce the level of uncertainty. The measure are likely to be: probability, possibility, necessity, belief and plausibility. However, as many classifiers that are combined produce soft outputs in a form of probabilities or fuzzy membership values it would be interesting to see whether the combination of such soft outputs has any benefits in comparison to the simple majority voting scheme.

GA in Weighted Combination of Soft-Output Classifier

Genetic Algorithm (GA) can be applied to find the optimal weights for linear weighted combination of the soft outputs of the classifiers. In the first of the model, it is referred to as soft linear combiner, a single weight $\{w_1,\ldots w_c\}$ is assigned to each of the classifiers with the optimization problem defined as finding the c optimal weights. And in second model, it is referred to as class independent soft linear combiner in which each of the c classifier are assigned with weights for each of the m classes. $W_i = \{w_{i1},\ldots,w_{im}\}$ for $i=1,\ldots c$ resulting in the optimizing problem. Based on this, soft output for the jth class of the Combined linearly weighted classifier based on the soft values y_{ij} given by each of the c individual classifiers as:

$$y_j^{comb} = \sum_{i=1}^{c} w_{ij} y_{ij} \, for \, j = 1,\ldots,m \qquad (1)$$

The winning class is selected on the basis of finding the maximum value of:

$$y_j^{comb} := d = \max ind(y_j^{comb}) \qquad (2)$$

The optimisation criterion that has also been used as a fitness function driving the genetic algorithm's search for optimal combination weights is given as:

$$J = \sum_{i=1}^{n} (d_i - t_i) \qquad (3)$$

where d_i are the labels of the winning class as given by Equation 2 and t_i are the known target class labels from the validation set on samples used for the estimation of the weights.

Fuzzy Integrals

Fuzzy integrals aim at searching for the maximal agreement between the real possibilities relating to objective evidence and the expectation g which defines the level of importance of a subset of sources. The concept of fuzzy integrals arises from the λ –fuzzy measure. It generalises the probability by adding parameter to the additive probability measure with respect to disjoint objects of measure:

$$\underset{\substack{A,B \subset X \\ A \cap B = 0}}{\forall} g(A \cup B) = g(A) + g(B) + \lambda_g(A)_g(B)$$

$$(4)$$

From the normalization $g(X)=1$ we can derive value by solving the equation:

$$\lambda + 1 = \prod_{i=1}^{a} (1 + \lambda g^i) \qquad (5)$$

where g^i are fuzzy densities which could be chosen subjectively or estimated through a training process. Thus, knowing the fuzzy densities g^i, $i = 1,\ldots\ldots\ldots, n$, one can construct the fuzzy measures g_λ are a subclass of belief (for $\lambda \geq 0$) and plausibility ($\lambda \leq 0$) measures defined by Shafer.

Class Ranking Based Techniques

Majority Voting

Voting technique is majority voting straight forward technique used for ranking. It considers only the most likely class provided by each classifier and chooses the most frequent class label among this crisp output set. A trainable variant of majority voting is weighted majority voting, which multiplies each vote by a weight before the actual voting. The weight for each classifier can be obtained; e.g., by estimating the classifiers' accuracies on a validation set. Another voting technique that takes the entire n-best list of a classifier into account, and not only the crisp 1-best candidate class, is Borda count. For BC the overall rank count for class i is computed as:

$$r_i = \sum_{j=1}^{N} w_j r_i^j \qquad (6)$$

Here, the weights can be the performance of each individual classifier measured on training or validation set.

Logistic Regression

Logistic response function is possible to use if the responses from m classifiers are highest for the classes ranked at the top. The function is implied as:

$$\pi(x) = \frac{\exp(\alpha + \beta_1 x_2 + \ldots + \ldots \beta_m x_m)}{1 + \exp(\alpha + \beta_1 x_1 + \beta_2 x_2 \ldots + \ldots \beta_m x_m)} \qquad (7)$$

where $\alpha, \beta_1 \ldots \ldots \beta_m$ are parameters, which are constant. The output of the transformation:

$$L(x) = \log \frac{\pi(x)}{1 - \pi(x)} = (\alpha + \beta_1 x_1 + \ldots \ldots + \beta_m x_m) \qquad (8)$$

The model parameters can be estimated using data fitting methods based on maximum likelihood. The $\pi(x)$ values can be additionally treated as confidence measures. It is possible to determine a threshold value so that classes with confidence value below the threshold are rejected.

Fusing single class labels

Bagging

Bagging is a parallel algorithm in both its training and operational phases. The L ensemble members can be trained on different processors if needed. Bagging intends at developing independent classifiers by taking bootstrap replicates as the training sets. The samples are pseudo-independent because they are taken from the same Z. If classifier outputs were independent and classifiers had the same individual accuracy p, then the majority vote is guaranteed to improve on the individual performance. The bagging algorithm is as follows:

Training phase

Step 1: Initialize the parameters
- $D = \phi$ the ensemble.
- L, the number of classifiers to train.

Step 2: For k=1,.....L
- Take a bootstrap sample S_k from Z.
- Build a classifier D_k using S_k as the training set.
- Add the classifier to the current ensemble, $D = D \cup D_k$

Step 3: Return D

Classification phase

Step 1: Run $D_1 \ldots D_L$ on the input x.
Step 2: The class with the maximum number of votes is chosen as the label for x.

Boosting

Boosting is a prediction rule which is produced by combing rough and moderate inaccurate rule of thumb. Boosting works in an incremental concept by adding one classifier at a time to develop a classifier team. The algorithm used for this typical fusion is called adaptive boosting (ada boost). There are two implementations of AdaBoost: with reweighting and with resampling. The resampling implementation algorithm is shown below:

Training phase

Step 1: Initialize the parameters

- Set the weights $w^1 = [w_1,\ldots\ldots w_N]$, $w_j^1 \in [0,1], \sum_{j=1}^{N} w_j^1 = 1$ (Usually $w_j^1 = \frac{1}{N}$)
- Initialize the ensemble $D = \phi$
- Pick L, the number of classifiers to train

Step 2: For $k = 1,\ldots., L$

- Take a sample S_k from Z using distribution w^k
- Build a classifier D_k using S_k as the training set.
- Calculate the weighted ensemble error at step k by:

$$\varepsilon_k = \sum_{j=1}^{N} w_j^k l_k^j \qquad (9)$$

$l_k^j = 1$ - if D_k misclassifies z_j and $l_k^j = 0$ otherwise

- If $\in_k = 0$ or $\in_k \geq 0.5$, ignore D_k, reinitialize the weights w_j^k to $\frac{1}{N}$ and continue
- Else, calculate $\beta_k \frac{\in_k}{1- \in_k}, where \in_k \in (0, 0.5)$
- Update the individual weights

Step 3: Return D and $\beta_1 \ldots\ldots..,\beta_L$

Classification Phase

Step 1: Calculate the support for class ω_t by:

$$\mu_t(x) = \sum_{D_k(x)=\omega_t} In(\frac{1}{\beta_k}) \qquad (10)$$

Step 2: The class with the maximum support is choosen as the label for x

Combination of Classifiers

Classification is nothing but assigning labels to objects with a set of measurements so called features. But features are not all equally relevant. The feature sets are always in form of relations and noise in the exact context. Two main segments like feature selection and feature extraction can be used to locate the quality of the datasets. Hence if a adequate solution was achieved, it is there in passes to further recognition application.

Classifiers Selection

A classifier is any function which is defined in Equation (1):

$$D = \Re^n \to \Omega \qquad (11)$$

In the canonical model of a classifier a set of c discriminant functions $G = \{g_1(x),\ldots, g_c(x)\}$,

$$g_i : \Re^n \to \Re, i = 1,\ldots.. c \qquad (12)$$

each yielding a score for the respective class. The discriminant functions partition the feature space $\Re^n$ into c decision regions or classification regions denoted by $R_1 \ldots\ldots R_c$

$$R_i = \left\{ x \mid x \in \Re^n, g_i(x) = \max_{k=1\ldots\ldots c} g_k(x)\right\}, i = 1,\ldots.. c \qquad (13)$$

D specifies the decision regions or equivalently, by the discriminant functions G. The boundaries of the decision regions are called classification boundaries, and contain the points for which the highest discriminant function votes tie. It is important to know how well the classifier performs. The performance of a classifier is a compound characteristic, whose most important component is the classification accuracy.

Testing Classifier Accuracy

Every time we make a classification based on a test score, we should expect some number of misclassifications. The accuracy of a test is usually gauged by summing across all possible scores, e.g., root mean square and goodness-of-fit. The main methods of accuracy evaluations are:

- Resubstitution (N; N)
- Holdout ($2N/3$; $N/3$)
- x-fold cross-validation ($N-N/x$; N/x)

where N is the number of records (instances) in the dataset. The basic concepts behind the evaluation are (*i*) Success: instance (record) class is predicted correctly (*ii*) Error: instance class is predicted incorrectly (*iii*) Error rate: a percentage of errors made over the whole set of instances (records) used for testing (*iv*) Predictive Accuracy: a percentage of well classified data in the testing data set.

Phase 1: Resubstitution (N; N)

Testing the classification model using the given dataset in Figure 1.

Re-substitution Error Rate:

- Re-substitution error rate is obtained from training data.

- Training Data Error: uncertainty of the rules.
- The error rate is not always 0%, but usually (and hopefully) very low.
- Resubstitution error rate indicates only how good (bad) are our results (rules, patterns, *NN*) on the TRAINING data; expresses some knowledge about the algorithm used.

Phase 2: Holdout (2N/3; N/3)

Train-and-Test (for large sample sizes) (>1000)) dividing the given data set in:

- A training sample for generating the classification model.
- A test sample to test the model on independent objects with given classifications (randomly selected, 20-30% of the complete data set).

The holdout method reserves a certain amount of data for testing and uses the remainder for training, hence they are called disjoint. Usually, one third (N/3) of data is used for testing, and the rest (2N/3) for training. Here the choice of records for the train and test data is essential.

Phase 3: x-Fold Cross-Validation (N-N/x; N/x)

The cross-validation is used to prevent the overlap of the test sets. It is therefore followed in two steps:

Figure 1. Resubstitution (N; N)

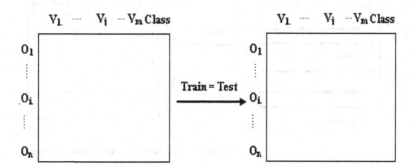

Figure 2. Holdout (2N/3; N/3)

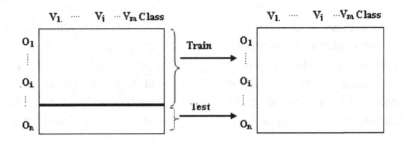

- first step: split data into x subsets of equal size
- second step: use each subset in turn for testing, the remainder for training

The error (predictive accuracy) estimates are averaged to yield an overall error (predictive accuracy) estimate.

A particular form of cross-validation which is called "leave-one–out" expressed as Cross-Validation → Sampling without replacement, then,

- dividing the given data set into subsamples of equal size,
- each subsample is tested by using a model generated from the remaining (m-1) subsamples. The m is represented as number of objects.

The leave-one-out procedure is as follows:

- Let $C(i)$ be the classifier (rules, patterns) built on all data except record x_i
- Evaluate $C(i)$ on x_i, and determine if it is correct or in error
- Repeat for all $i = 1, 2,..., n$.

The total error is the proportion of all the incorrectly classified x_i. The final set of rules (patterns) is a union of all rules obtained in the process.

Drawbacks of Single Classifiers

When solving a classification problem, we would like to choose the best classifier. However, the determination of the best classifier is a time-consuming process. This is because a classification algorithm may form different decision functions based on different initialization, different parameter settings, different training sets, or different feature selections. For instance, different initializa-

Figure 3. x-fold cross-validation (N-N/x; N/x)

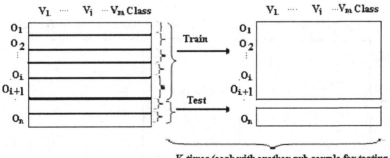

tion may result in different neural network classifiers. Different parameter choices can also result in different classifiers, such as kernel functions and regularization parameter in the SVM algorithm, and the number of neighbors in the *k*-NN algorithm. Even if the best classifier is identified, it might not necessarily be an "ideal" choice. A classification algorithm is designed internally based on some classifier performance measure criteria, e.g., training accuracy or complexity of the classifier, and the "best" classifier is selected according to the criteria. Maybe more than one classifier has same training accuracy or meets the criteria. However, the learning algorithm simply selects one classifier and discards others. The discarded classifiers may correctly classify some data examples which are misclassified by the selected best classifier. Potentially valuable information might be lost by discarding the classification results from less-successful classifiers.

Need for Classifier Combination

Classifier combination methods have proved to be an effective tool to increase the performance of pattern recognition applications. There are different categories of classifier combinations which attempts to put forward more specific directions for future theoretical research. Such effects have significant influence on the performance of combinations, and their study is necessary for complete theoretical understanding of combination algorithms. There are many methods available for classification. When faced with a new problem, where one has little prior knowledge, it is tempting to try many different classifiers in the hope that combining their predictions would give good performance. This had lead to the proliferation of classifier combination, which is therefore called ensemble learning methods.

There are well-known techniques for classifier combination, so called ensemble methods, such as bagging, boosting, and dagging. These methods try to make individual classifiers different by training

them with different training sets or weighting data points differently. This is because it is important to make the individual classifiers as independent as possible for ensemble methods to work well.

Another powerful and general method, called stacked generalisation can be used to combine lower-level models. Stacking methods for classifier combination use another classifier which has as inputs both the original inputs and the output of the individual classifiers. Stacking can be combined with bagging and dagging. Therefore, classifier combination deals with a different problem from those which are usually handled using ensemble and stacking methods.

Combining Classifiers

The key component of any ensemble system is the strategy employed in combining classifiers. Combination rules are often grouped as (*i*) trainable *vs.* non-trainable combination rules, or (*ii*) combination rules that apply to class labels *vs.* class-specific continuous outputs. In trainable combination rules, the parameters of the combiner, usually called *weights*, are determined through a separate training algorithm. The EM algorithm used by the mixture-of-experts model is such an example. The combination parameters created by trainable rules are usually instance specific, and hence are also called dynamic combination rules. Conversely, there is no separate training involved in non-trainable rules beyond that used for generating the ensembles.

In the second taxonomy, combination rules that apply to class labels need the classification decision only (that is, one of $\omega j, j = 1,..., C$), whereas others need the continuous-valued outputs of individual classifiers.

Combining Class Labels

Classifiers producing crisp, single class labels (SCL) provide the least amount of useful information for the combination process. However, they are still well performing classifiers, which could be applied to a variety of real-life problems. If some training data are available, it is possible to upgrade the outputs of these classifiers to the group operating on class rankings or even fuzzy measures. There are a number of methods to achieve this goal, for instance by performing an empirical probability distribution over a set of training data.

Here, we assume that only the class labels are available from the classifier outputs. Let us define the decision of the tth classifier as $d_{t,j} \varepsilon \{0, 1\}$, $t = 1..., T$ and $j = 1,... C$, where T is the number of classifiers and C is the number of classes. If t^{th} classifier chooses class ω_j, then $d_{t,j} = 1$, and 0, otherwise.

Voting Method

Voting strategies can be applied to a multiple classifier system assuming that each classifier gives a single class label as an output and no training data are available. There are a number of approaches to combination of such uncertain information units in order to obtain the best final decision. Let binary characteristic function be defined as follows:

$$B_j(C_j) \begin{cases} 1, & \text{if } d_i = c_i \\ 0, & \text{if } d_i \neq c_i \end{cases} \tag{14}$$

Then the general voting routine can be defined as Equation 15 shown in Box 1.

Majority Voting

There are three versions of majority voting, where the ensemble choose the class (*i*) on which all classifiers agree (unanimous voting), (*ii*) predicted by at least one more than half the number of classifiers (simple majority), or (*iii*) that receives the highest number of votes, whether or not the sum of those votes exceeds 50% (plurality voting or just majority voting). The ensemble decision for the plurality voting can be defined as choose class ω_J, if:

$$\sum_{t=1}^{T} d_{t,J} = \max_{j=1}^{c} \sum_{t=1}^{T} d_{t,j} \tag{16}$$

Majority voting is an optimal combination rule under the minor assumptions of: (1) we have an odd number of classifiers for a two class problem; (2) the probability of each classifier choosing the correct class is p for any instance x; and (3) the classifier outputs are independent.

Given a set of classifier $H = \{h_1........, h_T\}$ for a binary classification problem such that each individual classifier assigns a data example $x_i \in R^n$ into a class label w_1 or w_2, $h_i: R^n \rightarrow \Omega$ where $\Omega = \{w_1, w_2\}$

Class-Indifferent Combiners

The degrees of support for a given input x can be interpreted in different ways, the two most common being confidences in the suggested labels and estimates of the posterior probabilities for the classes.

Box 1.

$$E(D) \begin{cases} c_i, & \text{if } \underset{1 \subset \{1,...m\}}{\forall} \sum_{j=1}^{n} B_j(C_t) \leq \sum_{j=1}^{n} B_j(c_t) \geq \alpha..m + k(d) \\ r & \text{otherwise} \end{cases} \tag{15}$$

Let $x_t \in R^n$ be a feature vector and $\Omega = \{\omega_1, \omega_2, \ldots, \omega_c\}$ be the set of class labels. Each classifier D_i in the ensemble $D = \{D_1 \ldots \ldots D_t\}$ outputs c degree of support. The L classifier outputs for a particular input x can be organized in a decision profile ($DP(x)$) as the matrix. The combiners in this group derive $\mu(x)$ using all $L \times c$ degrees of support in $DP(x)$. Each vector in the intermediate feature space is an expanded version of $DP(x)$ obtained by concatenating its L rows. Any classifier can be applied at this point, from a simple linear regression to a neural network.

Decision Templates

The idea of the decision templates (DT) combiner is to remember the most typical decision profile for each class ω_j, called the decision template, DT_j, and then compare it with the current decision profile $DP(x)$ using some similarity measure S. The closest match will label x.

Two measures of similarity are based upon:
The Squared Euclidean distance ($DT(E)$). The Ensemble support for ω_j is:

$$\mu_j(x) = 1 - \frac{1}{Lxc} \sum_{i=1}^{L} \sum_{k=1}^{c} [DT_j(i,k) - d_{i,k}(x)]^2 \tag{17}$$

where $DT_j(i, k)$ is the (i, k)th entry in decision template DT_j. The output μ_j are scaled to span the interval $[0,1]$. The class with the maximal support would be the same.

The training and operation of the decision templates is given as:

Step 1: Decision templates (training): For $j = 1, \ldots \ldots \ldots c$. calculate the mean of the decision profiles $DP(z_k)$ of all members of ω_j from the data set Z. Call the mean a decision template DT_j

$$DT_j = \frac{1}{N_j} \sum_{\substack{z_i \in \omega_j \\ z_k \in Z}} DP(z_k) \tag{18}$$

where N_j in the number of elements of Z from ω_j.

Step 2: Decision templates (operation): Given the input $x_t \in R^n$, construct DP(x). Calculate the similarity S between $DP(x)$ and each DT_j

$$\mu_j(x) = S(DP(x), DT_j) j = 1, \ldots \ldots \ldots c \tag{19}$$

Classifier Combination Using Soft-Outputs

It is a mixture of expert outputs which represents supervised learning techniques. It is a tree like structure in which each leaf represents individual network, which given the input vector x tries to solve a local supervised learning problem.

Simple Bayes

The Bayesian methods can be applied to the classifier fusion under the condition that the outputs of the classifier are expressed in posterior probabilities. Effectively combination of given likelihoods is also a probability of the same type, which is expected to be higher than the probability of the best individual classifier for the correct class. Two basic Bayesian fusion methods are introduced. The first one named *Bayes Average* is a simple average of posterior probabilities. The second method uses Bayesian methodology to provide a belief measure associated with each classifier output and eventually integrates all single beliefs resulting in a combined final belief.

If the outputs of the multiple classifier system are given as posterior probabilities that an input sample x comes from a particular class C_1, $i = 1, \ldots, m$: $P(x \in C_i/x)$, it is possible to calculate an average posterior probability taken from all classifiers:

$$P_t(x \in C_1 \, / \, x) = \frac{1}{K} \sum_{k=1}^{K} P_K(x \in C_i \, / \, x) \qquad (20)$$

where i = 1,.., *m*. Such a Bayes decision, based on the newly estimated posterior probabilities is called an average Bayes classifier. This approach can be applied for the Bayes classifiers. For other classifiers there is a number of methods to estimate posterior probability. As an example for the *k*-NN classifier the transformation is given in the following form:

$$P_t(x \in C_1 \, / \, x) = \frac{k_i}{k_m} \qquad (21)$$

where k_i denotes the number of prototype samples from class C_i out of all k_{nn} nearest prototype samples. The quality of the Bayes average classifier depends on how the posterior probabilities are estimated and the diversity of used classifiers.

Algebraic Combiners

The continuous output provided by a classifier for a given class is interpreted as the degree of support given to that class, and it is usually accepted as an estimate of the posterior probability for that class. The posterior probability interpretation requires access to sufficiently dense training data, and that the outputs be appropriately normalized to add up to 1 over all classes. Usually, the *softmax* normalization is used for this purpose.

Simple algebraic combiners are, in general, non-trainable combiners of continuous outputs. The total support for each class is obtained as a simple function of the supports received by individual classifiers. Representation can be the total support received by class ω_j, the *j* th column of the decision profile *DP(x)*, as:

$$\mu_j(X) = \Im[d_1, j(X), \ldots \ldots, d_T, j(X)] \qquad (22)$$

where $\Im(.)$ is the combination function.

Product Rule

In product rule, supports provided by the classifiers are multiplied. This rule is very sensitive to the most pessimistic classifiers: a low support (close to 0) for a class from any of the classifiers can effectively remove any chance of that class being selected. However, if individual posterior probabilities are estimated correctly at the classifier outputs, then this rule provides the best estimate of the overall posterior probability of the class selected by the ensemble.

$$\mu_j(x) = \frac{1}{T} \prod_{t=1}^{T} d_{t,j}(x) \qquad (23)$$

Experiments on Biomedical Data

The emergence of information and communication technologies has drastically changed biomedical scientific processes. Experimental data and results today are easy to share and repurpose by enabling connection to databases containing such information. As a consequence, the variety of biomedical data available in the public domain is now very diverse and ranges from genomic-level high-throughput data.

Computational intelligence methods refer to fuzzy logic, neural networks, and evolutionary algorithms. These methods are able to handle nonlinear separable data, deal with uncertainties and imprecision, search solutions in large spaces, and provide probabilistic or continuous rather than discrete classification results. The advantage of fusion approaches makes them particularly suitable for solving complex biological problems.

Experimental Design

The experiment is based on Holdout design. A dataset *S* is first divided into *n* subsets. One subset is used as a group of testing data and all the other subsets used as training data. So, there are *n* groups of testing data and training data. Each data example is either in testing dataset or in training dataset in one group. The performance of the model is estimated by the average of *n* accuracies from *n* different testing data.

In the process, the validation data are prepared and the accuracies of the validation data are used as the three accuracy inputs of the fuzzy system. The validation data are classified to get the validation accuracies. The average of *m* validation accuracies from Holdout classification will be used as the SVM accuracy inputs in the fuzzy fusion model.

Experimental Data Description

Two datasets from UCI Data Set Repository are used to estimate the performance of the fuzzy SVM fusion models and MLP. All the three datasets are classification data. The data have been normalized before the classification.

- **Heart Data:** The dataset describes diagnosing of cardiac Single Proton Emission Computed Tomography (SPECT) images. Each of the patients is classified into two categories, either normal or abnormal. The database of 267 SPECT image sets (patients) was processed to extract features that summarize the original SPECT images. As a result, 44 continuous feature pattern was created for each patient. The pattern was further processed to obtain 22 binary feature patterns.
- **Breast Cancer:** The dataset is a clinical data. The Dataset is with electrical impedance measurements of freshly excised tissue samples from the breast. It contains 683 data.
- **Dermatology data:** This database contains 34 attributes, 33 of which are linear valued and one of them is nominal.

They all share the clinical features of erythema and scaling, with very little differences. The diseases in this group are psoriasis, seboreic dermatitis, lichen planus, pityriasis rosea, cronic dermatitis, and pityriasis rubra pilaris. Patients were first evaluated clinically with 12 features. Afterwards, skin samples were taken for the evaluation of 22 histopathological features. The values of the histopathological features are determined by an analysis of the samples under a microscope.

Experimental Results and Analysis

All the datasets are classified in Holdout patronizing method and each training data are further divided in order to obtain the validation accuracies. Table 1 shows the training and testing accuracies of the datasets in MLP and SVM networks for heart disease, breast cancer and dermatitis datasets.

From Table 2 the results explore that the SVM and MLP classifiers achieve high accuracy when it is in the combination method of decision templates. One more important result is classifier fusion model of DT outperforms the best of its for three datasets composing SVM classifiers and MLP and achieves higher accuracies.

EVALUATION OF FUSION MODEL

The terms expert, classifier and hypothesis are used interchangeably: the goal of an expert is to make a decision, by choosing one option from a previously defined set of options. This process

Table 1. Accuracy of datasets in (%) in MLP and SVM

No	Data sets	Training accuracy (%)	Testing accuracy (%)
1.	Heart data	66.00	55.00
2.	Breast data	100.00	95.61
3.	Dermatitis data	99.20	84.25

Table 2. Average accuracy of datasets

No.	Data sets	Combination methods	Average accuracy	Elapsed time (in seconds)
1.	Heart data	Majority vote	0.5556	0.405288
2.	Heart data	Decision Template	0.9136	0.398645
3.	Heart data	Bayes	0.4444	0.449540
4.	Heart data	Algebraic combiners (Product rule)	0.8642	0.397320
5.	Breast data	Majority vote	0.9561	0.571200
6.	Breast data	Decision Template	0.9610	0.473299
7.	Breast data	Bayes	0.9561	0.512573
8.	Breast data	Algebraic combiners (Product rule)	0.9561	0.497109
9.	Dermatitis data	Majority vote	0.8433	2.06747
10.	Dermatitis data	Decision Template	0.8796	2.006766
11.	Dermatitis data	Bayes	0.8426	1.990007
12.	Dermatitis data	Algebraic combiners (Product rule)	0.8426	1.596804

can be cast as a classification problem: the expert (classifier) makes a hypothesis about the classification of a given data instance into one of predefined categories that represent different decisions. The decision is based on prior training of the classifier, using a set of representative training data, for which the correct decisions are a priori known.

The classifier fusion model follows the below points:

a. The number of individual classifiers used.
b. The type of the individual classifiers. Some combination scheme use classifiers of the same types, e.g., neural networks, linear classifiers, nearest neighbor classifiers, and other schemes use sets of different classifier models.
c. The feature subsets used by the individual classifiers.
d. The aggregation of the individual decisions. Examples of these are majority vote; naive Bayes; behavior-knowledge space (BKS); simple aggregation connectives like average, product, minimum, maximum; fuzzy integral; trained linear combinations; neural network aggregation; Dempster–Shafer aggregation, etc.
e. The training data sets for the individual classifiers.
f. The type of training of the two-level scheme:
  i. Training of the individual classifiers and applying aggregation that does not require further training (e.g., aggregation techniques like average, minimum, product, maximum, etc.);
  ii. Training of the individual classifiers followed by training the aggregation;
  iii. Simultaneous training of the whole scheme.

Usually the individual classifiers are chosen ad hoc on the basis of their accuracy (the higher the better). When the paradigm is trained as a whole, the parameters of the individual classifiers are varied along with the parameters of the aggregation scheme.

Classifier Fusion

Classifiers such as multi-layer perceptron (MLP), radial basis function neural networks (RBFNN), Gaussian mixture models (GMM), learning vector quantisation (LVQ) and support vector machines (SVM) were tested on the benchmark datasets. Results achieved by testing against one classifier at a time indicate that MLP and SVM emerged as best single classifiers in the current case, with high classification accuracy.

Fusion at the classifier level in the current work has been achieved by training another classifier (MLP) using the output of the single best classifiers (MLP and SVM in the current case) as new features, with the aim of achieving more reliable and robust results. This is due to the fact that every classifier makes a different kind of error on a different region of the input space. Hence it is hoped that combining the information of more than one classifier might result in better classification rates for a given problem.

MLP Classifier

The MLP is a special kind of Artificial Neural Network (ANN). MLP has been chosen because of its well-known learning and generalization abilities, which is necessary for dealing with imprecision in input patterns. Architecturally, an MLP is a feed-forward layered network of artificial neurons. Each artificial neuron in the MLP computes a sigmoid function of the weighted sum of all its inputs. An MLP consists of one input layer, one output layer and a number of hidden or intermediate *layers*, as shown in Figure 4. When used without quali-fication, the terms "Neural Network" (NN) and "Artificial Neural Network" (ANN) usually refer to a Multilayer Perceptron Network.

The output from every neuron in a layer of the MLP is connected to all inputs of each neuron in the immediate next layer of the same. Neurons in the input layer of the MLP are all basically dummy neurons as they are used simply to pass on the input to the next layer just by computing an identity function each. The numbers of neurons in the input and the output layers of an MLP are chosen depending on the problem to be solved. The number of neurons in other layers and the number of layers in the MLP are all determined by a trial and error method at the time of its *train-ing*. An ANN requires training to learn an unknown input-output relationship to solve a problem.

- **Input Layer:** A vector of predictor vari-able values $(x_1...x_p)$ is presented to the input layer. The input layer (or processing before the input layer) standardizes these values so that the range of each variable is -1 to 1. The input layer distributes the values to

Figure 4. A block diagram of an MLP

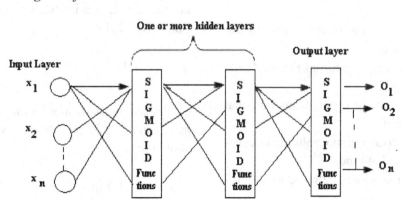

each of the neurons in the hidden layer. In addition to the predictor variables, there is a constant input of 1.0, called the *bias* that is fed to each of the hidden layers; the bias is multiplied by a weight and added to the sum going into the neuron.

- **Hidden Layer:** Arriving at a neuron in the hidden layer, the value from each input neuron is multiplied by a weight (w_{ji}), and the resulting weighted values are added together producing a combined value u_j. The weighted sum (u_j) is fed into a transfer function, σ, which outputs a value h_j. The outputs from the hidden layer are distributed to the output layer.

- **Output Layer:** Arriving at a neuron in the output layer, the value from each hidden layer neuron is multiplied by a weight (w_{kj}), and the resulting weighted values are added together producing a combined value v_j. The weighted sum (v_j) is fed into a transfer function, σ, which outputs a value y_k. The *y* values are the outputs of the network.

Training: Multilayer Perceptron Networks

The goal of the training process is to find the set of weight values that will cause the output from the neural network to match the actual target values as closely as possible. There are several issues involved in designing and training a multilayer perceptron network:

- Selecting how many hidden layers to use in the network.
- Deciding how many neurons to use in each hidden layer.
- Finding a globally optimal solution that avoids local minima.
- Converging to an optimal solution in a reasonable period of time.
- Validating the neural network to test for overfitting.

Depending on the models of ANNs, training is performed either under supervision of some teacher (i.e., with labeled data of known input-output responses) or without supervision. The MLP to be used for the present work requires supervised training. During training of an MLP *weights* or strengths of neuron-to-neuron connections, also called *synapses*, are iteratively tuned so that it can respond appropriately to all training data and also to other data, not considered at the time of training. Learning and generalization abilities of an ANN are determined on the basis of how best it can respond under these two respective situations. The MLP classifier designed for the present work is trained with the Back Propagation (BP) algorithm. It minimizes the *sum of the squared errors* for the training samples by conducting a *gradient descent* search in the *weight space*. The number neurons in a hidden layer in the same are also adjusted during its training. The problem of *pattern classification* involves two successive transformations as follows:

$$M \rightarrow F \rightarrow D$$

where, M, F and D stand for the measurement space, the feature space and the decision space respectively. Once a feature set is fixed up, it is left with the design of a mapping (δ) as follows:

$$\delta: F \rightarrow D$$

ANNs with their learning and generalization abilities can approximate a general class of functions given below:

$$f: \Re^n \rightarrow \Re$$

Pattern classification with ANNs requires approximating δ, as a discrete valued function shown below:

$$\delta: \Re^n \rightarrow \{1, 2 \ldots m\}$$

where, n and m denotes the number of features and the number of pattern classes respectively. So an ANN based pattern classifier requires n number of neurons in the input layer and m number of neurons in the output layer. Conventionally 1-out-of-m representation is used for its output.

Training: Support Vector Machine

Support Vector Machine has been used successfully for pattern recognition and regression tasks formulized under the concept of structural risk minimization rule. It was mainly designed for binary classification, in order to construct an optimal hyper-plane, to maximize the margin of separation between the negative and positive data set. Although, SVM is used for two class pattern classification problem but multi-class problem can also be solved by extending the binary classification to multi class classification. For the Support Vector Machine classifier, an open source software LibSVM tool can be used. In general, a classification task usually involves with training and testing data which consist of some data instances. Each instance in the training set contains one "target value" (class labels) and several "attributes" (features). The goal of SVM is to produce a model which predicts target value of data instances in the testing set which are given only the attributes. Before considering the data directly from the linearly scaling each attribute to the range [-1,+1] or [0,1]. Given a training set of instance-label pairs (x_i, y_i); i= 1 where $x_i \in R^n$ and $y \in \{1,-1\}^l$, the support vector machines (SVM) require the solution of the following optimization problem subject to:

$$\min_{w,b,\xi} \frac{1}{2} w^T w + C \sum_{i=1}^{l} \xi_i \qquad (24)$$
$$y_i(w^T \varphi(x_i) + b) \geq 1 - \xi_i, \xi_i \geq 0$$

Here training vectors x_i are mapped into a higher dimensional space by the function ϕ. Then

SVM finds a linear separating hyper plane with the maximal margin in this higher dimensional space. $C > 0$ is the penalty parameter of the error term. Futhermore, $K(x_i, x_j) \equiv \phi(x_i)^T \phi(x_j)$ is called the kernel function.

Support Vector Machine (SVM) models are closely related to classical multilayer perceptron neural networks. Using a kernel function, SVM's are an alternative training method for polynomial, radial basis function and multi-layer perceptron classifiers in which the weights of the network are found by solving a quadratic programming problem with linear constraints, rather than by solving a non-convex, unconstrained minimization problem as in standard neural network training. In SVM, a predictor variable is called an attribute, and a transformed attribute that is used to define the hyperplane is called a feature. The task of choosing the most suitable representation is known as feature selection. A set of features that describes one case (i.e., a row of predictor values) is called a vector. So the goal of SVM modeling is to find the optimal hyperplane that separates clusters of vector in such a way that cases with one category of the target variable are on one side of the plane and cases with the other category are on the other side of the plane.

Classifier Evaluation and ROC-Based Fusion Model

Evaluation of a classifier performance is done by minimizing an estimation of a generalization error or some other related measures. However, accuracy or error of a classifier is not necessarily a good one. In fact, when the data distribution is strongly unbalanced, accuracy may be misleading since the *all-positive* or *all-negative* classifier may achieve a very good classification rate. A ROC graph is a plot with the false positive rate on the *X* axis and the true positive rate on the *Y* axis. The point (0,1) is the perfect classifier: it classifies all positive cases and negative cases correctly. It is (0,1) because the false positive rate is 0 (none), and the true positive rate is 1 (all). The point (0,0) represents a classifier that predicts all cases to be negative, while the point (1,1) corresponds to a classifier that predicts every case to be positive. Point (1,0) is the classifier that is incorrect for all classifications. In many cases, a classifier has a parameter that can be adjusted to increase *TP* at the cost of an increased *FP* or decrease *FP* at the cost of a decrease in *TP*. Each parameter setting provides a (*FP*, *TP*) pair and a series of such pairs can be used to plot an ROC curve. A non-parametric classifier is represented by a single ROC point, corresponding to its (*FP*,*TP*) pair. It can also be viewed as a tradeoff between benefits (true positives) and costs (false positives).

Confusion Matrix

A confusion matrix summarizes the types of errors that a classification model is likely to make. The confusion matrix is calculated by applying the model to test data in which the target values are already known. These target values are compared with the predicted target values. A confusion matrix shown in the Table 3 is a square with n dimensions, where n is the number of target classes. For example, a multiclass classification model with the target values small, medium, and large would have a three-by-three confusion matrix. A binary classification model has two-by-two confusion matrix. The rows of a confusion matrix identify the known target values. The columns indicate the predicted values. The entries in the confusion matrix have the following meaning in the context of the present study:

Table 3 Confusion matrix

		Predicted	
		Negative	Positive
Actual	Negative	*a*	*b*
	Positive	*c*	*d*

- *a* is the number of correct predictions that an instance is negative,
- *b* is the number of incorrect predictions that an instance is positive,
- *c* is the number of incorrect of predictions that an instance negative, and
- *d* is the number of correct predictions that an instance is positive.

Several standard terms have been defined for the 2 class matrix:

The accuracy (AC) is the proportion of the total number of predictions that are correct. It is determined using the below equation:

$$AC = \frac{a+d}{a+b+c+d} \tag{25}$$

The recall or true positive rate (TP) is the proportion of positive cases that are correctly identified, as calculated using the formula:

$$TP = \frac{d}{c+d} \tag{26}$$

The false positive rate (FP) is the proportion of negatives cases that are incorrectly classified as positive, as calculated using the below equation:

$$FP = \frac{b}{a+b} \tag{27}$$

The true negative rate (TN) is defined as the proportion of negatives are that were classified correctly, as:

$$TN = \frac{a}{a+b} \tag{28}$$

The false negative rate (FN) is the proportion of positives cases that are incorrectly classified as negative, as:

$$FN = \frac{c}{c + d} \qquad (29)$$

Finally, precision (P) is the proportion of the predicted positive cases that are correct, as:

$$P = \frac{d}{b + d} \qquad (30)$$

The accuracy determined using equation may not be an adequate performance measure when the number of negative cases is much greater than the number of positive cases.

For a set of testing examples, a confusion matrix can be constructed as shown in Table 4. If the number of positives and negatives are denoted by N + and N - respectively, where N + = TP + FN and N - = FP + TN, then, the true positive rate (TPR) and the false positive rate (FPR) are defined as follows:

$TPR = TP/N^+$

$FPR = FP/N^-$

and the classification accuracy is defined as:

$$Accuracy = \frac{TP + TN}{N^+ + N^-} \qquad (31)$$

Table 4. Confusion matrix of a classifier

	Predicated Positive	Predicated Negative	Total Examples
Actual Positive	(TP) True Positives	(FN) False Negatives	N
Actual Negative	(FP) False Positives	(TN) True Negatives	N

Experiments on Biomedical Data

Method

The model construction and testing are based on Holdout method. Given a dataset *S*, it is first divided into *n* subsets. Each subset is treated as a group of testing data and all the other subsets together form a group of training data.

Environment

The dataset is loaded with raw input and target data. The repliation used is 1 with base classifiers of 3 and the identified classifiers are MLP and SVM. Partitioning of data is done using Holdout and four combination methods are used for comparison based on average accuracy. All code is executed under a PC running the windows OS with MATLAB 2010.

Results

Figure 5, 6, 7, 8, 9, 10 show the testing and training accuracies of the datasets in MLP and SVM networks.

Figure 11 the average accuracy of the combination method and the time graph for the respective methods.

Figures 12, 13 and 14 depicts the accuracy (recognition rate) for each fold of the respective datasets taken based of decision template combination method.

Discussion

When there are many competing approaches to a problem, an effort to determine a winning one is inevitable. The best algorithm depends on the structure of the available data and prior knowledge. The typical consensus is that boosting, which usually achieves better generalization performances, but it is also more sensitive to noise and outliers. The best combination method, just as the best

Figure 5. ROC curve for heart dataset based on MLP

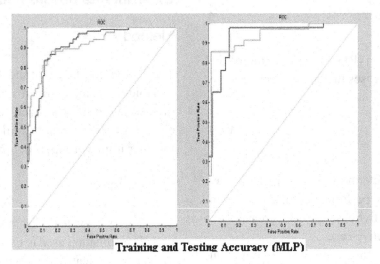

Training and Testing Accuracy (MLP)

Figure 6. ROC curve for heart dataset based on SVM

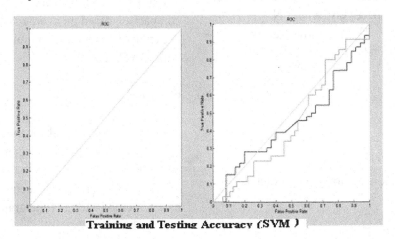

Training and Testing Accuracy (SVM)

Figure 7. ROC curve for breast cancer dataset based on MLP

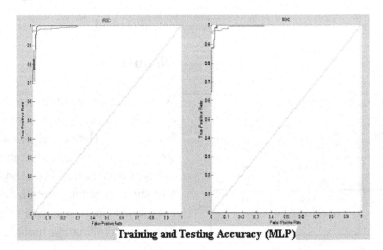

Training and Testing Accuracy (MLP)

Figure 8. ROC curve for breast cancer dataset based on SVM

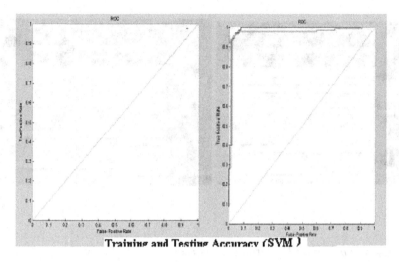

Figure 9. ROC curve for dermatitis dataset based on MLP

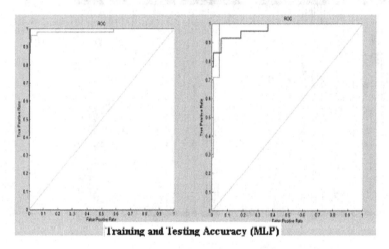

Figure 10. ROC curve for dermatitis dataset based on SVM

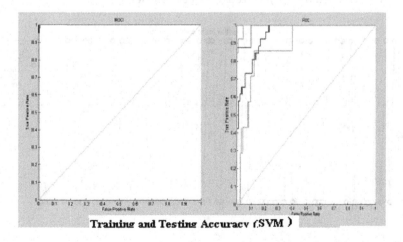

Figure 11. Accuracy and the time taken for combination methods

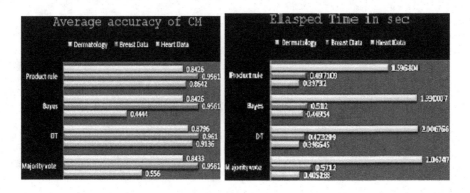

Figure 12. Accuracy rate based on DT for heart dataset

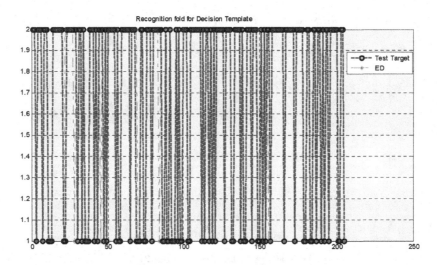

Figure 13. Accuracy rate based on DT for breast cancer dataset

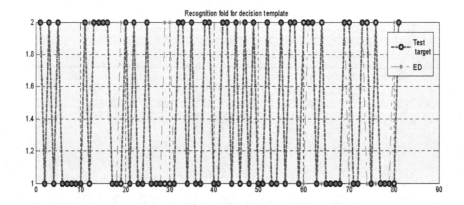

Figure 14. Accuracy rate based on DT for dermatitis dataset

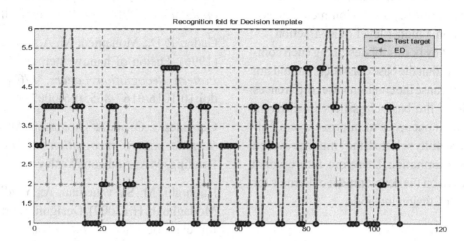

ensemble method, depends much on the particular problem. However, there is a growing consensus on using the Decision template due to its consistent performance over a broad spectrum of applications. If the accuracies of the classifiers can be reliably estimated, then the majority approaches may be considered. Hence the classifier outputs correctly estimate the posterior probabilities, by considering the decision template combination method.

CONCLUDING REMARKS

Conclusion

Today, coping with problems of complexity in diagnosis of hereditary diseases, a hybrid intelligent system can be developed as a tool for recognizing patterns of potential diseases in human beings. This ability is built through the development of intelligent classifier fusion.

It has been well-recognized that in many situations, combining outputs of several classifiers leads to improved classification results. This occurs because each classifier produces error on a different area of the input space. In other words, the subset of input space that each classifier

labels correctly will differ from one classifier to another. This implies that by using information from more than one classifier, it is probable that a better overall accuracy is obtained for a given problem. On the other hand, instead of picking up just one classifier, a better approach would be to use more than one classifier while averaging their outputs.

In this work, the classifier fusion model is developed as an ensemble of soft-output classifiers that are combined using prime fusion methods, i.e., majority vote, decision template, Bayes, and Algebraic combiners (or product rule). The fusion model is trained through supervised learning, i.e., multilayer perceptron (MLP) and support vector machine (SVM), to recognize genes and protein patterns of hereditary diseases. The application of the combined classifiers for recognizing heart disease, dermatitis, and breast cancer produces good and prospective results.

Future Works

Results obtained based on benchmark data exhibits that the new ensemble classifier works more efficient than the individual classifiers. There are many studies and researches focused on designing classifiers and classifier fusion. Surprisingly, there have been very few attempts to research on the combination of several fusion methods as a combination on a higher level of abstraction.

One of the key points for designing such combiner system is that the base classifiers should not be identical because the combiner uses differences in behavior of the base classifiers in different regions of the input space to improve overall efficiency. If carefully selected, they might provide a reduction of information. Therefore, future works will be focused on the development of kernels for combination of fusion methods.

REFERENCES

Acharya, T., & Ray, A. K. (2005). *Image processing: Principles and applications.* New Jersey., Alexandre, L., Campihlo, A. and& Kamel, M. (2001). On combining classifiers using sum and product rules. *Pattern Recognition Letters, 22,* 1283–1289.

Bezdek, J. (1999). *Fuzzy models and algorithms for pattern recognition and image processing. J.* Boston: Kluwer Academic.

Cevikalp, H., & Polikar, R. (2008). Local classifier weighting by quadratic programming. *Neural Networks, 9*(10).

Cho, S. B., & Kim, J. H. (1995). Combining multiple neural networks by fuzzy integral for robust classification. *IEEE Transactions on Systems, Man, and Cybernetics, 25*(2), 380–384. doi:10.1109/21.364825

Duda, R. O. Hart, P. E., and& Stork, D. G. (2000). *Pattern classification.*2nd ed., New York, NY: Wiley.

Freund, Y., & Schapire, R. (1996). Experiments with a new boosting algorithm. *In proceedings of the 13th International Conference on Machine Learning,* (pp. 149–156).

Fu, K. S. (1982). *Syntatic pattern recognition and applications.* Cliffs, NJ: Prentice-Hall.

Gader, P. D., Mohamed, M. A., & Keller, J. M. (1996). Fusion of handwritten word classifiers. *Pattern Recognition Letters, 17*(6), 577–584. doi:10.1016/0167-8655(96)00021-9

Gonzales, r. C. and& Thomason, M. G. (1978). *Syntatic pattern recognition: An introduction.* Reading, MA: Addison-Wesley.

Haghighi, M. S., Vahedian, A., Yazdi, H. S., & Modaghegh, H. (2009). Designing kernel scheme for classifier fusion. *International Journal of Computer Science and Information Security, 6*(2), 239–248.

Hinton, G. E. (1999). Products of experts. *Artificial Neural Networks Conf., 470,* 1-9.

Ho, T. H., Hull, J. J., & Srihari, S. N. (1994). Decision combination in multiple classifier system. *IEEE Transactions on Pattern Analysis and Machine Intelligence, 16*(1), 66–75. doi:10.1109/34.273716

Ho, T. K. (2002). Multiple classifier combination: Lessons and the next steps. *Hybrid Methods in Pattern Recognition,* 171-198.

Huang, Y., Liu, K., & Suen, C. (1995). The combination of multiple classifiers by a neural network approach. *J. Pattern Recognition Artif Intell, 9,* 579–597. doi:10.1142/S0218001495000547

Huang, Y. S., & Suen, C. Y. (1995). A method of combining multiple experts for the recognition of unconstrained handwritten numerals. *IEEE Transactions on Pattern Analysis and Machine Intelligence, 17*(1), 90–94. doi:10.1109/34.368145

Jia, K., & Lu, Y. (2007). A new method of combined classifier design based on fuzzy integral and support vector machines. *In ICCCAS International Conference on Communications, Circuits and Systems.*

Jordan, M. I., & Jacobs, R. A. (1994). Hierarchical mixtures of experts and the EM algorithms. *Neural Computation, 6*, 181–214. doi:10.1162/neco.1994.6.2.181

Kamel, M., & Wanas, N. (2003). Data dependence in combining classifiers. In *proceedings of the Fourth International Workshop on MCS*, No. 2709 Lecture Notes in Computer Science, (pp. 1-14).

Keller, J. M., Gader, P., Tahani, H., Chiang, J. H., & Mohamed, M. (1994). Advances in fuzzy integration for pattern recognition. *Fuzzy Sets and Systems, 65*, 273–283. doi:10.1016/0165-0114(94)90024-8

Kuncheva, L. (Ed.). (2005). Diversity in multiple classifier systems. *Information Fusion, 6*(1). doi:10.1016/j.inffus.2004.04.009

Kuncheva, L., Bezdek, J., & Duin, R. (2001). Decision templates for multiple classifier fusion: An experimental comparison. *Pattern Recognition, 34*, 299–314. doi:10.1016/S0031-3203(99)00223-X

Kuncheva, L. I. (2004). *Combining pattern classifiers: Methods and algorithms*. New York, NY: Wiley. doi:10.1002/0471660264

Kuncheva, L. I., Bezdek, J. C., & Sutton, M. A. (1998). On combining multiple classifiers by fuzzy templates. *Proc. NAFIPS Conf. EDS*, 193-197.

Lam, L. (2000). *Classifier combinations: Implementations and theoretical issues. Multiple Classifier Systems, No. 1857 of Lecture Notes in Computer Science* (pp. 78–86). Cagliari, Italy: Springer.

Mehta, M. (2007). *Classification of hereditary and genetic disorders*. Retrieved March 21, 2011, from http://pharmaxchange.info/notes/clinical/genetic_disorders.html.

Nayer, M, Wanas, Rozita A. Dara, Mohamed S. Kamel. (2006). Adaptive fusion and co-operative training for classifier ensembles Pattern Recognition. *Pattern Recognition, 39*(9), 1781–1794. doi:10.1016/j.patcog.2006.02.003

Pavlidis, T. (1977). *Structural pattern recognition*. New York, NY: Springer-Verlag.

Pedrycz, W., Bezdek, J. C., Hathaway, R. J., & Rogers, G. W. (1998). Two nonparametric models for fusing heterogenous fuzzy data. *IEEE Transactions on Fuzzy Systems, 6*(3), 411–425. doi:10.1109/91.705509

Perner, P., Wang, P., and& Rosenfeld. (Eds.). (1996). *Advances in structural and syntactical pattern recognition*. New York, NY: Springer-Verlag.

Ruta, D., & Gabrys, B. (2000). An overview of classifier fusion method. *Computing and Information Systems, 7*, 1–10.

Sharkey, A. J. C. (1999). *Combining artificial neural nets: Ensemble and modular multi-net systems. London*. London: Springer-Verlag.

Tahani, H., & Keller, J. M. (1990). Information fusion in computer vision using fuzzy integral. *IEEE Transactions on Systems, Man, and Cybernetics, 20*(3), 733–741. doi:10.1109/21.57289

Tax, D., Van Breukelen, M., Duin, R., & Kittler, J. (2000). Combining multiple classifiers by averaging or by multiplying? *Pattern Recognition, 33*, 1475–1485. doi:10.1016/S0031-3203(99)00138-7

Ueda, N. (2000). Optimal linear combination of neural networks for improving classification performance. *IEEE Transactions on Pattern Analysis and Machine Intelligence, 22*(2), 207–215. doi:10.1109/34.825759

Ueda, N., Nakano, R., Ghahramani, Z. and & Hinton, G. E. (2000). SMEM algorithm for mixture models., to appear in *Neural Computations, 12* (9), 2109-2128.

Valentini, G. and & Masulli, F. (2002). Ensembles of learning machines. *Neural Nets*, No. 2486 of Lecture Notes in Computer Science, 3-19.

Wang, D., Keller, J. M., Carson, C. A., McAdoo-Edwards, K. K., & Bailey, C. W. (1998). Use of fuzzy-logic-inspired features to improve bacterial recognition through classifier fusion. *IEEE Transactions on Systems, Man, and Cybernetics*, *28*(4), 583–591. doi:10.1109/3477.704297

Wolpert, D. (1992). Stacked generalization. *Neural Networks*, 5241–5259.

Woods, K., Kegelmeyer, W. P., & Bowyer, K. (1997). Combination of multiple classifiers using local accuracy estimates. *IEEE Transactions on Pattern Analysis and Machine Intelligence*, *19*(4), 405–410. doi:10.1109/34.588027

Woods, K., Philip Kegelmeyer Jr, W., & Bowyer, K. (1997). Combination of multiple classifiers using local accuracy estimates. *IEEE Transactions on Pattern Analysis and Machine Intelligence*, *19*(4), 405–410. doi:10.1109/34.588027

Xu, L., Krzyzak, A., & Suen, C. Y. (1992). Methods of combining multiple classifiers and their applications to handwriting recognition. *IEEE Transactions on Systems, Man, and Cybernetics*, *22*(3), 418–435. doi:10.1109/21.155943

Xu, L., Krzyzak, A., & Suen, C. Y. (1992). Methods of combining multiple classifiers and their application to handwriting recognition. *IEEE Transactions on Systems, Man, and Cybernetics*, *22*, 418–435. doi:10.1109/21.155943

Chapter 11
Connecting the Bench with the Bedside:
Translating Life Science Discoveries to Disease Treatments and Vice Versa

Yue Wang Webster
Eli Lilly and Company

Ernst R Dow
Eli Lilly and Company & Indiana University, USA

Mathew J Palakal
Indiana University, USA & Purdue University, USA

ABSTRACT

Translational research is a branch of researches that attempts to break the barrier between basic science and medical practice, enabling a knowledge flow cycle: basic science discoveries → preclinical/clinical studies → medical practice → health care policy and public awareness → molecular level understanding of disease. In this work, the authors analyze and summarize three aspects of translational research: (1) use cases and opportunities; (2) data types and challenges; and (3) available tools and technologies. They believe that both the opportunities and the challenges of translational research are due to the need to enable knowledge translation between life science and health care domains.

Even though numerous tools and technologies have been developed to meet this need with various degrees of success, a conceptual framework is needed to fully realize the value of those tools and technologies. The authors propose Complex System (CS) to be the logical foundation of such a framework. Since translational research is a spiral and dynamic process. With the CS mindset, they designed a multi-layer architecture called HyGen (Hypotheses Generation Framework) to address the challenges faced by translational researchers. In order to evaluate the framework, the authors carried out heuristic and quantitative tests in the Colorectal Cancer disease area. The results demonstrate the potential of this hybrid approach to bridge silos and to identify hidden links among clinical observations, drugs, genes and diseases, which may eventually lead to the discovery of novel disease targets, biomarkers and therapies.

DOI: 10.4018/978-1-61350-435-2.ch011

Copyright © 2012, IGI Global. Copying or distributing in print or electronic forms without written permission of IGI Global is prohibited.

INTRODUCTION

A vision of future medicine shared by many researchers is "3R"—to provide the Right treatment to the Right patient at the Right time, in other words, to predict the risk of a clinical event during the course of an individual's lifetime, diagnose the event as early as possible and apply the most effective treatment (Webb CP, 2004). To achieve this goal, scientific discoveries must be translated into practical applications. Such discoveries typically start from "lab bench", where basic researches are conducted at a molecular or cellular level, then progress to the patient's "bedside" as therapies (Pizzo, 2002). On the other hand, knowledge gained by "bedside" is important for the researchers at "lab bench" to future their understanding of human disease and pre-clinical models (Dauphinée 2000).

Over the past decade, the fields of "bedside" and "lab bench" have generated extremely large amount of data. As life science and medical practice continue their exponential growth in complexity and scope, the need for collaboration among experts across different disciplines becomes inevitable. Investigators from worldwide have been trying to establish knowledge mappings and sharing between discovery researchers, practitioners, and end users (Robert Molidor AS, 2003; Ruttenberg, 2007). One solution, translational research, is a branch of research that attempts to develop insight into such cross-disciplinary knowledge transformation and collaboration (Ruttenberg et al., 2007). Translational research provides a systematic way to identify implicit associations and insights "hidden" in large and heterogeneous datasets. Recent decades have witnessed many examples of the important roles that translational research plays in life science and health care practice.

One example is the use of translational approach in drug repositioning. Identifying new indications for existing drugs is an important strategy of drug discovery. For example, Atorv-astatin is an FDA approved drug used to lower cholesterol (Refolo et al., 2001). An investigator may want to find other possible diseases that might be treated by Atorvastatin. Using a non-translational approach, the investigator would query for pathways related to Atorvastatin in KEGG and would retrieve no result from KEGG. Using a translational approach, the drug hunter would first search for the indications of Atorvastatin. The drug hunter would then search for genes that are associated with those indications. Next the drug hunter would look for pathways associated with those genes in KEGG and would find one of the pathways to be the Alzheimer's Disease (AD) pathway. He may consider AD as a possible new indication for Atorvastatin. This hypothesis is supported by other studies that show clinical benefit of Atorvastatin in AD patients (Blain & Poirier, 2004; Sparks et al., 2005). The drug hunter can rapidly identify such opportunities because clinical and genomic disciplines are effectively connected in a translational approach.

Discovering novel disease targets is another application of translational research. Identifying the disease gene is often the first step towards discovering the cure. For example, a scientist, looking for AD treatment, may first search for all drug-able genes associated with AD. A non-translational approach is to search against various biological databases for drug-able genes associated with AD. Since the disease has few known pathway steps, this approach yields limited success and no drug-able GPCR target can be identified. Qu et al. described a translational approach in (Qu et al., 2007). They first retrieved all genes participating in the AD pathway. Next they searched for all pathways associated with those genes. Then they repeated the first two steps by searching for genes participated in all pathways found in the previous iteration. Using this approach, the authors reported that they could identify more novel targets. For instance, they found eight GPCR targets that are implicitly associated with AD at the second iteration. Those associations are supported by evidence found in multiple studies (Beek et al., 2003; Xiong et al., 2003). One of the genes, SLIT2, is found to be involved in neuron recombination and axonogenesis (Ozdinler & Erzurumlu, 2002; Xu et al., 2004; Yeo et al., 2004). AD-related deficits have been observed for the functionally related RNA messages encoding the SLIT2 axon guidance receptor factor and the neuroglycan C precursor (Vittorio et al., 2002).

BACKGROUND

Data Sources Involved in Translational Research

A wide variety of data types and artifacts from different sources is involved in translational research. They range from data that describe molecular-level events, to data describing complex biological processes at cellular or organism level, and to information about an individual or a group. In Table 1, we summarized many biomedical sources that contain a wide spectrum of data types across multiple levels: molecule→pathway→cell → organ → individual → population segments, subgroups → society. It is easy to see that the data sources are heterogeneous and often maintained by different organizations.

Semantic Web

Knowledge in life science and healthcare sources can be represented by semantic graphs, which provide the ability to aggregate and connect loosely linked disease and molecular level information into a formal knowledge structure. Semantic Web (SW) technologies have shown great promise in navigating and drawing sophisticated inference from diverse data sources (Mukherjea, 2005; Robu et al., 2006; Ruttenberg, Clark, Bug, Samwald, Bodenreider, Chen, et al., 2007).;

SW has four building blocks: a mechanism to uniquely identify the web resources; a framework to describe web resources; a query language; and an ontology language. Each building block can be implemented differently. Here, we only discuss the standards recommended by the World Wide Web Consortium (www.w3.org). Uniform Resource Identifier (URI) is "a compact sequence of characters that identifies an abstract or physical resource". It distinguishes one resource from all others. It is the foundation of SW. Resource Description Framework (RDF) is a format that describes web resources by triples (subject-predicate-object). The subject and object are the resources, and the predicate is the relationship between the subject and the object. A subject or object can be an organic compound, a gene, a pathway or a patient. Predicate (a.k.a. property) can be any relationship between the subject and the object (i.e. causes, regulates, transcribes, etc.) For instance, "drug A causes disorder B" can be represented as <A treats B>, where A is the subject, B is the object, and "treat" is the property. Simple Protocol and RDF Query Language (SPARQL) is a SQL-like query language for query SW. It essentially consists of a standard query language, a data access protocol and a data model. Using SPARQL, users can form semantic queries that otherwise require lengthy and complex SQL statements in a relational database. RDF Schema (RDFS) and Web Ontology Language (Bayardo et al.) have both been used in SW applications to encode ontologies. OWL is more expressive than RDFS. The data described by OWL ontology is interpreted as a set of "individuals" or "classes" and a set of "property assertions" which relate these individuals to each other. The axioms in OWL ontology define constraints on the individuals and the types of relationships permitted between them. A SW system, therefore, can infer additional information based on the axioms.

Graph Analysis

Graph analysis has drawn much interest among bioinformatics researchers due to the rapid growth

Table 1. Data sources involved in translational research

Data Sources	Domain	Content	Data Level
PubMed http://medlineplus.gov	biological, clinical	Biomedical literature publications	all levels
Clinical Trials http://clinicaltrials.gov	clinical	basic information on federally and privately supported clinical trials	population
MedlinePlus http://medlineplus.gov	clinical	Health information of patient and health care providers	organ, individual
TOXNET http://toxnet.nlm.nih.gov	chemical	toxicology, hazardous chemicals, environmental health, and toxic releases	small molecule
Entrez http://www.ncbi.nlm.nih.gov/sites/gquery	chemical, biological, clinical	Multiple databases, including PubMed, Nucleotide and Protein Sequences, Protein Structures, Complete Genomes, Taxonomy, and others. disease corresponding gene associations	large molecule
GenBank http://www.ncbi.nlm.nih.gov/genbank/	biological	an annotated collection of all publicly available DNA sequences	molecular (sequence)
OMIM http://www.ncbi.nlm.nih.gov/omim	biological, clincial	human genes and genetic disorders, links to MEDLINE and sequence records in the Entrez Gene, and additional resources at NCBI	cell, organ, individual, population
KEGG Pathway http://www.genome.jp/kegg/	biological	Molecular interaction and reaction networks for metabolism, various cellular processes, and human diseases	molecule, pathway
Reactome http://www.reactome.org/	biological	curated core pathways and reactions in human biology	pathway
PDSPki http://pdsp.med.unc.edu/pdsp.php	chemical, biological	Ki, (affinity) values of compounds at various molecular targets	molecule
AlzSWAN http://hypothesis.alzforum.org		information on AD research, including scientists, experiments, data, publications, etc.	molecule, cell, organ, individual
AlzGene [Bertram et al. 2007]	biological, clinical	genetic association studies performed on Alzheimer's disease phenotypes	molecule, individual
Homologene http://www.ncbi.nlm.nih.gov/homologene	biological, clinical	homologs among the annotated genes of different eukaryotic genomes	molecule, organism
Allen Brain Atlas http://www.brain-map.org/	biological, clinical	genes found to have a high level of expression within certain brain structure	organ, molecule,
BAMS [Bota M. 2005]	biological	connections between different brain structures	cell, organ
PubChem http://pubchem.ncbi.nlm.nih.gov/	chemical, biological	biological activities of small molecules	molecule
Entrez Gene http://www.ncbi.nlm.nih.gov/gene/	biological	genes	molecule
UniPort [Wu CH 2006]	biological	protein sequence and function, including data from Swiss-Prot, TrEMBL, and PIR	molecule
senseLab http://senselab.med.yale.edu/		six related databases on pathological mechanisms related to AD	
BIND [Bader et al. 2003]	biological	biomolecular interaction, complex and pathway information	molecule, cell
BioCyc http://biocyc.org	biological	genome and metabolic pathways of organisms	molecule, pathway, organism
STRING http://string.embl.de/	biological	protein-protein interactions	molecule

continues on following page

Table 1. Continued

Data Sources	Domain	Content	Data Level
BioCarta http://www.biocarta.com/		gene-pathway association	molecule, pathway
DrugBank http://www.drugbank.ca/	chemical, biological	drug linked to drug target (sequence, structure, and pathway) information.	small molecule, large molecule pathway,

of publicly available high throughput data (Braun et al., 2008; Feldman et al., 2008; Hopkins, 2007; Lage et al., 2007; Lee et al., 2008; Ma'ayan et al., 2007; Xu & Li, 2006; Yildirim et al., 2007). Such data have provided linkages among chemical, biological, and clinical entities. After SW technologies are used to integrate information-silos into a common semantic graph, conventional graph algorithms can be extended to mine such graphs, where biomedical entities are modeled as nodes and the relationships as edges (links). Some common terminologies and methods in graph analysis are defined as following.

A graph G = (V,E) is a collection of nodes (V) and edges (E) connecting those nodes. An edge e = (u, v) ∈ E connects two nodes u and v. The nodes u and v are said to be incident with the edge e and adjacent to each other. The degree d(v) of a node (a.k.a. vertex) v is the number of its incident edges. Let (e1, ..., ek) be a sequence of edges in a graph G = (V,E). This sequence is called a path if there are nodes v0, ..., vk such that ei = (vi−1, vi) for i = 1, ..., k and the edges ei are pair-wise distinct and the nodes vi are pair-wise distinct. The length of a path is given by its number of edges, k = |(e1, ..., ek)|. A shortest path between two nodes u, v is a path with minimal length. The diameter is the maximum shortest path length amongst all pairs of nodes in a graph.

Average degree, diameter, and average shortest path are topology measurements often used in graph analysis. Average degree reflects the "connectivity" of a graph. Diameter and average shortest path reflect the "compactness" of a graph. A small diameter or a low average shortest path length indicates that all the nodes are in proximity to each other. A highly connected, compact graph often represents a dense knowledge space where concepts are closely related to each other. In such a graph, the changes of one node have greater impact on other nodes than it would be in a loosely connected graph.

Common approaches of ranking graph nodes (Chen et al., 2009; Ding et al., 2005; Harith & Christopher, 2005; Scardoni & Laudanna, 2009] include concept structure analysis, PageRank, and Hyperlink-Induced Topic Search (HITS). PageRank with Priors proposed by White and Smyth (White & Smyth, 2003) simulates the steps of a Web surfer, who starts from any of the root nodes on the Internet and follows a random link at each step with β as the probability of returning to the root nodes. A score is computed for each node on the Internet to reflect its probability of being reached by the surfer. This score is used to measure the relative "closeness" of a node to the root nodes. K-Step Markov method simulates a similar Web surfing scenario as in PageRank, except that the surfer returns to the root nodes after K steps and restarts the process. K-Step Markov algorithm estimates the relative probability that a surfer will spend time at a node given that the surfer starts in a set of root nodes and stops after K steps. HITS with Priors proposed by Kleinberg measures two properties of a node: (1) authority score estimates the importance of the node itself; and (2) hub score measures the importance of other nodes linked to the current node (Kleinberg, 1998). Therefore, HITS with Priors not only considers the number of links to and from a node but also its neighbors'.

CONNECTING INFORMATION SILOS AND PEOPLE SILOS

Challenges in Translational Research

The goal of translational research is to achieve effective knowledge transformation between life science domains and medical practice. However, new discoveries are often stored in their discipline sources that form information-silos; and experts tend to interact within their own circles which are social-silos. The two types of silos form the two major challenges in translational research.

Information Silos

Multi-disciplinary and multi-level data involved in biomedical research present the first challenge for a translational framework: integration of vast amount of information in disparate silos. Figure 1 summarizes the wide variety of data types and artifacts from different discipline sources involved in translational research, such as chemical, biological, clinical, and public health data. The main subject of chemical data is molecules and their interactions both with each other and with the environment. Such information (physical properties, chemical properties, and reactions) can often be captured in basic data types (numbers and strings). 2D or 3D structure information can be expressed in special text format. Graphical representation is used mostly in visualizing structures, studying molecular dynamics, and protein-ligand docking. Biological data are more heterogeneous because it encompasses many domains of knowledge (molecular and cell biology, genetics, structural biology, pharmacology, physiology, etc.). Clinical data is concerned with or based on the actual observation and treatment of diseases in patients rather than experiment or theory (Dictionary.com (accessed in Feb. 2009)). Different from chemical and biological data, temporal information is an intrinsic component of clinical data. It is often probabilistic or fuzzy in nature. Most clinical data

are concerned with a single patient (individual level data), such as laboratory test results, patient demographics, discharge summaries, and progress notes. On the other hand, public health data is often concerned with a group of people (high-level aggregated data) who have common characteristics, such as data used to study disease outbreaks and epidemics. Since the focus of public health is to promote healthy behaviors and to prevent diseases through surveillance of cases. Social context is an important part of public health data.

The challenge here is how to connect data from different levels. For example, how to link molecular data such as gene sequence with data specific to an individual such as a patient's Electronic Health Record, and with data collected at population level such as genome-wide association study of patients from a certain ethnical group.

People Silos

Many stakeholders are involved in translational research, including scientist, physicians and patients. People tend to interact within their own social or academic circles. Communications and share-learning among experts from different domains is essential for translational approach. Ruttenberg proposed in (Ruttenberg, Clark, Bug, Samwald, Bodenreider, Chen, et al., 2007) that knowledge should be shared among specialists in different disease areas. One success story of cross-disease research is the discovery of NST-729 as a cross-disease biomarker for neurodegeneration and as the first molecular probe for Amyotrophic Lateral Sclerosis (Shirvan et al., 2009). Based on the knowledge that Parkinson's Disease (PD), AD, Huntington's Disease [Dauphinée], and ALS share common features at the clinical (Royall et al., 2002), neural (Levy et al., 2005; Planells-Cases et al., 2006), cellular (Dawson & Dawson, 2003; Sauer et al., 2005), and molecular levels (Bertram & Tanzi, 2005), Shirvan et al. studied and compared the performance of NST-729 cross the transgenic models of two neurodegenerative

Figure 1. Data involved in translational research

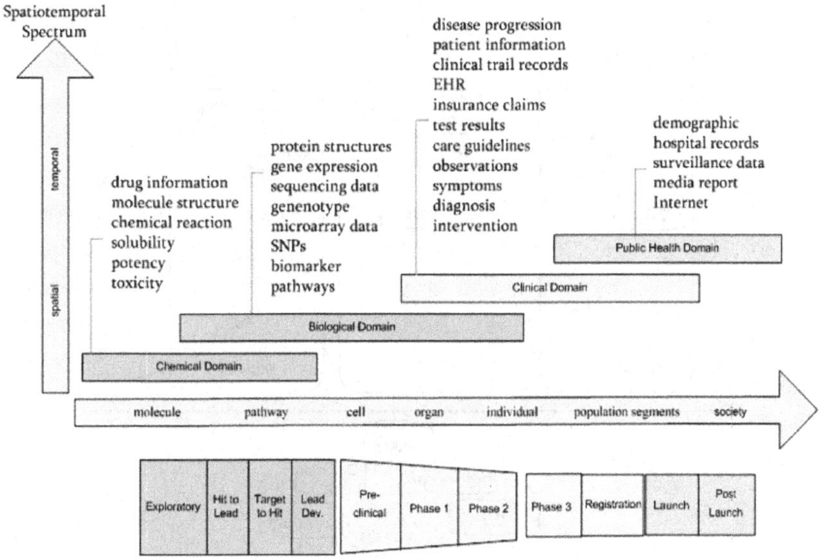

disorders, AD and ALS. Without an effective bridge between the people silos, such comparison will not be possible.

Establishing such bridges, however, has always been difficult. Studies have shown that the discover made by experts in one domain has not been efficiently shared and adopted by key players in the other domain (Gaughan, 2006). Part of the reason, we believe, is that each stakeholder is interested in different aspect of biomedical research. For example, considering the knowledge about a disease gene:

- chemists are interested in molecules that are active against the target gene;
- molecular biologists care for the epigenetic regulators for the gene;
- in-vivo biologists are interested in the animal species with the closest genome for this gene;
- systems physiologists want to know whether gene variations exists in sub populations;
- physicians are worried about whether the variations affect treatment outcome;

- patients ask whether the variations of their individual genes will increase their risk of suffering from a certain disease;

People silos have direct impact on translational research in both knowledge production and dissemination (Eysenbach, 2008; Swan, 2009). As shown in Figure 2, a successful translational research framework has to accomplish at least two tasks: (1) to bridge the silos and discover novel associations; and (2) to deliver the results to the users based on their specific needs.

Solutions and Recommendations

To overcome the above challenges in translational research, we recommend a hybrid framework, combining SW, graph algorithm and user profiling. We believe this hybrid approach is advantageous in discovering hidden associations across disciplines and tailoring the results for individual user. The reasons are as following. An association can be modeled as two nodes linked by an edge in a graph. Therefore, we may model discipline silos as a large, connected graph. Conventional

Figure 2. Bridging the information-silos and the people-silos

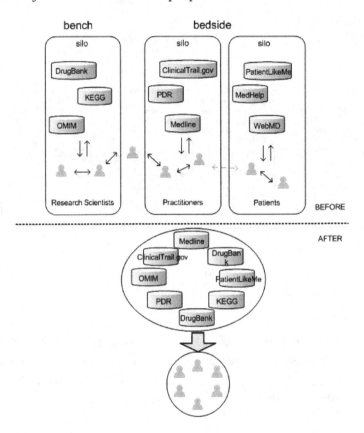

graph algorithms can be extended to mine the graph based on user profiles, which allows us to deliver the mining results in a user-centric manner to the respective stakeholder. It is expensive to conduct graph analyses on a large-scale graph and may encounter too many the false positives. Therefore, we propose to use sub graphs to reduce the cost of the analyses and increase precision. The sub graphs also capture the personalized views of the full knowledge space. Such views are specific to each user and are part of the strategy to tailor search results for different stakeholders of translational research.

To demonstrate this approach and to evaluate its feasibility, we designed and implemented a knowledge discovery framework called HyGen. In (Webster et al., 2010), we described the design and implementation details of HyGen. Here we intend to highlight three key design decisions and

explain why those decisions were made to address the unique challenges in translational research.

Merge Terms and Alias into Unique Graph Nodes

To insure that a clinical term and its synonyms are merged to the same node in the semantic graph, we normalized the terms against UMLS. MetaMap (http://mmtx.nlm.nih.gov) was used to map clinical-relevant terms from short phrases in titles and clinical synopses sections to UMLS concepts. For the long free-text fields of OMIM records, our experiments showed that our customized Pipeline Pilot protocols have a higher recall rate (75% to 80%) than MetaMap (less than 25%) when mining large OMIM text fields. We use similar approach to normalize the drug indications of DrugBank records, as well as disease terms of PharmGKB and GAD.

The chemical compounds in OMIM record, DrugBank, PharmGKB, and KEGG are normalized against CHEMLIST, a dictionary for identifying chemical information in the literature (Hettne et al., 2009). From the normalized compound list, marketed drugs or drug candidates in clinical trials phase-II or later are extracted. Each drug or drug candidate is then connected with its target genes based on PharmGKB and DrugBank records. All gene names and alias were mapped to EntrezGene Id. Other types of associations from genomic, pharmacological, and proteomic sources are also incorporated in the full graph.

The mapping program was coded in Java. It interacts with MetaMap and Pipeline Pilot's Text Analytics Collection to recognize and map source-dependent terms to standard dictionaries. It uses Jena API (www.jena.sourceforge.net) to create and manipulate the associations as RDF triples. The associations harvested were loaded into AllegroGraph RDFStore (http://www.franz. com/agraph/allegrograph) based on a custom-built top-level ontology developed in Protégé.

Since a UMLS concept Id or a CHEMLIST Id defines the URI of a node, a term and its aliases are uniquely mapped to the same node that represents the clinical concept or chemical substance in the full graph. To establish mappings of instance-level terms is the key to connect various biomedical data sources. Biomedical ontologies and thesaurus such as UMLS and their companion linguistic tools have made it possible to automate a large part of the mapping process.

Refine Network by Iterative Feedback

A full semantic web built using the above approach may easily have millions of triples. Directly querying such graph will result in too many false positives. We propose an iterative process inspired by the pseudo-relevance feedback used in some document retrieval systems. Based on the full graph, different virtual sub graphs are constructed for different user profiles. Given a user profile, HyGen begins by traversing the full graph to find all the neighbors of the seeds and marking them as discovered. Numerical weights (from 0 to 1) are assigned to the edges based on the data sources where the associations are originated. Users can adjust the data source weight based on their own experience and needs in the user profiles. For example, if a user is very familiar with database A and would like to search for novel information beyond the scope of A, then the user can assign a lower score to A. Next, HyGen performs graph analysis to rank all the discovered nodes based on the criteria defined in the user profile. Any low ranking node is turned back to undiscovered. This counts as one step.

In the subsequent iterations, HyGen searches for undiscovered nodes that are neighbors of the discovered nodes; ranks all the discovered nodes; and re-labels them discovered or undiscovered according to the ranks. If the user specified the maximum number of steps X in the profile, then HyGen stops searching after X steps. Otherwise, HyGen stops after it has exhausted all nodes in the full graph. At the end of the final iteration, all the discovered nodes and their edges form the virtual sub graph specific to the given user profile.

In other words, HyGen's exploration radiates out slowly from the original seeds, acquiring or disowning nodes at each iteration. We named the process of re-ranking discovered nodes pseudo-relevance feedback. The term was borrowed from document retrieval systems. However, instead of using pseudo- relevance feedback for query expansion, HyGen applies this strategy to re-rank and re-arrange the nodes that have already been discovered. Adopting pseudo-relevance feedback in this novel way, HyGen can quickly construct a user-specific view of the full knowledge space with high sensitivity and selectivity.

Case Studies in Colorectal Cancer

Colorectal Cancer (CRC) also called colon cancer or large bowel cancer, is the second leading cause of cancer-related death (Markowitz & Bertagnolli, 2009). CRC disease progression is believed to be a step-wise process, where cells change from normal epithelium through polyp form to carcinoma. Mutations in two classes of genes: tumor-suppressor genes and proto-oncogenes, are found to increase the risk of developing CRC. Studies have also shown that CRC is related to at least one of three different pathways: termed chromosomal instability, microsatellite instability, and the CpG island methylator phenotype (Boland, 2002). Different pathways tend to affect different sets of tumor suppressor genes and are characterized by different biological behaviors.

Early and accurate detection of different types of colorectal cancer may greatly improve the chances of survival. Medical interventions should be tailored for individual patient. However, this is not the case. Even though great progress was made in understanding the molecular basis of CRC, it has translated into few genetic biomarkers that are currently used in clinical practice (De Roock et al., 2009). We believe a translational approach is needed to help transform the biological discoveries into clinically diagnostic tools and personalized CRC medicine.

Scientific discoveries can help practitioners to provide better care to patients. In this case study, we simulated the user profile of a medical doctor who is a CRC specialist and is interested in other disorders and complications related to CRC. The profile, P_{doc}, contained 32 known genes related to CRC. Since the user is an expert looking for knowledge applicable to medical practices, we set up P_{doc} to award fresh but medium-length associations and nodes with higher degree of connectivity, because highly connected nodes are more likely to be organizing functional modules and critical for survival. The maximum iteration X was set to 2 and the sub graph finished with 4591 edges

Table 2. Disorders suggested to a practitioner (5% cutoff)

Disorder	Score	# Paper
neural tube defects	1.00	5
rippling muscle disease	0.97	0
polydactyly, preaxial IV	0.88	0
vitamin d-dependent rickets, type I	0.85	0
mismatch repair cancer syndrome	0.82	11
dyssegmental dysplasia, silverman-handmaker type	0.82	0
osteoporosis	0.81	29
spondylometaphyseal dysplasia, kozlowski type	0.78	0
premature chromatid separation trait	0.77	0
neurofibromatosis, type I	0.76	3
meningioma, familial	0.73	1
otospondylomegaepiphyseal dysplasia	0.68	0

and 2392 nodes. The top disorders associated with CRC are listed in Table 2.

To judge the novelty of the results, we searched PubMed for original papers where the new disorder name and CRC occurred together in the same titles or abstracts. The number of co-occurrences is listed in Table 2 as well. The low numbers seem to indicate that some suggestions are quite novel, assuming novel information will be less known and appear in fewer papers.

The high-ranking disorders may shine lights on the common disease mechanisms of CRC and other disorders. For example, we have found that the link between CRC and Neural Tube Defects (NTD) is scientifically possible. Folate supplements have been used to prevent NTD (Pitkin, 2007; Ray et al., 2007). There are studies claiming that folate may also lower CRC risk (Duthie, 1999; Guerreiro et al., 2008). The initial full graph has no direct links between CRC and NTD. Zooming into the sub graph, we noticed that mutation in TP53 is linked to increase risk of CRC; TP53 is a gene encoding tumor protein p53, which is involved in DNA repair and changes in metabolism; TP53 connects to MTHFR via a drug that is a pyrimidine analogue and inhibits the cell's ability to synthesize DNA; and MTHFR polymorphism is linked to an increased risk for NTD. Those links suggest that CRC and NTD pathways may share some common components. By comparing of their pathways and biological process, an expert may arrive at new hypnoses about the disease mechanisms of CRC and NTD.

The next high-ranking association identified by HyGen, Rippling muscle disease (RMD), is a rare autosomal dominant disorder that may occur sporadically (Arimura, 2002). It was reported that sporadic RMD could be treated by thymectomy or immunosuppression (Muller-Felber et al., 1999; Steven, 2004). Some RMD patients' symptoms were reduced after treated with anti-cancer drugs (Takagi et al., 2002). Experts suggest that sporadic RMD may be a new paraneoplastic or autoimmune disease, characterized by certain antibodies response against self (Steven, 2004). Similar antibodies can also sometimes be found in patients with CRC (Akira et al., 1974; Ditzel, 2000).

The third high-ranking association in Table 2 is preaxial polydactyly. It is a congenital anomaly characterized by the presence of more than the normal number of fingers. Many believe it is part of a complex genetic syndrome (Lettice & Hill, 2005; Temtamy et al., 2003). The gene or set of genes responsible for preaxial polydactyly have been localized to chromosome 7q36 (Radhakrishna et al., 1996; Tsukurov et al., 1994). A homeobox gene HB9 is within the critical region of 7q36 and is also expressed in pancreas, small intestine, and colon (Zguricas et al., 1999). The association seems to suggest that the two phenotypes, preaxial polydactyly and CRC, are linked through HB9.

The last example we discuss here is the possible link between CRC and type I vitamin D-resistant rickets, VDDRI (ranked 4th in Table 2). Even though no PubMed paper contains those two disorders in the same abstract, the practitioner, being an experienced physician, may realize that

vitamin D is recommended to lower the risks of both diseases. Further research may show him that VDDRI is associated with mutations in the gene of the vitamin D receptor (VDR) (Nicolaidoua et al., 2007). Meanwhile, colorectal cells contain vitamin D Receptors and are able to convert 25(OH) vitamin D into 1,25(OH)2 vitamin D, which may prevent tumor progression in colon. The practitioner may follow up on this interesting connection by comparing the lab results of VDDRI and CRC patients, especially their 1,25(OH)2 VD level tests. This finding may eventually lead to novel diagnosis tools or therapies.

FUTURE RESEARCH DIRECTIONS

Web2.0 and Emerging Sources for Translational Research

Web2.0 refers to web applications that facilitate interactive information sharing, interoperability, user-centered design, and collaboration on the World Wide Web, such as YouTube, Facebook, and Twitter. From 2005 to 2009, participation in such social networking sites more than quadrupled (Chou et al., 2009). Such sites are emerging sources for translational research. First, the folksonomy constructed by Web2.0 user can elicit new health care concepts, coding sets, and classifications. In the future, we may see adoption of consumer-professional vocabulary mapping technologies by translational research systems. Certain translational approaches may need to completely replace the research-driven taxonomy with consumer-drive folksonomy.

Second, there are large cohorts of online patients groups who share similar health conditions and come from diverse background. Access to their individual-level data is critical for identifying disease causing factors and for translating biological knowledge into personalized medicine. Openness may become an emerging theme in translational research community. From technical perspectives, transparency, interoperability, open source, and open programming interfaces will become important design philosophies for translational research systems. From social perspectives, individuals are more open in sharing information when seeking solutions for their health problems (Allison, 2009). Therefore, translational research community needs to increase the effort in engaging and empowering health care consumers. Historically translational research tools were designed for professionals. In the future, we may see growing demands for consumer-centric translational research tools and services.

Thirdly, the collective wisdom of common users and professionals in social networks will contribute to the knowledge of treating diseases, as well as preventing them. Historically, translational studies concentrated on developing therapies; the focus of future translational research may shift toward earlier stages of health care cycle. For example, translational researcher may be able to identify risk factors and predict health outcome specific for an individual by analyzing the online member profiles and the corresponding health-related information.

Agent-Based Information Extraction

HyGen's current data extraction layer is not fully automated. We propose the use of intelligent mining agents in the future. A mining agent extracts data from a data source and converts the information into triples $\{c_1, r_{12}, c_2\}$. New triples that have been validated will be posted on a "blackboard" to share with other mining agents. Each agent decides whether the new triples are relevant and takes actions accordingly, for example one agent may decide to retrieve additional data, and another agent may decide to re-evaluate some conflicting data. There are two key requirements for the agents: (a) they shall be able to adjust the discovery process as more information becomes available; and (b) they shall be able to influence the discovery process of each other.

The major challenge of designing an agent-based information extraction layer for HyGen is caused by the complex and transient interrelationships among biomedical data sources. Agents need to know the rules for processing the information and rules for interacting with each other. Some data sources publish the metadata that can be used to derive processing rules. There are also techniques for deriving metadata based on the data in the data sources (Bayardo, et al., 1997; Patel et al., 2010). However, automatic generation of interaction rules for agents attached to diverse data sources is still a difficult problem (Walczak, 2009). In the case of HyGen, the interaction rules are especially complex due to the heterogeneous nature of translational data sources.

Edge Properties

HyGen's graphs are matrix-based graphs. The edges have only one property: a numerical weight assigned according to the data sources. In the future, to reflect the complex relationships exist in life science and health care knowledge space, we should enable property-based graphs, where properties can be attached to the edges. In property-based graphs, edges can have any number of key-value pairs as their properties. Today, we analyze the graphs based on their topological features. Having edge properties will give us the ability to analyze the graph using property-based algorithm.

Another advantage of a property-based graph is in delivering more user-specific views. In a property-based graph, two neighboring nodes may be connected by multiple edges. In other words, any types of relationships (edges) can exist between the same pair of concept. Some relationships may be present in one view but not in the other based on the different user profiles.

Profile-Driven Ranking Criteria

One of the key steps of pseudo-relevance feedback algorithm mentioned earlier is to rank and re-rank nodes based on graph analysis. The rank of a node v can be computed as the weighted mean of different criteria, each of which has a normalized value between 0 and 1.

One of the limitations of this study is the selection of the ranking criteria. The criteria currently used by HyGen were selected based on experience and literature review (Bamba & Mukherjea, 2005; Moskovitch, 2007). Assuming an association discovered by HyGen contains a certain piece of information. We measure seven aspects of each piece of information: how relevant is the information; how specific is the information; how important is the source of the information; how fresh is the information; whether the information is directly or indirectly associated with the search terms; how rare is the concepts involved in this piece of information; and whether this piece of information occupies a central position in the knowledge space. Some of those criteria may not be necessary. Some criteria may even prevent HyGen from obtaining the optimal ranking. On the other hand, criteria that can provide better rankings may have been missed from the list of seven criteria. Therefore, the current ranking produced by HyGen may not be optimal.

To obtain the optimal set of criteria, we need to develop sets of ranked associations based on different user profiles and use them as the training sets or gold standards. We can then try different combinations of the criteria, compare the results with each gold standard, and identify the optimal criteria set for each type of profile. When starting a search, the user's profile will be populated with an optimal criteria set pre-tailored for the given user type. A guideline should also be provided indicating which set of criteria is suitable for the types of search questions the user wants to address.

To establish optimal criteria for different stakeholders and to reduce personal bias, a user study of large number of pilot users, preferably consumers and professionals interested in multiple disease areas, is needed. We may pursue this study in the future; however it is outside the scope of the current dissertation.

CONCLUSION

Modeling life science and health care knowledge as semantic graph enable us to aggregate and connect loosely associated disease and molecular level information into a formal structure. Graph-based pseudo- relevance feedback strategy can be used to discover and prioritize associations relevant to users' interests. Case study in Colorectal Cancer demonstrated that starting from knowledge gained in the "bench", the proposed hybrid approach can discover novel connections and suggest possible hypotheses to users at the "bedside", and vice versa. We believe the knowledge model and approach described here can be applied to other diseases.

Although SW concepts and technologies have been studied by many researchers, fewer reports have been published on applying user profiling technologies to rank multi-level and cross-disciplinary biomedical data based on graph attributes. With a few exceptions (Gudivada et al. 2008), most existing life science networks (graphs) have few types of nodes. This hybrid approach is able to integrate many types of nodes and discovers associations among different types of biomedical entities.

REFERENCES

Akira, B. M., Akira, S., Tetsuo, A., Yasuyuki, E., Michiyoshi, S., Iwao, O., & Tsutomu, W. (1974). Autoimmune hemolytic anemia associated with colon cancer. *Cancer*, *33*, 111–114. doi:10.1002/1097-0142(197401)33:1<111::AID-CNCR2820330117>3.0.CO;2-9

Allison, M. (2009). Can web 2.0 reboot clinical trials? *Nature Biotechnology, 27,* 895–902. doi:10.1038/nbt1009-895

Arimura, K. (2002). Rippling muscle syndrome. *Internal Medicine (Tokyo, Japan), 41,* 325–326. doi:10.2169/internalmedicine.41.325

Bader, G. D., Betel, D., & Hogue, C. W. V. (2003). BIND: the Biomolecular Interaction Network Database. *Nucleic Acids Research, 31,* 248–250. doi:10.1093/nar/gkg056

Bamba, B., & Mukherjea, S. (2005). Utilizing Resource Importance for Ranking Semantic Web Query Results In *Semantic Web and Databases,* 185-198. Berlin: Springer Berlin.

Bayardo, R. J., Jr., Bohrer, W., Brice, R., Cichocki, A., Fowler, J., Helal, A., et al. (1997). InfoSleuth: agent-based semantic integration of information in open and dynamic environments. In *Proceedings of the Proceedings of the 1997 ACM SIGMOD international conference on Management of data,* Tucson, USA 1997.

Beek, J., Elward, K., & Gasque, P. (2003). Activation of Complement in the Central Nervous System. *Annals of the New York Academy of Sciences, 992,* 56–71. doi:10.1111/j.1749-6632.2003.tb03138.x

Bertram, L., Mcqueen, M. B., Mullin, K., Blacker, D., & Tanzi, R. E. (2007). Systematic meta-analyses of Alzheimer disease genetic association studies: the AlzGene database. *Nature Genetics, 39,* 17. doi:10.1038/ng1934

Bertram, L., & Tanzi, R. E. (2005). The genetic epidemiology of neurodegenerative disease. *The Journal of Clinical Investigation, 115,* 1449–1457. doi:10.1172/JCI24761

Blain, J.-F., & Poirier, J. (2004). Cholesterol homeostasis and the pathophysiology of Alzheimer's disease. *Expert Review of Neurotherapeutics, 4,* 823–829. doi:10.1586/14737175.4.5.823

Boland, C. (2002). Molecular basis for stool-based DNA tests for colorectal cancer: a primer for clinicians. *Reviews in Gastroenterological Disorders, 1,* 12–19.

Bota, M., D.H.-W.S.L.W. (2005). Brain Architecture Management System. *Neuroinformatics, 3,* 15–48. doi:10.1385/NI:3:1:015

Braun, P., Rietman, E., & Vidal, M. (2008). Networking metabolites and diseases. *Proceedings of the National Academy of Sciences of the United States of America, 105,* 9849–9850. doi:10.1073/pnas.0805644105

Chen, J., Aronow, B., & Jegga, A. (2009). Disease candidate gene identification and prioritization using protein interaction networks. *BMC Bioinformatics, 10,* 1–2.

Chou, W.-Y. S., Hunt, Y. M., Beckjord, E. B., Moser, R. P., & Hesse, B. W. (2009). Social Media Use in Use in the United States: Implications for Health Communication. *Journal of Medical Internet Research, 11,* 48–50. doi:10.2196/jmir.1249

Dauphinée, D.M.M., & Joseph, B. Md, Phd. (2000). Breaking Down the Walls: Thoughts on the Scholarship of Integration. *Journal of Medical Education, 75,* 5.

Dawson, T. M., & Dawson, V. L. (2003). Molecular Pathways of Neurodegeneration in Parkinson's Disease. *Science, 302,* 819–822. doi:10.1126/science.1087753

De Roock, W., Biesmans, B., De Schutter, J., & Tejpar, S. (2009). Clinical biomarkers in oncology: focus on colorectal cancer. *Molecular Diagnosis & Therapy, 13,* 103–114.

Ding, L., Pan, R., Finin, T., Joshi, A., Peng, Y., & Kolari, P. (2005). Finding and Ranking Knowledge on the Semantic Web. In *4th International Semantic Web Conference,* Galway, Ireland.

Ditzel, H. (2000). Human antibodies in cancer and autoimmune disease. *Immunologic Research, 21*, 185–193. doi:10.1385/IR:21:2-3:185

Duthie, S. J. (1999). Folic acid deficiency and cancer: mechanisms of DNA instability. *British Medical Bulletin, 55*, 578–592. doi:10.1258/0007142991902646

Eysenbach, G. (2008). Medicine 2.0: Social Networking, Collaboration, Participation, Apomediation, and Openness. *Journal of Medical Internet Research, 10*, 5–6. doi:10.2196/jmir.1030

Feldman, I., Rzhetsky, A., & Vitkup, D. (2008). Network properties of genes harbouring inherited disease mutations. *Proceedings of the National Academy of Sciences of the United States of America, 105*, 4323–4328. doi:10.1073/pnas.0701722105

Gaughan, A. (2006). Bridging the divide: the need for translational informatics. *Pharmacogenomics, 7*, 117–122. doi:10.2217/14622416.7.1.117

Gudivada, R. C., Qu, X. A., Chen, J., Jegga, A. G., Neumann, E. K., & Aronow, B. J. (2008). Identifying disease-causal genes using Semantic Web-based representation of integrated genomic and phenomic knowledge. *Journal of Biomedical Informatics, 41*, 717–729. doi:10.1016/j.jbi.2008.07.004

Guerreiro, C. S., Carmona, B., Goncalves, S., Carolino, E., Fidalgo, P., & Brito, M. (2008). Risk of colorectal cancer associated with the C677T polymorphism in 5,10-methylenetetrahydrofolate reductase in Portuguese patients depends on the intake of methyl-donor nutrients. *The American Journal of Clinical Nutrition, 88*, 1413–1418.

Harith, A., & Christopher, B. (2005). Ontology ranking based on the analysis of concept structures. In *Proceedings of the Proceedings of the 3rd international conference on Knowledge capture*, Banff, Canada2005.

Hettne, K. M., Stierum, R. H., Schuemie, M. J., Hendriksen, P. J., Schijvenaars, B. J., & Van Mulligen, E. M. (2009). A Dictionary to Identify Small Molecules and Drugs in Free Text. *Bioinformatics (Oxford, England), 25*, 2983–2991. doi:10.1093/bioinformatics/btp535

Hopkins, A. L. (2007). Network pharmacology. *Nature Chemical Biology, 4*, 682–690. doi:10.1038/nchembio.118

Kleinberg, J. M. (1998). Authoritative sources in a hyperlinked environment. In *Proceedings of the ninth ACM-SIAM symposium on Discrete algorithms*, San Francisco, USA.

Lage, K., Karlberg, E. O., Storling, Z. M., Olason, P. I., Pedersen, A. G., & Rigina, O. (2007). A human phenome-interactome network of protein complexes implicated in genetic disorders. *Nature Biotechnology, 25*, 309. doi:10.1038/nbt1295

Lee, D.S., Park, J., Kay, K.A., Christakis, N.A., & Oltvai, Z.N. & Barabä¡Si, A.L. (2008). The implications of human metabolic network topology for disease comorbidity. *Proceedings of the National Academy of Sciences of the United States of America, 105*, 9880–9885. doi:10.1073/pnas.0802208105

Lettice, L. A., & Hill, R. E. (2005). Preaxial polydactyly: a model for defective long-range regulation in congenital abnormalities. *Current Opinion in Genetics & Development, 15*, 294–300. doi:10.1016/j.gde.2005.04.002

Levy, Y., Gilgun-Sherki, Y., Melamed, E., & Offen, D. (2005). Therapeutic potential of neurotrophic factors in neurodegenerative diseases. *BioDrugs, 19*, 97–127. doi:10.2165/00063030-200519020-00003

Ma'ayan, A., Jenkins, S. L., Goldfarb, J., & Iyengar, R. (2007). Network analysis of FDA approved drugs and their targets. *The Mount Sinai Journal of Medicine, New York, 74*, 27–32. doi:10.1002/msj.20002

Markowitz, S. D., & Bertagnolli, M. M. (2009). Molecular Basis of Colorectal Cancer. *The New England Journal of Medicine, 361*, 2449–2460. doi:10.1056/NEJMra0804588

Moskovitch, R. (2007). A Comparative Evaluation of Full-text, Concept-based, and Context-sensitive Search. *Journal of the American Medical Informatics Association, 14*, 164–174. doi:10.1197/jamia.M1953

Mukherjea, S. (2005). Information retrieval and knowledge discovery utilising a biomedical Semantic Web. *Briefings in Bioinformatics, 6*, 252–262. doi:10.1093/bib/6.3.252

Muller-Felber, W., Ansevin, C. F., Ricker, K., Muller-Jenssen, A., Töpfer, M., Goebel, H. H., & Pongratz, D. E. (1999). Immunosuppressive treatment of rippling muscles in patients with myasthenia gravis. *Neuromuscular Disorders, 9*, 604–607. doi:10.1016/S0960-8966(99)00065-6

Nicolaidoua, P., Papadopouloua, A., Matsinosb, Y. G., Georgoulic, H., Fretzayasa, A., & Papadimitrioua, A. (2007). Vitamin D Receptor Polymorphisms in Hypocalcemic Vitamin D-Resistant Rickets Carriers. *Hormone Research, 67*, 179–183. doi:10.1159/000097014

Ozdinler, P. H., & Erzurumlu, R. S. (2002). Slit2, a Branching-Arborization Factor for Sensory Axons in the Mammalian CNS. *The Journal of Neuroscience, 22*, 4540–4549.

Patel, S., Thakkar, T., Swaminarayan, P., & Sajja, P. (2010). Development of Agent-Based Knowledge Discovery Framework to Access Data Resource Grid. *Advances in Computational Sciences and Technology, 3*, 23–31.

Philip, P. (2002). Letter from the Dean. In *Standford Medicine Magazine*.

Pitkin, R. M. (2007). Folate and neural tube defects. *The American Journal of Clinical Nutrition, 85*, 285–288.

Planells-Cases, R., Lerma, J., & Ferrer-Montiel, A. (2006). Pharmacological intervention at ionotropic glutamate receptor complexes. *Current Pharmaceutical Design, 12*, 3583–3596. doi:10.2174/138161206778522092

Qu, X., Gudivada, R. C., Jegga, A., Neumann, E., & Aronow, B. (2007). Semantic Web-based Data Representation and Reasoning Applied to Disease Mechanism and Pharmacology. In *IEEE International Conference on Bioinformatics & Biomedicine*, Freemont, USA, 131-143.

Radhakrishna, U., Blouin, J. L., Solanki, J. V., Dhoriani, G. M., & Antonarakis, S. E. (1996). An autosomal dominant triphalangeal thumb: polysyndactyly syndrome with variable expression in a large Indian family maps to 7q36. *American Journal of Medical Genetics, 66*, 209–215. doi:10.1002/(SICI)1096-8628(19961211)66:2<209::AID-AJMG17>3.0.CO;2-X

Random House Unabridged Dictionary. (n.d.). Retrieved from http://www.dictionary.com (accessed in Feb. 2009).

Ray, J. G., Wyatt, P. R., Thompson, M. D., Vermeulen, M. J., Meier, C., & Wong, P.-Y. (2007). Vitamin B12 and the Risk of Neural Tube Defects in a Folic-Acid-Fortified Population. *Epidemiology (Cambridge, Mass.), 18*, 362–366. doi:10.1097/01.ede.0000257063.77411.e9

Refolo, L., Pappolla, M., Lafrancois, J., Malester, B., Schmidt, S., & Thomas-Bryant, T. (2001). A cholesterol-lowering drug reduces beta-amyloid pathology in a transgenic mouse model of Alzheimer's disease. *Neurobiology of Disease, 8*, 890–899. doi:10.1006/nbdi.2001.0422

Robert Molidor As, M. M. A. Z. T. (2003). New trends in bioinformatics: from genome sequence to personalized medicine. *Experimental Gerontology, 38*, 4.

Robu, I., Robu, V., & Thirion, B. (2006). An introduction to the Semantic Web for health sciences librarians. *Journal of the Medical Library Association*, *94*, 198–205.

Royall, D. R., Lauterbach, E. C., Cummings, J. L., Reeve, A., Rummans, T. A., & Kaufer, D. I. (2002). Executive Control Function: A Review of Its Promise and Challenges for Clinical Research. A Report From the Committee on Research of the American Neuropsychiatric Association. *The Journal of Neuropsychiatry and Clinical Neurosciences*, *14*, 377–405. doi:10.1176/appi.neuropsych.14.4.377

Ruttenberg, A, C.T., Bug W, Samwald M, Bodenreider O, Chen H, Doherty D, Forsberg K, Gao Y, Kashyap V, Kinoshita J, Luciano J, Marshall Ms, Ogbuji C, Rees J, Stephens S, Wong Gt, Wu E, Zaccagnini D, Hongsermeier T, Neumann E, Herman I, Cheung Kh. (2007). Advancing translational research with the Semantic Web. *BMC Bioinformatics*, (Suppl 3), S2. doi:10.1186/1471-2105-8-S3-S2

Ruttenberg, A., Clark, T., Bug, W., Samwald, M., Bodenreider, O., & Chen, H. (2007). Advancing translational research with the Semantic Web. *BMC Bioinformatics*, *8*, 1–2. doi:10.1186/1471-2105-8-S3-S2

Sauer, S. W., Okun, J. G., Schwab, M. A., Crnic, L. R., Hoffmann, G. F., & Goodman, S. I. (2005). Bioenergetics in Glutaryl-Coenzyme A Dehydrogenase Deficiency: A Role For Glutaryl-Coenzyme A. *The Journal of Biological Chemistry*, *280*, 21830–21836. doi:10.1074/jbc.M502845200

Scardoni, G., & Laudanna, C. (2009). Analyzing biological network parameters with CentiScaPe. *Bioinformatics (Oxford, England)*, *25*, 2857–2859. doi:10.1093/bioinformatics/btp517

Shirvan, A., Reshef, A., Yogev-Falach, M., & Ziv, I. (2009). Molecular imaging of neurodegeneration by a novel cross-disease biomarker. *Experimental Neurology*, *219*, 274–283. doi:10.1016/j.expneurol.2009.05.032

Sparks, D. L., Sabbagh, M. N., Connor, D. J., Jean Lopezn, C., Launer, L. J., & Browne, P. (2005). Atorvastatin for the Treatment of Mild to Moderate Alzheimer Disease. *Archives of Neurology*, *62*, 753–757. doi:10.1001/archneur.62.5.753

Steven, A. G. (2004). Acquired rippling muscle disease with myasthenia gravis. *Muscle & Nerve*, *29*, 143–146. doi:10.1002/mus.10494

Swan, M. (2009). Emerging Patient-Driven Health Care Models: An Examination of Health Social Networks, Consumer Personalized Medicine and Quantified Self-Tracking. *International Journal of Environmental Research and Public Health*, *6*, 492–525. doi:10.3390/ijerph6020492

Takagi, A., Kojima, S., Watanabe, T., Ida, M., & Kawagoe, S. (2002). Rippling Muscle Syndrome Preceding Malignant Lymphoma. *Internal Medicine (Tokyo, Japan)*, *41*, 147–150. doi:10.2169/internalmedicine.41.147

Temtamy, S.A., Aglan, M.S., & Nemat, A. & M., E. (2003). Expanding the phenotypic spectrum of the Baller-Gerold syndrome. *Genetic Counseling (Geneva, Switzerland)*, *14*, 299–312.

Tsukurov, O., Boehmer, A., Flynn, J., Nicolai, J.-P., Hamel, B. C. J., & Traill, S. (1994). A complex bilateral polysyndactyly disease locus maps to chromosome 7q36. *Nature Genetics*, *6*, 282–286. doi:10.1038/ng0394-282

Vittorio, C., Jill, S., Melvyn, J. B., Ricardo Palacios, P., Nicolas, G. B., & Walter, J. L. (2002). Gene expression profiling of 12633 genes in Alzheimer hippocampal CA1: Transcription and neurotrophic factor down-regulation and up-regulation of apoptotic and pro-inflammatory signaling. *Journal of Neuroscience Research*, *70*, 462–473. doi:10.1002/jnr.10351

Walczak, S. (2009). Managing personal medical knowledge: agent-based knowledge acquisition. *International Journal of Technology Management, 47*, 22–36. doi:10.1504/IJTM.2009.024112

Webb Cp, P. H. (2004). Translation research: from accurate diagnosis to appropriate treatment. *Journal of Translational Medicine, 2*, 35. doi:10.1186/1479-5876-2-35

Webster, Y., Gudivada, R., Dow, E., Koehler, J., & Palakal, M. (2010). A Framework for Cross-Disciplinary Hypothesis Generation. In *ACM 25th Symposium on Applied Computing*, Sierre, Switzerland.

White, S., & Smyth, P. (2003). Algorithms for estimating relative importance in networks. In *Proceedings of the ninth ACM SIGKDD international conference on Knowledge discovery and data mining*, Washington, D.C., USA.

Wu Ch, A.R., & Bairoch, A, Natale Da, Barker Wc, Boeckmann B, Ferro S, Gasteiger E, Huang H, Lopez R, Magrane M, Martin Mj, Mazumder R, O'donovan C, Redaschi N & Suzek B. (2006). The Universal Protein Resource (UniProt): an expanding universe of protein information. *Nucleic Acids Research, 34*, D187–D191. doi:10.1093/nar/gkj161

Xiong, Z.-Q., Qian, W., Suzuki, K., & Mcnamara, J. O. (2003). Formation of Complement Membrane Attack Complex in Mammalian Cerebral Cortex Evokes Seizures and Neurodegeneration. *The Journal of Neuroscience, 23*, 955–956.

Xu, H., Yuan, X., Guan, C., Duan, S., Wu, C., & Feng, L. (2004). Calcium signaling in chemorepellant Slit2-dependent regulation of neuronal migration. *Proceedings of the National Academy of Sciences of the United States of America, 101*, 4296–4301. doi:10.1073/pnas.0303893101

Xu, J., & Li, Y. (2006). Discovering disease-genes by topological features in human protein-protein interaction network. *Bioinformatics (Oxford, England), 22*, 2800–2805. doi:10.1093/bioinformatics/btl467

Yeo, S.-Y., Miyashita, T., Fricke, C., Little, M. H., Yamada, T., & Kuwada, J. Y. (2004). Involvement of Islet-2 in the Slit signaling for axonal branching and defasciculation of the sensory neurons in embryonic zebrafish. *Mechanisms of Development, 121*, 315–324. doi:10.1016/j.mod.2004.03.006

Yildirim, M. A., Goh, K. I., Cusick, M. E., Barabasi, A. L., & Vidal, M. (2007). Drug-target network. *Nature Biotechnology, 25*, 1119–1126. doi:10.1038/nbt1338

Zguricas, J., Heus, H., Morales-Peralta, E., Breedveld, G., Kuyt, B., & Mumcu, E. F. (1999). Clinical and genetic studies on 12 preaxial polydactyly families and refinement of the localisation of the gene responsible to a 1.9 cM region on chromosome 7q36. *Journal of Medical Genetics, 36*, 33–40.

ADDITIONAL READING

Allison, M. (2009). Can Web 2.0 Reboot Clinical Trials? *Nature Biotechnology, 27*(10), 895–902. doi:10.1038/nbt1009-895

Campillos, M., Kuhn, M., Gavin, A.C., et al., (n.d.). Drug Target Identification Using Side-Effect Similarity. *Science, 321*(5886): p. 263-266.

Chen, H., Ding, L., & Wu, Z. (2009). Semantic Web for Integrated Network Analysis in Biomedicine. *Briefings in Bioinformatics, 10*(2), 177–192. doi:10.1093/bib/bbp002

Chen, J., Aronow, B., & Jegga, A. (2009). Disease Candidate Gene Identification and Prioritization Using Protein Interaction Networks. *BMC Bioinformatics, 10*(73), 1–2.

Feldman, I., Rzhetsky, A., & Vitkup, D. (2008). Network Properties of Genes Harbouring Inherited Disease Mutations. *Proceedings of the National Academy of Sciences of the United States of America, 105*(11), 4323–4328. doi:10.1073/pnas.0701722105

Goh, K.-I., Cusick, M. E., & Valle, D. (2007). The Human Disease Network. *Proceedings of the National Academy of Sciences of the United States of America, 104*(21), 8685–8690. doi:10.1073/pnas.0701361104

Gudivada, R. C., Qu, X. A., & Chen, J. (2008). Identifying Disease-Causal Genes Using Semantic Web-Based Representation of Integrated Genomic and Phenomic Knowledge. *Journal of Biomedical Informatics, 41*(5), 717–729. doi:10.1016/j.jbi.2008.07.004

Hopkins, A. L. (2007). Network Pharmacology. *Nature Chemical Biology, 4*(11), 682–690. doi:10.1038/nchembio.118

Lee, D. S., Park, J., & Kay, K. A. (2008). The Implications of Human Metabolic Network Topology for Disease Comorbidity. *Proceedings of the National Academy of Sciences of the United States of America, 105*(29), 9880–9885. doi:10.1073/pnas.0802208105

Ma'ayan, A., Jenkins, S. L., & Goldfarb, J. (2007). Network Analysis of Fda Approved Drugs and Their Targets. *The Mount Sinai Journal of Medicine, New York, 74*(1), 27–32. doi:10.1002/msj.20002

Nacher, J. C., & Schwartz, J. M. (2008). A Global View of Drug-Therapy Interactions. *BMC Pharmacology, 8*(1), 5. doi:10.1186/1471-2210-8-5

Ortutay, C., & Vihinen, M. (2009). Identification of Candidate Disease Genes by Integrating Gene Ontologies and Protein-Interaction Networks: Case Study of Primary Immunodeficiencies. *Nucleic Acids Research, 37*(2), 622–628. doi:10.1093/nar/gkn982

Ruttenberg, A., Clark, T., & Bug, W. (2007). Advancing Translational Research with the Semantic Web. *BMC Bioinformatics, 8*(3), 1–2. doi:10.1186/1471-2105-8-S3-S2

Stelzl, U. (2005). A Human Protein-Protein Interaction Network: A Resource for Annotating the Proteome. *Cell, 122*(1), 957. doi:10.1016/j.cell.2005.08.029

Stojanovic, N., Studer, R., & Stojanovic, L. (2003). *An Approach for the Ranking of Query Results in the Semantic Web in 2nd International Semantic Web Conference.* Sanibel Island, USA.

Webster, Y., Gudivada, R., Dow, E., et al. (2010). *A Framework for Cross-Disciplinary Hypothesis Generation.* In ACM 25th Symposium on Applied Computing. Sierre, Switzerlan.

Yildirim, M. A., Goh, K. I., & Cusick, M. E. (2007). Drug-Target Network. *Nature Biotechnology, 25*(10), 1119–1126. doi:10.1038/nbt1338

Compilation of References

Aarhus, M., Helland, C. A., Lund-Johansen, M., Wester, K., & Knappskog, P. M. (2010). Microarray-based gene expression profiling and DNA copy number variation analysis of temporal fossa arachnoid cysts. *Cerebrospinal Fluid Research, 7*(6).

Abrams, P. A. (1999). Is predator-mediated coexistence possible in unstable systems? *Ecology, 80,* 608–621.

Acharya, T., & Ray, A. K. (2005). *Image processing: Principles and applications*. New Jersey., Alexandre, L., Campihlo, A. and& Kamel, M. (2001). On combining classifiers using sum and product rules. *Pattern Recognition Letters, 22,* 1283–1289.

Agnolet, S., Jaroszewski, J. W., Verpoorte, R., & Staerk, D. (2010). H NMR-based metabolomics combined with HPLC-PDA-MS-SPE-NMR for investigation of standardized Ginkgo biloba preparations. *Metabolomics, 6*(2), 292–302. doi:10.1007/s11306-009-0195-x

Akira, B. M., Akira, S., Tetsuo, A., Yasuyuki, E., Michiyoshi, S., Iwao, O., & Tsutomu, W. (1974). Autoimmune hemolytic anemia associated with colon cancer. *Cancer, 33,* 111–114. doi:10.1002/1097-0142(197401)33:1<111::AID-CNCR2820330117>3.0.CO;2-9

Albert, R. (2007). Network Inference, Analysis, and Modeling in Systems Biology. *The Plant Cell, 19,* 3327–3338. doi:10.1105/tpc.107.054700

Albert, R., Jeong, H., & Barabási, A. L. (2000). Error and attack tolerance of complex networks. *Nature, 406,* 378–381. doi:10.1038/35019019

Alberts, J. B., & Odell, G. M. (2004). In silico reconstitution of listeria propulsion exhibits nanosaltation. *PLoS Biology, 2,* 2054–2066. doi:10.1371/journal.pbio.0020412

Allen, T. F. H., & Starr, T. B. (1982). *Hierarchy: Perspectives for Ecological Complexity*. Chicago, IL: University of Chicago Press.

Allesina, S., Alonso, D., & Pascual, M. (2008). A General Model for Food Web Structure. *Science, 320*(5876), 658–661. doi:10.1126/science.1156269

Allesina, S., & Bodini, A. (2004). Who dominates whom in the ecosystem? Energy flow bottlenecks and cascading extinctions. *Journal of Theoretical Biology, 230,* 351–358. doi:10.1016/j.jtbi.2004.05.009

Allesina, S., & Bodini, A. (2005). Food web networks: Scaling relation revisited. *Ecological Complexity, 2,* 323–338. doi:10.1016/j.ecocom.2005.05.001

Allison, M. (2009). Can web 2.0 reboot clinical trials? *Nature Biotechnology, 27,* 895–902. doi:10.1038/nbt1009-895

Altmaier, E., Ramsay, S. L., & Graber, A. (2008). Bioinformatics analysis of targeted metabolomics – uncovering old and new tales of diabetic mice under medication. *Endocrinology, 149,* 3478–3489. doi:10.1210/en.2007-1747

Altschul, S. F., Gish, W., Miller, W., Myers, E. W., & Lipman, D. J. (1990). Basic local alignment search tool. *Journal of Molecular Biology, 215*(3), 403–410.

Alves, R., Antunes, F., & Salvador, A. (2006). Tools for kinetic modeling of biochemical networks. *Nature Biotechnology, 24*(6), 667–672. doi:10.1038/nbt0606-667

Anand, A., & Suganthan, P. N. (2009). Multiclass cancer classification by support vector machines with class-wise optimized genes and probability estimates. *Journal of Theoretical Biology, 259*(3), 533–540. doi:10.1016/j.jtbi.2009.04.013

Ando, S., & Tanaka, Y. (2005). Mass spectrometric studies on brain metabolism, using stable isotopes. *Mass Spectrometry Reviews*, *24*(6), 865–886. doi:10.1002/mas.20045

Andrews, J., Bouffard, G. G., Cheadle, C., Lü, J., Becker, K. G., & Oliver, B. (2000). Gene discovery using computational and microarray analysis of transcription in the Drosophila melanogaster testis. *Genome Research*, *10*(12), 2030–2043. doi:10.1101/gr.10.12.2030

Andronescu, M., Zhang, Z. C., & Condon, A. (2005). Secondary structure prediction of interacting RNA molecules. *Journal of Molecular Biology*, *345*(5), 987–1001. doi:10.1016/j.jmb.2004.10.082

Andronescu, M. (2003). Algorithms for predicting the secondary structure of pairs and combinatorial sets of nucleic acid strands. *Master thesis*, University of British Columbia, BC, Canada.

Andronescu, M. S. (2008). Computational approaches for RNA energy parameter estimation. *PhD thesis*, University of British Columbia, BC, Canada.

Arimura, K. (2002). Rippling muscle syndrome. *Internal Medicine (Tokyo, Japan)*, *41*, 325–326. doi:10.2169/internalmedicine.41.325

Arkin, A., & Ross, J. (1995). Statistical construction of chemical reaction mechanisms from measured time-series. *Journal of Physical Chemistry*, *99*, 970–979. doi:10.1021/j100003a020

Arkin, A., Shen, P., & Ross, J. (1997). A Test Case of Correlation Metric Construction of a Reaction Pathway from Measurements. *Science*, *277*(29), 1275–1279. doi:10.1126/science.277.5330.1275

Arreguin-Sanchez, F., Arcos, E., & Chavez, E. A. (2002). Flows of biomass and structure in an exploited benthic ecosystem in the gulf of California, Mexico. *Ecological Modelling*, *156*, 167–183. doi:10.1016/S0304-3800(02)00159-X

Askenazi, M., Driggers, E. M., Holtzman, D. A., Norman, T. C., Iverson, S., & Zimmer, D. P. (2003). Integrating transcriptional and metabolite profiles to direct the engineering of lovastatin-producing fungal strains. *Nature Biotechnology*, *21*(2), 150–156. doi:10.1038/nbt781

Assfalg, M., Bertini, I., & Colangiuli, D. (2008). Evidence of different metabolic phenotypes in humans. *Proceedings of the National Academy of Sciences of the United States of America*, *105*, 1420–1424. doi:10.1073/pnas.0705685105

Bader, G. D., Betel, D., & Hogue, C. W. V. (2003). BIND: the Biomolecular Interaction Network Database. *Nucleic Acids Research*, *31*, 248–250. doi:10.1093/nar/gkg056

Baeten, J. C. M. (2005). A brief history of process algebra. *Theoretical Computer Science*, *335*(2–3), 131–146. doi:10.1016/j.tcs.2004.07.036

Baird, D., Luczkovich, J. J., & Christian, R. R. (1998). Assessment of spatial and temporal variability in ecosystem attributes of the St Marks National Wildlife Refuge, Apalachee Bay, Florida. *Estuarine, Coastal and Shelf Science*, *47*, 329–349. doi:10.1006/ecss.1998.0360

Baird, D., & Ulanowicz, R. E. (1989). The seasonal dynamics of the Chesapeake Bay ecosystem. *Ecological Monographs*, *59*, 329–364. doi:10.2307/1943071

Bajic, V. B., Tan, S. L., Christoffels, A., Schönbach, C., Lipovich, L., & Yang, L. (2006, Apr). Mice and men: their promoter properties. *PLOS Genetics*, *2*(4), e54. doi:10.1371/journal.pgen.0020054

Bamba, B., & Mukherjea, S. (2005). Utilizing Resource Importance for Ranking Semantic Web Query Results In *Semantic Web and Databases*, 185-198. Berlin: Springer Berlin.

Banavar, J. R., Maritan, A., & Rinaldo, A. (1999). Size and form in efficient transportation networks. *Nature*, *399*, 130–132. doi:10.1038/20144

Bansal, M., Belcastro, V., Ambesi-Impiombato, A., & di Bernardo, D. (2007). How to infer gene networks from expression profiles. *Molecular Systems Biology*, *3*(78).

Barantin, L., Le Pape, A., & Akoka, S. (1997). A new method for absolute quantitation of MRS metabolites. *Magnetic Resonance in Medicine*, *38*(2), 179–182. doi:10.1002/mrm.1910380203

Barnes, M., Freudenberg, J., Thompson, S., Aronow, B., & Pavlidis, P. (2005). Experimental comparison and cross-validation of the Affymetrix and Illumina gene expression analysis platforms. *Nucleic Acids Research*, *33*(18), 5914–5923. doi:10.1093/nar/gki890

Bascompte, J.,[REMOVED HYPERLINK FIELD] & Jordano, P. (2007). Plant-Animal Mutualistic Networks: The Architecture of Biodiversity. *Annual Review of Ecology Evolution and Systematics*, *38*, 567–593. doi:10.1146/annurev.ecolsys.38.091206.095818

Bashi, K., Forrest, A., & Ramanathan, M. (2005). SPLIN-DID: a semi-paramteric, model based method for obtaining transcription rates and gene regulation paramters from genomic and proteomic expression profiles. *Bioinformatics (Oxford, England)*, *21*(20), 3873–3879. doi:10.1093/bioinformatics/bti624

Bauer, B., Jordán, F., & Podani, J. (in press). Node centrality indices in food webs: rank orders versus distributions. *Ecological Complexity*.

Bayardo, R. J., Jr., Bohrer, W., Brice, R., Cichocki, A., Fowler, J., Helal, A., et al. (1997). InfoSleuth: agent-based semantic integration of information in open and dynamic environments. In *Proceedings of the Proceedings of the 1997 ACM SIGMOD international conference on Management of data*, Tucson, USA1997.

Beckoners, O. (2007). Metabolic profiling, metabolomic and metabonomic procedures for NMR spectroscopy of urine, plasma, serum and tissue extracts. *Nature Protocols*, *2*, 2692–2703. doi:10.1038/nprot.2007.376

Beckonert, O., Bollard, M. E., & Ebbels, T. M. D. (2003). NMR-based metabonomic toxicity classification: hierarchical cluster analysis and k-nearest neighbor approaches. *Analytica Chimica Acta*, *490*, 3–15. doi:10.1016/S0003-2670(03)00060-6

Beckonert, O., Keun, H. C., Ebbels, T. M., Bundy, J., Holmes, E., & Lindon, J. C. (2007). Metabolic profiling, metabolomic and metabonomic procedures for NMR spectroscopy of urine, plasma, serum and tissue extracts. *Nature Protocols*, *2*(11), 2692–2703. doi:10.1038/nprot.2007.376

Beckonert, O., Monnerjahn, J., Bonk, U., & Leibfritz, D. (2003). Visualizing metabolic changes in breast-cancer tissue using 1H-NMR spectroscopy and self-organizing maps. *NMR in Biomedicine*, *16*(1), 1–11. doi:10.1002/nbm.797

Beebe, K., Pell, R. J., & Seasholtz, M. B. (1998). *Chemometrics: A practical guide*. New York: John Wiley & Sons.

Beek, J., Elward, K., & Gasque, P. (2003). Activation of Complement in the Central Nervous System. *Annals of the New York Academy of Sciences*, *992*, 56–71. doi:10.1111/j.1749-6632.2003.tb03138.x

Belacel, N., Wang, C., & Cuperlovic-Culf, M. (2010). *"Clustering". Invited book chapter in Statistical Bioinformatics*. New York: John Wiley & Sons.

Berkes, F. (2004). Rethinking community-based conservation. *Conservation Biology*, *18*, 621–630. doi:10.1111/j.1523-1739.2004.00077.x

Berlow, E. L. (1999). Strong effects of weak interactions in ecological communities. *Nature*, *398*, 330–334. doi:10.1038/18672

Berlow, E. L., Dunne, J. A., Martinez, N. D., Stark, P. B., Williams, R. J., & Brose, U. (2008). Simple prediction of interaction strengths in complex food webs. *Proceedings of the National Academy of Sciences of the United States of America*, *106*, 187–191. doi:10.1073/pnas.0806823106

Berlow, E. L., Neutel, A.-M., Cohen, J. E., de Ruiter, P. C., Ebenman, B., & Emmerson, M. (2004). Interaction strengths in food webs: issues and opportunities. *Journal of Animal Ecology*, *73*, 585–598. doi:10.1111/j.0021-8790.2004.00833.x

Bersier, L.F., Banašek-Richter, C., & Cattin, M.F. (2002). Quantitative descriptors of food-web matrices. *Ecology*, *83*, 2394–2407. doi:10.1890/0012-9658(2002)083[2394:QDOFWM]2.0.CO;2

Bersier, L.-F., Dixon, P., & Sugihara, G. (1999). Scale-invariant or scale-dependent behavior of the link density property in food webs: A matter of sampling effort? *American Naturalist*, *153*, 676–682. doi:10.1086/303200

Bertness, M. D., & Callaway, R. (1994). Positive interaction in communities. *Trends in Ecology & Evolution*, *9*, 191–193. doi:10.1016/0169-5347(94)90088-4

Bertram, L., Mcqueen, M. B., Mullin, K., Blacker, D., & Tanzi, R. E. (2007). Systematic meta-analyses of Alzheimer disease genetic association studies: the AlzGene database. *Nature Genetics*, *39*, 17. doi:10.1038/ng1934

Bertram, L., & Tanzi, R. E. (2005). The genetic epidemiology of neurodegenerative disease. *The Journal of Clinical Investigation*, *115*, 1449–1457. doi:10.1172/JCI24761

Bezdek, J. (1999). *Fuzzy models and algorithms for pattern recognition and image processing. J.* Boston: Kluwer Academic.

Bictash, M., Ebbels, T. M., Chan, Q., Loo, R. L., & Yap, I. K. S. (2009). Opening up the "Black Box": Metabolic phenotyping and metabolomie-wide association studies in epidemiology. *Journal of Clinical Epidemiology, 63,* 970–979. doi:10.1016/j.jclinepi.2009.10.001

Bijlsma, S., Bobeldijk, I., Verheij, E. R., Ramaker, R., Kochhar, S., & Macdonald, I. A. (2006). Large-scale human metabolomics studies: a strategy for data (pre-) processing and validation. *Analytical Chemistry, 78*(2), 567–574. doi:10.1021/ac051495j

Björnstad, O. N., Fromentin, J. M., Stenseth, N. C., & Gjøsæter, J. (1999). Cycles and trends in cod populations. *Proceedings of the National Academy of Sciences of the United States of America, 96,* 5066–5071. doi:10.1073/pnas.96.9.5066

Blain, J.-F., & Poirier, J. (2004). Cholesterol homeostasis and the pathophysiology of Alzheimer's disease. *Expert Review of Neurotherapeutics, 4,* 823–829. doi:10.1586/14737175.4.5.823

Blossey, R., Cardelli, L., & Phillips, A. (2008). Compositionality, stochasticity and cooperativity in dynamic models of gene regulation. *HFSP (Human Frontier Science Program Organization). Journal, 2*(1), 17–28.

Boccard, J., Veuthey, J. L., & Rudaz, S. (2010). Knowledge discovery in metabolomics: an overview of MS data handling. *Journal of Separation Science, 33*(3), 290–304. doi:10.1002/jssc.200900609

Bodini, A., Bellingeri, M., Allesina, S., & Bondavalli, C. (2009). Using food web dominator trees to catch secondary extinctions in action. *Philosophical Transactions of the Royal Society of London. Series B, Biological Sciences, 364*(1524), 1725–1731. doi:10.1098/rstb.2008.0278

Bogdanova, G. T., Brouwer, A. E., Kapralov, S. N., & Östergård, P. R. J. (2001). Error-correcting codes over an alphabet of four elements. *Designs, Codes and Cryptography, 23*(3), 333–342. doi:10.1023/A:1011275112159

Boland, C. (2002). Molecular basis for stool-based DNA tests for colorectal cancer: a primer for clinicians. *Reviews in Gastroenterological Disorders, 1,* 12–19.

Bondavalli, C., Bodini, A., Rossetti, G., & Allesina, S. (2006). Detecting stress at a whole ecosystem level. The case of a mountain lake: Lake Santo (Italy). *Ecosystems (New York, N.Y.), 9,* 1–56. doi:10.1007/s10021-005-0065-y

Bondavalli, C., & Ulanowicz, R. E. (1999). Unexpected effects of predators upon their prey: The case of the American alligator. *Ecosystems (New York, N.Y.), 2,* 49–63. doi:10.1007/s100219900057

Bonsall, M. B., & Hastings, A. (2004). Demographic and environmental stochasticity in predator-prey metapopulation dynamics. *Journal of Animal Ecology, 73,* 1043–1055. doi:10.1111/j.0021-8790.2004.00874.x

Boogerd, F., Bruggeman, J. F., Hofmeyr, J.-H. S., & Westerhoff, H. V. (Eds.). (2007). *Systems Biology: Philosophical Foundations.* New York: Elsevier.

Borrvall, C., Ebenman, B., & Jonsson, T. (n.d.). (200). Biodiversity lessens the risk of cascading extinction in model food webs. *Ecology Letters, 3,* 131–136. doi:10.1046/j.1461-0248.2000.00130.x

Bota, M., D.H.-W.S.L.W. (2005). Brain Architecture Management System. *Neuroinformatics, 3,* 15–48. doi:10.1385/NI:3:1:015

Botter, G., Settin, T., Marani, M., & Rinaldo, A. (2006). A stochastic model of nitrate transport and cycling at basin scale. *Water Resources Research, 42,* W04415. doi:10.1029/2005WR004599

Boys, R. J., Wilkinson, D. J., & Kirkwood, T. B. (2008). *Bayesian inference for a discretely observed stochastic kinetic model.* Springer Netherlands.

Bozdech, Z., Zhu, J., Joachimiak, M. P., Cohen, F. E., Pulliam, B., & DeRisi, J. L. (2003). Expression profiling of the schizont and trophozoite stages of Plasmodium falciparum with a long-oligonucleotide microarray. *Genome Biology, 4,* R9. doi:10.1186/gb-2003-4-2-r9

Brahmachary, M., Schönbach, C., Yang, L., Huang, E., Tan, S. L., & Chowdhary, R. (2006, Dec). Computational Promoter Analysis of Mouse, Rat and Human Antimicrobial Peptide-coding Genes. *BMC Bioinformatics, 18*(7Suppl 5), S8. doi:10.1186/1471-2105-7-S5-S8

Braich, R., Johnson, C., Rothermund, P., Hwang, D., Chelyapov, N., & Leman, L. (2001). Solution of a satisfiability problem on a gel-based DNA computer. *Lecture Notes in Computer Science, 2054*, 27–42. doi:10.1007/3-540-44992-2_3

Braun, P., Rietman, E., & Vidal, M. (2008). Networking metabolites and diseases. *Proceedings of the National Academy of Sciences of the United States of America, 105*, 9849–9850. doi:10.1073/pnas.0805644105

Brelauer, K. J., Frank, R., Blöcher, H., & Marky, L. A. (1986). Predicting DNA duplex stability from the base sequence. *Proceedings of the National Academy of Sciences of the United States of America, 83*(11), 3746–3750. doi:10.1073/pnas.83.11.3746

Brenner, S., & Lerner, R. A. (1992). Encoded combinatorial chemistry. *Proceedings of the National Academy of Sciences of the United States of America, 89*(12), 5381–5383. doi:10.1073/pnas.89.12.5381

Brouwer, A. E., Shearer, J. B., Sloane, N. J. A., & Smith, W. D. (1990). A new table of constant weight codes. *IEEE Transactions on Information Theory, 36*, 1334–1380. doi:10.1109/18.59932

Brown, M., Dunn, W. B., Dobson, P., Patel, Y., Winder, C. L., & Francis-McIntyre, S. (2009). Mass spectrometry tools and metabolite-specific databases for molecular identification in metabolomics. *Analyst (London), 134*(7), 1322–1332. doi:10.1039/b901179j

Browne, M. (2007). A geometric approach to non-paramteric density estimation. *Pattern Recognition, 40*, 134–140. doi:10.1016/j.patcog.2006.05.012

Bustelo, X. R., Sauzeau, V., & Berenjeno, I. M. (2007). GTP-binding proteins of the Rho/Rac family: Regulation, effectors and function in vivo. *BioEssays, 29*, 356–370. doi:10.1002/bies.20558

Bylesjo, M., Rantalainen, M., & Cloarec, O. (2006). OPLS discriminant analysis combining the strength of PSL-DA and SIMCA classification. *Journal of Chemometrics, 20*, 341–351. doi:10.1002/cem.1006

Camacho, J., Guimerà, R., & Amaral, L. A. N. (2002). Robust patterns in food web structure. *Physical Review Letters, 88*, 228102. doi:10.1103/PhysRevLett.88.228102

Cambon, A. C., Khalyfa, A., Cooper, N. G., & Thompson, C. M. (2007). Analysis of probe level patterns in Affymetrix microarray data. *BMC Bioinformatics, 8*(146).

Cardelli, L., Caron, E., Gardner, P., Kahramanoğulları, O., & Phillips, A. (2009). A process model of Rho GTP-binding proteins. *Theoretical Computer Science, 410*(33-34), 3166–3185. doi:10.1016/j.tcs.2009.04.029

Cardelli, L., & Zavattaro, G. (2010). Turing universality of the Biochemical Ground Form. *Mathematical Structures in Computer Science, 20*(1), 45–73. doi:10.1017/S0960129509990259

Cardelli, L. (2009). Artificial biochemistry. In Condon, A., Harel, D., Kok, J. N., Salomaa, A., & Winfree, E. (Eds.), *Algorithmic Bioprocesses. Natural Computing Series, Part 7* (pp. 429–462). Springer.

Cardelli, L. (2005). Abstract machines of systems biology. In Priami, C., Merelli, E., Gonzalez, P. P., & Omicini, A. (Eds.), *Transactions on Computational Systems Biology. III, Lecture Notes in Bioinformatics 3737* (pp. 145–168). New York: Springer.

Cardelli, L. (2008). From processes to ODEs by chemistry. In Ausiello, G. & Karhumäki J. & Mauri G. & Ong C.-H. L. (Eds.). *Fifth IFIP International Conference On Theoretical Computer Science* - TCS 2008, IFIP 20th World Computer Congress, International Federation for Information Processing 273, (pp. 261-281). New York: Springer.

Cardelli, L., & Zavattaro, G. (2008). Termination problems in chemical kinetics. In Breugel, F. v. & Chechik, M. (Eds.), *CONCUR 2008 - Concurrency Theory, 19th International Conference,* Proceedings, Lecture Notes in Computer Science 5201, (pp. 477-491), Springer.

Cardelli, L., Caron, E., Gardner, P., Kahramanoğulları, O., & Phillips, A. (2009b). A process model of actin polymerization. In Cannata N. & Merelli E. & Ulidowski, I. (Eds.). *From Biology To Concurrency and Back, Sattelite Workshop of ICALP '08.* Electronic Notes in Theoretical Computer Science 229, (pp. 127-144). New York: Elsevier.

Carey, M. F., Peterson, C. L., & Smale, S. T. (2009). *Transcriptional Regulation in Eukaryotes: Concepts, Strategies, and Techniques.* CSHL Press.

Case, T. J., & Mark, L. (2000). Taper Interspecific Competition, Environmental Gradients, Gene Flow, and the Coevolution of Species' Borders. *American Naturalist, 155*(5), 583–605. doi:10.1086/303351

Caspi, R., & Karp, P. D. (2007). Using the MetaCyc pathway database and the BioCyc database collection. *Curr Protoc Bioinformatics, Chapter 1*, Unit1 17.

Castrillo, J. I., Hayes, A., Mohammed, S., Gaskell, S. J., & Oliver, S. G. (2003). An optimized protocol for metabolome analysis in yeast using direct infusion electrospray mass spectrometry. *Phytochemistry, 62*(6), 929–937. doi:10.1016/S0031-9422(02)00713-6

Cattin, M. F., & Bersier, L.-F., Banašek-Richter, C., Baltensperger, R., & Gabriel, J.-P. (2004). Phylogenetic constraints and adaptation explain food-web structure. *Nature, 427*, 835–839. doi:10.1038/nature02327

Cavill, R., Keun, H. C., & Holmes, E. (2009). Genetic algorithms for simultaneous variable and sample selection in metabolomics. *Bioinformatics (Oxford, England), 25*, 112–118. doi:10.1093/bioinformatics/btn586

Cevikalp, H., & Polikar, R. (2008). Local classifier weighting by quadratic programming. *Neural Networks, 9*(10).

Chalcraft, K. R., Lee, R., Mills, C., & Britz-McKibbin, P. (2009). Virtual quantification of metabolites by capillary electrophoresis-electrospray ionization-mass spectrometry: predicting ionization efficiency without chemical standards. *Analytical Chemistry, 81*(7), 2506–2515. doi:10.1021/ac802272u

Charbonnier, Y., Gettler, B., Francois, P., Bento, M., Renzoni, A., & Vaudaux, P. (2005). A generic approach for the design of whole-genome oligoarrays, validated for genomotyping, deletion mapping and gene expression analysis on Staphylococcus aureus. *BMC Genomics, 6*(1), 95. doi:10.1186/1471-2164-6-95

Chee, Y. M., & Ling, S. (2008). Improved lower bounds for constant GC-content DNA codes. *IEEE Transactions on Information Theory, 54*(1), 391–394. doi:10.1109/TIT.2007.911167

Chen, H., & Sharp, B. M. (2002). Oliz, a suite of Perl scripts that assist in the design of microarrays using 50mer oligonucleotides from the 3' untranslated region. *BMC Bioinformatics, 3*(27).

Chen, J., Aronow, B., & Jegga, A. (2009). Disease candidate gene identification and prioritization using protein interaction networks. *BMC Bioinformatics, 10*, 1–2.

Cheng, C., Yun, K-Y., Ressom, H., Mohanty, B., Bajic, V.B., Jia, Y., Yun, S.J. & de los Reyes, B.G. (2007, Jun). An early response regulatory cluster induced by low temperature and hydrogen peroxide in chilling tolerant japonica rice. *BMC Genomics, 18*, 8:175.

Chimini, G., & Chavrier, P. (2000). Function of Rho family proteins in actin dynamics during phagocytosis and engulfment. *Nature Cell Biology, 2*, 191–196. doi:10.1038/35036454

Chipman, H., Hastie, T. J., & Tibshirani, R. (2008). *Clustering microarray data of Gene Expression Microarray Dat. (T. P. Speed, A cura di)*. Chapman & Hall.

Cho, S. B., & Kim, J. H. (1995). Combining multiple neural networks by fuzzy integral for robust classification. *IEEE Transactions on Systems, Man, and Cybernetics, 25*(2), 380–384. doi:10.1109/21.364825

Chou, H. H., Hsia, A. P., Mooney, D. L., & Schnable, P. S. (2004). Picky: oligo microarray design for large genomes. *Bioinformatics (Oxford, England), 20*, 2893–2902. doi:10.1093/bioinformatics/bth347

Chou, I. C., Martens, H., & Voit, E. O. (2006). Paramter estimation in biochemical systems models with alternating regression. *Theoretical Biology & Medical Modelling, 3*(25).

Chou, W.-Y. S., Hunt, Y. M., Beckjord, E. B., Moser, R. P., & Hesse, B. W. (2009). Social Media Use in Use in the United States: Implications for Health Communication. *Journal of Medical Internet Research, 11*, 48–50. doi:10.2196/jmir.1249

Christensen, V., & Walters, C. J. (2004). Ecopath with Ecosim: methods, capabilities and limitations. *Ecological Modelling, 172*, 109–139. doi:10.1016/j.ecolmodel.2003.09.003

Chu, C. Y., Xiao, X., & Zhou, X. G. (2006). Metabolomics and bioinformatic analysis in asphyxiated neonates. *Clinical Biochemistry, 39*, 203–209. doi:10.1016/j.clinbiochem.2006.01.006

Chu, W., Ghahramani, Z., Falciani, F., & Wild, D. L. (2005). Biomarker discovery in microarray gene expression data with Gaussian processes. *Bioinformatics (Oxford, England)*, *21*(16), 3385–3393. doi:10.1093/bioinformatics/bti526

Chung, W. H., Rhee, S.-K., Wan, X. F., Bae, J.-W., Quan, Z.-X., & Park, Y.-H. (2005). Design of long oligonucleotide probes for functional gene detection in a microbial community. *Bioinformatics (Oxford, England)*, *21*, 4092–4100. doi:10.1093/bioinformatics/bti673

Ciocchetta, F., & Hillston, J. (2008). Process Algebras in Systems Biology. Bernardo, M. & Degano, P. & Zavattaro G. (Eds.). *Formal Methods for Computational Systems Biology, 8th International School on Formal Methods for the Design of Computer, Communication, and Software Systems, SFM 2008,* Advanced Lectures. Lecture Notes in Computer Science 5016, (pp. 265-312). New York: Springer.

Ciocchetta, F., & Jordán, F. (2010). Modelling and analysing hierarchical ecological systems in BlenX. *Technical Report TR-1-2010*, CoSBi, Trento.

Ciocchetta, F., & Priami, C. (2007). Biological Transactions for Quantitative Models. Busi, N. & Zandron, C. (Eds.), *Proceedings of the First Workshop on Membrane Computing and Biologically Inspired Process Calculi, MeCBIC 2006*, Electronic Notes in Theoretical Computer Science 171(2), (pp. 55-67), Elsevier.

Clark, J. S. (2009). Beyond neutral science. *Trends in Ecology & Evolution*, *24*, 8–15. doi:10.1016/j.tree.2008.09.004

Clayton, T. A., Lindon, J. C., & Cloarec, O. (2006). Pharmaco-metabonomic phenotyping and personalized drug treatment. *Nature*, *440*, 1073–1077. doi:10.1038/nature04648

Cloarec, O., Campbell, A., & Tseng, L. H. (2007). Virtual chromatographic enhancement in clyoflow LC-NM experiment via statistical total correlation spectroscopy. *Analytical Chemistry*, *79*, 5682–5689. doi:10.1021/ac061928y

Cloarec, O., Dumas, M., & Craig, A. (2005). Statistical total correlation spectroscopy: an exploratory approach for latent biomarker identification from metabolic 1H NMR data sets. *Analytical Chemistry*, *77*, 1282–1289. doi:10.1021/ac048630x

Cohen, J. E. (1978). *Food Webs and Niche Space*. Princeton University Press.

Cohen, J. E., Beaver, R. A., Cousins, S. H., DeAngelis, D. L., Goldwasser, L., & Heong, K. L. (1993). Improving food webs. *Ecology*, *74*, 252–258. doi:10.2307/1939520

Cohen, J. E., Briand, F., & Newman, C. M. (Eds.). (1990). *Community Food Webs: Data and Theory. (Biomathematics)*. Springer-Verlag.

Cohen, J. E., & Newman, C. M. (1985). A stochastic theory of community food webs. I. Models and aggregated data. *Proceedings of the Royal Society of London. Series B. Biological Sciences*, *224*, 421–448. doi:10.1098/rspb.1985.0042

CoSBiLab. (2010). Retrieved from http://www.cosbi.eu.

Cousins, S. H. (1987). The decline of the trophic level concept. *Trends in Ecology & Evolution*, *2*, 312–316. doi:10.1016/0169-5347(87)90086-3

Crampin, E. J., Schnell, S., & McSharry, P. E. (2004). Mathematical and computational techniques to deduce complex biochemical reaction mechanisms. *Progress in Biophysics and Molecular Biology*, *86*, 72–112. doi:10.1016/j.pbiomolbio.2004.04.002

Crothers, D., & Zimm, B. (1964). Theory of the melting transition of synthetic polynucleotides: Evaluation of the stacking free energy. *Journal of Molecular Biology*, *116*, 1–9. doi:10.1016/S0022-2836(64)80086-3

Cuperlovic-Culf, M., Belacel, N., & Culf, A. (2009). NMR metabolomic analysis of samples using fuzzy K-means clustering. *Magnetic Resonance in Chemistry*, *47*, S96–S104. doi:10.1002/mrc.2502

Cuperlovic-Culf, M., Chute, I., & Barnett, D. (2010). Cell culture metabolomics. *Drug Discovery Today*, *15*, 610–621. doi:10.1016/j.drudis.2010.06.012

Curien, P.-L., Danos, V., Krivine, J., & Zhang, M. (2008). Computational self-assembly. *Theoretical Computer Science*, *404*(1-2), 61–75. doi:10.1016/j.tcs.2008.04.014

Cury, P., Bakun, A., Crawford, R. J. M., Jarre, A., Quiñones, R. A., Shannon, L. J., & Verheye, H. M. (2000). Small pelagics in upwelling systems: patterns of interaction and structural changes in "wasp-waist" ecosystems. *Journal of Marine Science*, *57*, 603–618.

Dale, V. H., & Beyeler, S. C. (2001). Challenges in the development and use of ecological indicators. *Ecological Indicators*, *1*, 3–10. doi:10.1016/S1470-160X(01)00003-6

Damian, D., Oresic, M., & Verheij, E. (2007). Applications of a new subspace clustering algorithm (COSA) in medical systems biology. *Metabolomics*, *3*, 69–77. doi:10.1007/s11306-006-0045-z

Danos, V., Feret, J., Fontana, W., Harmer, R., & Krivine, J. (2007). Rule-based modelling of cellular signalling. In Caires, L. & Vasconcelos, V. T. (Eds.). *CONCUR 2007 - Concurrency Theory, 18th International Conference*, Proceedings. Lecture Notes in Computer Science 4703, (pp. 17-41). New York: Springer.

Danos, V., Feret, J., Fontana, W., Harmer, R., & Krivine, J. (2008). Rule-based modelling, symmetries, refinements. In Fisher J. (Ed.). *Proceedings of the 1st international workshop on Formal Methods in Systems Biology*, Lecture Notes in Computer Science 5054, (pp 103 – 122). New York: Springer.

Dauphinée, D.M.M., & Joseph, B. Md, Phd. (2000). Breaking Down the Walls: Thoughts on the Scholarship of Integration. *Journal of Medical Education*, *75*, 5.

Dawson, T. M., & Dawson, V. L. (2003). Molecular Pathways of Neurodegeneration in Parkinson's Disease. *Science*, *302*, 819–822. doi:10.1126/science.1087753

De Roock, W., Biesmans, B., De Schutter, J., & Tejpar, S. (2009). Clinical biomarkers in oncology: focus on colorectal cancer. *Molecular Diagnosis & Therapy*, *13*, 103–114.

DeAngelis, D. L., & Gross, L. J. (1992). *Individual-based Models and Approaches in Ecology*. New York, NY: Chapman and Hall.

DeAngelis, D. L., & Mooij, W. M. (2005). Individual-based modeling of ecological and evolutionary processes. *Annual Review of Ecology Evolution and Systematics*, *36*, 147–168. doi:10.1146/annurev.ecolsys.36.102003.152644

Deaton, R., Murphy, R., Garzon, M., Franceschetti, D., & Stevens, S. (1999). Good encodings for DNA-based solutions to combinatorial problems. *DIMACS Series in Discrete Mathematics and Theoretical Computer Science*, *44*, 247–258.

Deaton, R., Garzon, M., Murphy, R., Rose, J., Franceschetti, D., & Stevens, S. (1996). Genetic search of reliable encodings for DNA- based computation. *Proceedings of the First Annual Conference on Genetic Programming*, 9–15.

Delcourt, S., & Blake, R. (1991). Stacking energies in DNA. *The Journal of Biological Chemistry*, *266*(23), 15160–15169.

Dematté, L., Priami, C., & Romanel, A. (2008). The Beta Workbench: a computational tool to study the dynamics of biological systems. *Briefings in Bioinformatics*, *9*(5), 437–449. doi:10.1093/bib/bbn023

Dematté, L., Larcher, R., Palmisano, A., Priami, C., & Romanel, A. (2010). Programming Biology in BlenX. In Choi, S. (Ed.), *Systems Biology for Signaling Networks 1* (pp. 777–820). New York: Springer. doi:10.1007/978-1-4419-5797-9_31

Dematté, L., Priami, C., & Romanel, A. (2007). BetaWB: modelling and simulating biological processes. In G.A. Wainer, & H. Vakilzadian (Eds.), *Proceedings of Summer Computer Simulation Conference (SCSC 2007)* (pp. 777-784). San Diego: Society for Computer Simulation International.

Denkert, C., Budczies, J., & Weichert, W. (2008). Metabolite profiling of human colon carcinoma – deregulation of TCA cycle and amino acid turnover. *Molecular Cancer*, *7*, 72–87. doi:10.1186/1476-4598-7-72

Denkert, C., Budczies, J., Kind, T., Weichert, W., Tablack, P., & Sehouli, J. (2006). Mass spectrometry-based metabolic profiling reveals different metabolite patterns in invasive ovarian carcinomas and ovarian borderline tumors. *Cancer Research*, *66*(22), 10795–10804. doi:10.1158/0008-5472.CAN-06-0755

Devoe, H., & Tinoco, L. (1962). The stability of helical polynucleotides: base contributions. *Journal of Molecular Biology*, *4*, 500–517. doi:10.1016/S0022-2836(62)80105-3

Dhar, P., Meng, T. C., Somani, S., Ye, L., Sairam, A., & Chitre, M. (2004). Cellware--a multi-algorithmic software for computational systems biology. *Bioinformatics (Oxford, England)*, *20*(8), 1319–1321. doi:10.1093/bioinformatics/bth067

Ding, L., Pan, R., Finin, T., Joshi, A., Peng, Y., & Kolari, P. (2005). Finding and Ranking Knowledge on the Semantic Web. In *4th International Semantic Web Conference*, Galway, Ireland.

Ditzel, H. (2000). Human antibodies in cancer and autoimmune disease. *Immunologic Research, 21*, 185–193. doi:10.1385/IR:21:2-3:185

Do, J.H & Choi, D.K. (2006). Computational approaches to gene prediction. *J Microbiol. Apr; 44*(2),137-44.

Doak, D., & Marvier, M. (2003). Predicting the effects of species loss on community stability. In Kareiva, P., & Levin, S. A. (Eds.), *The Importance of Species* (pp. 140–160). Princeton, NJ: Princeton University Press.

Doktycz, M. J., Goldstein, R. F., Paner, T. M., Gallo, F. J., & Benight, A. S. (1992). Studies of DNA dumbbells. I. Melting curves of 17 DNA dumbbells with different duplex stem sequences linked by T4 endloops: evaluation of the nearest neighbor stacking interactions in DNA. *Biopolymers, 32*(7), 849–864. doi:10.1002/bip.360320712

Down, T. A., Bergman, C. M., Su, J., & Hubbard, T. J. P. (2007). Large-Scale Discovery of Promoter Motifs in *Drosophila melanogaster. PLoS Computational Biology, 3*(1), e7..doi:10.1371/journal.pcbi.0030007

Dr, S., Sajda, P., Stoyanova, R., et al. (2005). *Recovery of metabolomics spectral sources using non-negative matrix factorization.* Proc 2005 IEEE.

Du, Q., & Grunzburger, M. (2002). Grid generation and optimization based on centroidal Voronoi tessellations. *Math. Comp., 133* (2-3).

Duarte, I. F., Marques, J., & Ladeirinha, A. F. (2009). Analytical approaches toward successful human cell metabolome studies by NMR spectroscopy. *Analytical Chemistry, 81*, 5023–5032. doi:10.1021/ac900545q

Duda, R. O. Hart, P. E., and& Stork, D. G. (2000). *Pattern classification.*2nd ed., New York, NY: Wiley.

Dufour, Y. S., Wesenberg, G. E., Tritt, A. J., Glasner, J. D., Perna, N. T., Mitchell, J. C., & Donohue, T. J. (2010). chipD: a web tool to design oligonucleotide probes for high-density tiling arrays. *Nucleic Acids Research, 38* Suppl(), W321-5.

Dunn, W. B., Broadhurst, D. I., & Atherton, H. J. (2010). Systems levels studies of mammalian metabolomes: the roles of mass spectrometry and nuclear magnetic resonance spectroscopy. *Chemical Society Reviews*. doi:. doi:10.1039/b906712b

Dunne, J. A. (2002). Network structure and biodiversity loss in food webs: robustness increases with connectance. *Ecology Letters, 5*, 558–567. doi:10.1046/j.1461-0248.2002.00354.x

Dunne, J. A., Williams, R. J., & Martinez, N. D. (2002a). Food-web structure and network theory: the role of connectance and size. *Proceedings of the National Academy of Sciences of the United States of America, 99*, 12917–12922. doi:10.1073/pnas.192407699

Dunne, J. A., Williams, R. J., & Martinez, N. D. (2004). Network structure and robustness of marine food webs. *Marine Ecology Progress Series, 273*, 291–302. doi:10.3354/meps273291

Duthie, S. J. (1999). Folic acid deficiency and cancer: mechanisms of DNA instability. *British Medical Bulletin, 55*, 578–592. doi:10.1258/0007142991902646

Ebenman, B., & Jonsson, T. (2005). Using community viability analysis to identify fragile systems and keystone species. *Trends in Ecology & Evolution, 20*, 568–575. doi:10.1016/j.tree.2005.06.011

Eklöf, A. & Ebenman, B. (2006). Species loss and secondary extinctions in simple and complex model

Elser, J. J., Sterner, R. W., Gorokhova, E., Fagan, W. F., Markow, T. A., & Cotner, J. B. (2000). Biological stoichiometry from genes to ecosystems. *Ecology Letters, 3*, 540–550. doi:10.1046/j.1461-0248.2000.00185.x

Elton, C. (1927). *Animal Ecology*. Chicago, IL: The University of Chicago Press.

Emmerson, M., & Yearsley, J. M. (2004). Weak interactions, omnivory and emergent food-web properties. *Proceedings. Biological Sciences, 271*, 397–405. doi:10.1098/rspb.2003.2592

Emrich, S. J., Lowe, M., & Delcher, A. L. (2003). PROBEmer: A web-based software tool for selecting optimal DNA oligos. *Nucleic Acids Research, 31*(13), 3746–3750. doi:10.1093/nar/gkg569

Estrada, E. (2007). Characterisation of topological keystone species: local, global and "meso-scale" centralities in food webs. *Ecological Complexity, 4*, 48–57. doi:10.1016/j.ecocom.2007.02.018

Etienne-Manneville, S., & Hall, A. (2002). Rho GTPases in cell biology. *Nature, 420*, 629–635. doi:10.1038/nature01148

Eysenbach, G. (2008). Medicine 2.0: Social Networking, Collaboration, Participation, Apomediation, and Openness. *Journal of Medical Internet Research, 10*, 5–6. doi:10.2196/jmir.1030

Fagan, A., Culhane, A. C., & Higgins, D. G. (2007). A multivariate analysis approach to the integration of proteomic and gene expression data. *Proteomics, 7*(13), 2162–2171. doi:10.1002/pmic.200600898

Faijes, M., Mars, A. E., & Smid, E. J. (2007). Comparison of quenching and extraction methodologies for metabolome analysis of Lactobacillus plantarum. *Microbial Cell Factories, 6*, 27. doi:10.1186/1475-2859-6-27

Faith, J. J., Hayete, B., Thaden, J. T., Mogno, I., Wierzbowski, J., & Cottarel, G. (2007). Large-scale mapping and validation of Escherichia coli transcriptional regulation from a compendium of expression profiles. *PLoS Biology, 5*(1), 54–66. doi:10.1371/journal.pbio.0050008

Fan, T. W., Lane, A. N., Higashi, R. M., Farag, M. A., Gao, H., & Bousamra, M. (2009). Altered regulation of metabolic pathways in human lung cancer discerned by (13)C stable isotope-resolved metabolomics (SIRM). *Molecular Cancer, 8*, 41. doi:10.1186/1476-4598-8-41

Fan, T. W., Yuan, P., Lane, A. N., Higashi, R. M., Wang, Y., & Hamidi, A. B. (2010). Stable isotope-resolved metabolomic analysis of lithium effects on glial-neuronal metabolism and interactions. *Metabolomics, 6*(2), 165–179. doi:10.1007/s11306-010-0208-9

Fath, B. D., & Patten, B. C. (1999). Review of the foundations of network environ analysis. *Ecosystems (New York, N.Y.), 2*, 167–179. doi:10.1007/s100219900067

Faulhammer, D., Cukras, A., Lipton, R., & Landweber, R. (2000). Molecular computation: RNA solutions to chess problems. *Proceedings of the National Academy of Sciences of the United States of America, 97*, 1385–1389. doi:10.1073/pnas.97.4.1385

Feest, A., Aldred, T. D., & Jedamzik, K. (2010). Biodiversity quality: a paradigm for biodiversity. *Ecological Indicators, 10*, 1077–1082. doi:10.1016/j.ecolind.2010.04.002

Feldkamp, U., Banzhaf, W., & Rauhe, H. (2000). A DNA sequence compiler. *In Proceedings of the 6th DIMACS Workshop on DNA Based Computers, 253.*

Feldman, I., Rzhetsky, A., & Vitkup, D. (2008). Network properties of genes harbouring inherited disease mutations. *Proceedings of the National Academy of Sciences of the United States of America, 105*, 4323–4328. doi:10.1073/pnas.0701722105

Fiehn, O., Kopka, J., & Dormann, P. (2000). Metabolite profiling for plant functional genomics. *Nature Biotechnology, 18*, 1157–1161. doi:10.1038/81137

Fiehn, O. (2001). Combining genomics, metabolome analysis, and biochemical modelling to understand metabolic networks. *Comparative and Functional Genomics, 2*(3), 155–168. doi:10.1002/cfg.82

Fiehn, O. (2002). Metabolomics--the link between genotypes and phenotypes. *Plant Molecular Biology, 48*(1-2), 155–171. doi:10.1023/A:1013713905833

Finn, J. T. (1976). Measures of ecosystem structure and function derived from analysis of flows. *Journal of Theoretical Biology, 56*, 363–380. doi:10.1016/S0022-5193(76)80080-X

Fisher, J., & Henzinger, T. (2007). Executable cell biology. *Nature Biotechnology, 25*, 1239–1249. doi:10.1038/nbt1356

FitzGerald, P. C., Sturgill, D., Shyakhtenko, A., Oliver, B., & Vinson, C. (2006). Comparative genomics of *Drosophila* and human core promoters. *Genome Biology, 7*, R53. doi:10.1186/gb-2006-7-7-r53

Flikka, K., Yadetie, F., Laegreid, A., & Jonassen, I. (2004). XHM: a system for detection of potential cross hybridizations in DNA microarrays. *BMC Bioinformatics, 27*(5), 117. doi:10.1186/1471-2105-5-117

Fraser, A. M., & Swinney, H. L. (1986). Independent coordinates for strange attractors from mutual information. *Physical Review A., 33*(2), 1134–1140. doi:10.1103/PhysRevA.33.1134

Freund, Y., & Schapire, R. (1996). Experiments with a new boosting algorithm. *In proceedings of the 13th International Conference on Machine Learning*, (pp. 149–156).

Friedman, J. H., & Meulman, J. J. (2004). Clustering objects on subsets of attributes. *Journal of the Royal Statistical Society. Series B. Methodological, 66*, 1–25. doi:10.1111/j.1467-9868.2004.02059.x

Friedman, N. (2004). Inferring cellular networks using probabilistic graphical models. *Science, 303*, 799–805. doi:10.1126/science.1094068

Friedman, N., Linial, M., Nacjman, I., & Pe'er, D. (2000). Using Bayesian networks to analyze expression data. *Journal of Computational Biology, 7*, 601–620. doi:10.1089/106652700750050961

Frutos, A. G., Liu, Q., Thiel, A. J., Sanner, A. M. W., Condon, A. E., Smith, L. M., & Corn, R. M. (1997). Demonstration of a word design strategy for DNA computing on surfaces. *Nucleic Acids Research, 25*, 4748–4757. doi:10.1093/nar/25.23.4748

Fu, K. S. (1982). *Syntatic pattern recognition and applications*. Cliffs, NJ: Prentice-Hall.

Fujivara, I., Vavylonis, D., & Pollard, T. D. (2007). Polymerization kinetics of ADP- and ADP-Pi actin determined by fluoresence microscopy. *Proceedings of the National Academy of Sciences of the United States of America, 104*(21), 8827–8832. doi:10.1073/pnas.0702510104

Funahashi, A., Jouraku, A., Matsuoka, Y., & Kitano, H. (2007). Integration of CellDesigner and SABIO-RK. *In Silico Biology, 7*(2Suppl), S81–S90.

Fussmann, G. F., Loreau, M., & Abrams, P.A. (2007). Eco-evolutionary dynamics of communities and ecosystems. *Functional Ecology, 21*(3), 465.477.

Gaborit, P., & King, O. D. (2005). Linear construction for DNA codes. *Theoretical Computer Science, 334*, 99–113. doi:10.1016/j.tcs.2004.11.004

Gader, P. D., Mohamed, M. A., & Keller, J. M. (1996). Fusion of handwritten word classifiers. *Pattern Recognition Letters, 17*(6), 577–584. doi:10.1016/0167-8655(96)00021-9

Gagneur, J., & Casari, G. (2005). From molecular networks to qualitative cell behavior. *FEBS Letters, 579*(8), 1867–1871. doi:10.1016/j.febslet.2005.02.007

Gallant, P. J., Morin, E. L., & Peppard, L. E. (1998). Feature-based classification of myoelectric signals using artificial neural networks. *Medical & Biological Engineering & Computing, 36*(4), 485–489. doi:10.1007/BF02523219

Gamal, A. A. E., Hemachandra, L. A., Shperling, I., & Wei, V. K. (1987). Using simulated annealing to design good codes. *IEEE Transactions on Information Theory, 33*(1), 116–123. doi:10.1109/TIT.1987.1057277

Garcia-Garcia, E., & Rosales, C. (2002). Signal transduction during Fc receptor-mediated phagocytosis. *Journal of Leukocyte Biology, 72*, 1092–1108.

Garlaschelli, D., Caldarelli, G., & Pietronero, L. (2003). Universal scaling relations in food webs. *Nature, 423*, 165–168. doi:10.1038/nature01604

Gaughan, A. (2006). Bridging the divide: the need for translational informatics. *Pharmacogenomics, 7*, 117–122. doi:10.2217/14622416.7.1.117

German, J. B., Roberts, M. A., Fay, L., & Watkins, S. M. (2002). Metabolomics and individual metabolic assessment: the next great challenge for nutrition. *The Journal of Nutrition, 132*(9), 2486–2487.

German, J. B., Roberts, M. A., & Watkins, S. M. (2003). Personal metabolomics as a next generation nutritional assessment. *The Journal of Nutrition, 133*(12), 4260–4266.

German, J. B., Watkins, S. M., & Fay, L. B. (2005). Metabolomics in practice: emerging knowledge to guide future dietetic advice toward individualized health. *Journal of the American Dietetic Association, 105*(9), 1425–1432. doi:10.1016/j.jada.2005.06.006

Ghiggi, A. (2010). *DNA strands design with thermodynamic constraints*. Master thesis, Università della Svizzera Italiana.

Gillespie, D. T. (1977). Exact stochastic simulation of coupled chemical reactions. *Journal of Physical Chemistry, 81*(25), 2340–2361. doi:10.1021/j100540a008

Giskeødegård, G. F., Grinde, M. T., & Sitter, B. (2010). Multivariate modeling and prediction of breast cancer prognostic factors using MR metabolomics. *Journal of Proteome Research, 9*, 972–979. doi:10.1021/pr9008783

Gizzatkulov, N. M., Goryanin, I. I., Metelkin, E. A., Mogilevskaya, E. A., Peskov, K. V., & Demin, O. V. (2010). DBSolve Optimum: a software package for kinetic modeling which allows dynamic visualization of simulation results. *BMC Systems Biology, 4*, 109. doi:10.1186/1752-0509-4-109

Godejohann, M., Tseng, L. H., Braumann, U., Fuchser, J., & Spraul, M. (2004). Characterization of a paracetamol metabolite using on-line LC-SPE-NMR-MS and a cryogenic NMR probe. *Journal of Chromatography. A, 1058*(1-2), 191–196.

Goldsmith, P., Fenton, H., Morris-Stiff, G., Ahmad, N., Fisher, J., & Prasad, K. R. (2010). Metabonomics: a useful tool for the future surgeon. *The Journal of Surgical Research, 160*(1), 122–132. doi:10.1016/j.jss.2009.03.003

Goldwasser, L., & Roughgarden, J. (1997). Sampling effects and estimation of food-web properties. *Ecology, 78*, 41–54. doi:10.1890/0012-9658(1997)078[0041:SEATEO]2.0.CO;2

Golightly, A., & Wilkinson, D. (2008). Bayesian inference for nonlinear multivariate diffusion models observed with error. *Computational Statistics & Data Analysis, 52*(3), 1674–1693. doi:10.1016/j.csda.2007.05.019

Gonzales, r. C. and& Thomason, M. G. (1978). *Syntatic pattern recognition: An introduction*. Reading, MA: Addison-Wesley.

Goodacre, R., & Broadhurst, D. (2007). Proposed minumum reporting standards for data analysis in metabolomics. *Metabolomics, 3*, 231–241. doi:10.1007/s11306-007-0081-3

Gordon, P. M. K., & Sensen, C. W. (2004). Osprey: a comprehensive tool employing novel methods for the design of oligonucleotides for DNA sequencing and microarrays. *Nucleic Acids Research, 32*(17), e133. doi:10.1093/nar/gnh127

Goryachev, A. B., & Pokhilko, A. V. (2006). *Computational model explains high activity and rapid cycling of Rho GTPases within protein complexes*. PLOS Computational Biology, 2, 151-1521. For the license terms of the figures adapted from this work, see http://creativecommons.org/licenses/by/2.5/.

Gotoh, O., & Tagashira, Y. (1981). Stabilities of nearest-neighbor doublets in double helical DNA determined by fitting calculated melting profiles to observed profiles. *Biopolymers, 20*, 1033–1042. doi:10.1002/bip.1981.360200513

Gottschalk, M.; Ivanova, G.& Collins, D.M. et al. (2008). *Metabolomic studies of human lung carcinoma cell lines using in vitro 1H NMR of whole cells and cellular extracts*. NMR Biomed.

Green, J. L. (2005). Complexity in ecology and conservation: mathematical, statistical, and computational challenges. *Bioscience, 55*, 501–510. doi:10.1641/0006-3568(2005)055[0501:CIEACM]2.0.CO;2

Griffin, J. L., Bollard, M., Nicholson, J. K., & Bhakoo, K. (2002). Spectral profiles of cultured neuronal and glial cells derived from HRMAS 1H NMR spectroscopy. *NMR in Biomedicine, 15*, 375–384. doi:10.1002/nbm.792

Griffin, J. L. (2003). Metabonomics: NMR spectroscopy and pattern recognition analysis of body fluids and tissues for characterisation of xenobiotic toxicity and disease diagnosis. *Current Opinion in Chemical Biology, 7*(5), 648–654. doi:10.1016/j.cbpa.2003.08.008

Griffin, J. L., & Bollard, M. E. (2004). Metabonomics: its potential as a tool in toxicology for safety assessment and data integration. *Current Drug Metabolism, 5*(5), 389–398. doi:10.2174/1389200043335432

Grimm, V. (1999). Ten years of individual-based modelling in ecology: what have we learned and what could we learn in the future? *Ecological Modelling, 115*, 129–148. doi:10.1016/S0304-3800(98)00188-4

Gudivada, R. C., Qu, X. A., Chen, J., Jegga, A. G., Neumann, E. K., & Aronow, B. J. (2008). Identifying disease-causal genes using Semantic Web-based representation of integrated genomic and phenomic knowledge. *Journal of Biomedical Informatics, 41*, 717–729. doi:10.1016/j.jbi.2008.07.004

Guerreiro, C. S., Carmona, B., Goncalves, S., Carolino, E., Fidalgo, P., & Brito, M. (2008). Risk of colorectal cancer associated with the C677T polymorphism in 5,10-methylenetetrahydrofolate reductase in Portuguese patients depends on the intake of methyl-donor nutrients. *The American Journal of Clinical Nutrition, 88,* 1413–1418.

Guler, I., & Ubeyli, E. D. (2007). Multiclass support vector machines for EEG-signals classification. *IEEE Transactions on Information Technology in Biomedicine, 11*(2), 117–126. doi:10.1109/TITB.2006.879600

Gullberg, J., Jonsson, P., Nordstrom, A., Sjostrom, M., & Moritz, T. (2004). Design of experiments: an efficient strategy to identify factors influencing extraction and derivatization of Arabidopsis thaliana samples in metabolomic studies with gas chromatography/mass spectrometry. *Analytical Biochemistry, 331*(2), 283–295. doi:10.1016/j.ab.2004.04.037

Guo, K., & Li, L. (2009). Differential 12C/13C-isitope dansylation labeling and fast liquid chromatography/MS for absolute and relative quantification of the metabolome. *Analytical Chemistry, 81,* 3919–3932. doi:10.1021/ac900166a

Gurry, T., Kahramanoğulları, O., & Endres, R. G. (2009). Biophysical mechanism for Ras-nanocluster formation and signaling in plasma membrane. *PLoS ONE, 4*(7). doi:10.1371/journal.pone.0006148

Haas, S. A., Hild, M., Wright, A. P. H., Hain, T., Talibi, D., & Vingron, M. (2003). Genome-scale design of PCR primers and long oligomers for DNA microarrays. *Nucleic Acids Research, 31*(19), 5576–5581. doi:10.1093/nar/gkg752

Haddad, I., Killer, K., Frimmersdorf, E., et al. (2009). An emergent self-organizing map based analysis pipeline for comparative metabolome studies. In *Silico Biol. 9,* 0014.

Hageman, J. A., van den Berg, R. A., & Westerhuis, J. A. (2006). Bagged K-means clustering of metabolome data. *Clinical Rev Anal Chem, 36,* 211–220. doi:10.1080/10408340600969916

Hageman, J.A.; van den Berg, R.A.& Westerhuis, J.A. et al. (2009). *Genetic algorithm based two-mode clustering of metabolomics data.* Metabolomics

Haghighi, M. S., Vahedian, A., Yazdi, H. S., & Modaghegh, H. (2009). Designing kernel scheme for classifier fusion. *International Journal of Computer Science and Information Security, 6*(2), 239–248.

Hall, A. B., Gakidis, M. A., Glogauer, M., Wilsbacher, J. L., Gao, S., Swat, W., & Brugge, J. S. (2006). Requirements for Vav guanine nucleotide exchange factors and Rho GTPases in FcγR- and complement-mediated phagocytosis. *Immunity, 24,* 305–316. doi:10.1016/j.immuni.2006.02.005

Halperin, A., Buhot, A., & Zhulina, E. B. (2006). On the hybridization isotherms of DNA microarrays: the Langmuir model and its extensions. *Journal of Physics Condensed Matter, 18,* S463. doi:10.1088/0953-8984/18/18/S01

Han, J., & Kamber, M. (2006). *Data Mining: Concepts and Techniques* (2nd ed.). San Francisco: Morgan Kaufmann.

Hanlon, S. E., & Lieb, J. D. (2004). Progress and challenges in profiling the dynamics of chromatin and transcription factor binding with DNA microarrays. *Current Opinion in Genetics & Development, 14,* 697–705. doi:10.1016/j.gde.2004.09.008

Hannon, B. (1973). The structure of ecosystems. *Journal of Theoretical Biology, 41,* 535–546. doi:10.1016/0022-5193(73)90060-X

Hannon, B. (1986). Ecosystem control theory. *Journal of Theoretical Biology, 121,* 417–437. doi:10.1016/S0022-5193(86)80100-X

Harary, F. (1961). Who eats whom? *General Systems, 6,* 41–44.

Harbig, J., Sprinkle, R., & Enkemann, S. A. (2005). A sequence-based identification of the genes detected by probesets on the Affymetrix U133 plus 2.0 array. *Nucleic Acids Research, 33*(3), e31. doi:10.1093/nar/gni027

Harith, A., & Christopher, B. (2005). Ontology ranking based on the analysis of concept structures. In *Proceedings of the Proceedings of the 3rd international conference on Knowledge capture,* Banff, Canada2005.

Harley, C. D. G. (2003). Species importance and context: spatial and temporal variation in species interactions. In Kareiva, P., & Levin, S. A. (Eds.), *The Importance of Species* (pp. 44–68). Princeton, NJ: Princeton University Press.

Harris, C., & Ghaffari, N. (2008). Biomarker discovery across annotated and unannotated microarray datasets using semi-supervised learning. *BMC Genomics, 9*(Suppl 2), S7. doi:10.1186/1471-2164-9-S2-S7

Hatzigeorgiou, A (2002). Translation initiation start prediction in human cDNAs with high accuracy. *Bioinformatics. Feb;18*(2),343-50.

Hayete, B., Garden, T. S., & Collins, J. J. (2007). Size matters: network inference tackles the genome scale. *Molecular Systems Biology, 3*(77).

Heiner, M., Gilbert, D., & Donaldson, R. (2008). Petri Nets for Systems and Synthetic Biology. Bernardo, M. & Degano, P. & Zavattaro G. (Eds.). *Formal Methods for Computational Systems Biology, 8th International School on Formal Methods for the Design of Computer, Communication, and Software Systems, SFM 2008*, Advanced Lectures. Lecture Notes in Computer Science 5016, (pp. 215-264), Springer.

Herrgard, M. J., Swainston, N., & Dobson, P. (2008). A consensus yeast metabolic network reconstruction obtained from a community approach to systems biology. *Nature Biotechnology, 26*, 1155–1160. doi:10.1038/nbt1492

Hettne, K. M., Stierum, R. H., Schuemie, M. J., Hendriksen, P. J., Schijvenaars, B. J., & Van Mulligen, E. M. (2009). A Dictionary to Identify Small Molecules and Drugs in Free Text. *Bioinformatics (Oxford, England), 25*, 2983–2991. doi:10.1093/bioinformatics/btp535

Heymans, J. J., Ulanowicz, R. E., & Bondavalll, C. (2002). Network analysis of the South Florida Everglades Gramminoid Marshes and comparison with nearby Cypress ecosystems. *Ecological Modelling, 149*, 5–23. doi:10.1016/S0304-3800(01)00511-7

Higashi, M., Burns, T. P., & Patten, B. C. (1989). Food network unfolding - an extension of trophic dynamics for application to natural ecosystems. *Journal of Theoretical Biology, 140*, 243–261. doi:10.1016/S0022-5193(89)80132-8

Hiller, K., Hangebrauk, J., Jager, C., Spura, J., Schreiber, K., & Schomburg, D. (2009). MetaboliteDetector: comprehensive analysis tool for targeted and nontargeted GC/MS based metabolome analysis. *Analytical Chemistry, 81*(9), 3429–3439. doi:10.1021/ac802689c

Hinton, G. E. (1999). Products of experts. *Artificial Neural Networks Conf., 470*, 1-9.

Hlavacek, W. S. & Faeder, J. R. & Blinov, M. L. & Posner, R. G. & Hucka M. & Fontana W. (2006). Rules for modeling signal-transduction systems. *Science Signaling* (STKE).

Ho, P. S., Frederick, C. A., Quigley, G. J., van der Marel, G. A., van Boom, J. H., Wang, A. H., & Rich, A. (1985). G.T wobble base-pairing in Z-DNA at 1.0 A atomic resolution: the crystal structure of d(CGCGTG). *The EMBO Journal, 4*(13A), 3617–3623.

Ho, M. R., Chen, C. H., & Lin, W. C. (2010). Gene-oriented ortholog database: a functional comparison platform for orthologous loci. *Database (Oxford), 2010*, baq002. Epub 2010 Feb 10. doi:10.1093/database/baq002

Ho, T. H., Hull, J. J., & Srihari, S. N. (1994). Decision combination in multiple classifier system. *IEEE Transactions on Pattern Analysis and Machine Intelligence, 16*(1), 66–75. doi:10.1109/34.273716

Ho, T. K. (2002). Multiple classifier combination: Lessons and the next steps. *Hybrid Methods in Pattern Recognition*, 171-198.

Holling, C. S. (2001). Understanding the complexity of economic, ecological and social systems. *Ecosystems (New York, N.Y.), 4*, 390–405. doi:10.1007/s10021-001-0101-5

Holling, C. S. (1965). The functional response of predator to prey density and its role in mimicry and population regulation. *Memoirs of the Entomological Society of Canada, 45*, 1–60. doi:10.4039/entm9745fv

Holloway, A. J., van Laar, R. K., Tothill, R. W., & Bowtell, D. (2002). Options available-from start to finish-for obtaining data from DNA microarrays II. *Nature Genetics, 32*(suppl. 2), 481–489. doi:10.1038/ng1030

Holmes, E., Loo, R. L., & Cloarec, O. (2007). Detection of urinary drug metabolite (xenometabolome) signatures in molecular epidemiology studies via statistical total correlation (NMR) spectroscopy. *Analytical Chemistry, 79*, 2629–2640. doi:10.1021/ac062305n

Holmes, E., Loo, R. L., & Stamler, J. (2008). Human metabolic phenotype diversity and its association with diet and blood pressure. *Nature, 453*, 396–401. doi:10.1038/nature06882

Hoops, S., Sahle, S., Gauges, R., Lee, C., Pahle, J., & Simus, N. (2006). COPASI--a COmplex PAthway SImulator. *Bioinformatics (Oxford, England)*, *22*(24), 3067–3074. doi:10.1093/bioinformatics/btl485

Hoos, H., & Stützle, T. (2004). *Stochastic Local Search: Foundations and Applications*. San Francisco: Morgan Kaufmann.

Hopkins, A. L. (2007). Network pharmacology. *Nature Chemical Biology*, *4*, 682–690. doi:10.1038/nchembio.118

Hoppe, A. D., & Swanson, J. A. (2004). Cdc42, Rac1, and Rac2 display distinct patterns of activation during phagocytosis. *Molecular Biology of the Cell*, *15*(8), 3509–3519. doi:10.1091/mbc.E03-11-0847

Hornshoj, H., Stengaard, H., Panitz, F., & Bendixen, C. (2004). SEPON, a Selection and Evaluation Pipeline for OligoNucleotides based on ESTs with a non-target Tm algorithm for reducing cross-hybridization in microarray gene expression experiments. *Bioinformatics (Oxford, England)*, *20*, 428–429. doi:10.1093/bioinformatics/btg434

Hu, J., Matzavinos, A., & Othmer, H. G. (2007). A theoretical approach to actin filament dynamics. *Journal of Statistical Physics*, *128*(1/2), 111–138. doi:10.1007/s10955-006-9204-x

Huang, Y., Liu, K., & Suen, C. (1995). The combination of multiple classifiers by a neural network approach. *J. Pattern Recognition Artif Intell*, *9*, 579–597. doi:10.1142/S0218001495000547

Huang, Y. S., & Suen, C. Y. (1995). A method of combining multiple experts for the recognition of unconstrained handwritten numerals. *IEEE Transactions on Pattern Analysis and Machine Intelligence*, *17*(1), 90–94. doi:10.1109/34.368145

Huang, E., Yang, L., Chowdhary, R., Kassim, A., & Bajic, V. B. (2005). *Information Processing and Living Systems*. World Scientific. An algorithm for *ab initio* DNA motif detection; pp. 611–614.

Hughes, A. R., Inouye, B. D., Johnson, M. T. J., Underwood, N., & Vellend, M. (2008). Ecological consequences of genetic diversity. *Ecology Letters*, *11*, 609–623. doi:10.1111/j.1461-0248.2008.01179.x

Huopaniemi, I., Suvitaival, T., & Nikkila, J. (2009). Two-way analysis of high-dimensional collinear data. *Data Mining and Knowledge Discovery*, *19*, 261–276. doi:10.1007/s10618-009-0142-5

Hurlbert, S. H. (1997). Functional importance vs keystoneness: reformulating some questions in theoretical biocenology. *Australian Journal of Ecology*, *22*, 369–382. doi:10.1111/j.1442-9993.1997.tb00687.x

Ibrahim, Z., Kurniawan, T. B., Khalid, N. K., Sudin, S., & Khalid, M. (2009). Implementation of an ant colony system for DNA sequence optimization. *Artificial Life and Robotics*, *14*, 293–296. doi:10.1007/s10015-009-0683-0

Idborg-Bjorkman, H., Edlund, P. O., Kvalheim, O. M., Schuppe-Koistinen, I., & Jacobsson, S. P. (2003). Screening of biomarkers in rat urine using LC/electrospray ionization-MS and two-way data analysis. *Analytical Chemistry*, *75*(18), 4784–4792. doi:10.1021/ac0341618

Ideker, T. (2004). A Systems Approach to Discovering Signaling and Regulatory Pathways – or, How to Digest Large Interaction Networks Into Relevant Pieces. *Advances in Experimental Medicine and Biology*, *547*, 21–30. doi:10.1007/978-1-4419-8861-4_3

Ihekwaba, A. E., Wilkinson, S. J., Broomhead, D. S., Waithe, D., Grimpley, R., & Benson, N. (2007). Bridging the gap between in silico and cell based analysis of the NF-kB signalling pathway by in vitro studies of IKK2. *The FEBS Journal*, *90*, 1678–1690. doi:10.1111/j.1742-4658.2007.05713.x

Irizarry, R. A., Hobbs, B., Collin, F., Beazer-Barclay, Y. D., Antonellis, K. J., Scherf, U., & Speed, T. P. (2003). Exploration, normalization, and summaries of high density oligonucleotide array probe level data. *Biostatistics (Oxford, England)*, *4*(2), 249–264. doi:10.1093/biostatistics/4.2.249

Ishii, N., Nakahigashi, K., Baba, T., Robert, M., Soga, T., & Kanai, A. (2007). Multiple high-throughput analyses monitor the response of E. coli to perturbations. *Science*, *316*(5824), 593–597. doi:10.1126/science.1132067

Iwasa, J. H., & Mullins, R. D. (2007). Spatial and temporal relationships between actin-filament nucleation, capping, and disassembly. *Current Biology*, *17*, 395–406. doi:10.1016/j.cub.2007.02.012

Izquierdo-Garcia, J. L., Rodriguez, I., Kyriazis, A., Villa, P., Barreiro, P., & Desco, M. (2009). A novel R-package graphic user interface for the analysis of metabonomic profiles. *BMC Bioinformatics*, *10*, 363. doi:10.1186/1471-2105-10-363

Jaffe, A. B., & Hall, A. (2005). Dynamic changes in the length distribution of actin filaments during polymerization can be modulated by barbed end capping proteins. *Cell Motility and the Cytoskeleton*, *61*, 1–8. doi:10.1002/cm.20061

Jaffe, A. B., & Hall, A. (2005). Rho GTPases: Biochemistry and biology. *Annual Review of Cell and Developmental Biology*, *21*, 247–269. doi:10.1146/annurev.cellbio.21.020604.150721

Jain, A. K., Murty, M. N., & Flynn, P. J. (1999). Data Clustering: A Review. *ACM Computing Surveys*, *31*(3), 264–323. doi:10.1145/331499.331504

Jang, H. J., Nde, C., Toghrol, F., & Bentley, W. E. (2008). Microarray analysis of toxicogenomic effects of orthophenylphenol in Staphylococcus aureus. *BMC Genomics*, *9*, 411. doi:10.1186/1471-2164-9-411

Jia, K., & Lu, Y. (2007). A new method of combined classifier design based on fuzzy integral and support vector machines. *In ICCCAS International Conference on Communications, Circuits and Systems*.

Jiang, D., Tang, C., & Zhang, A. (2004). Cluster Analysis for Gene Expression Data: A Survey. *IEEE Transactions on Knowledge and Data Engineering*, *16*(11), 1370–1386. doi:10.1109/TKDE.2004.68

Jordan, M. I., & Jacobs, R. A. (1994). Hierarchical mixtures of experts and the EM algorithms. *Neural Computation*, *6*, 181–214. doi:10.1162/neco.1994.6.2.181

Jordán, F., Benedek, Zs., & Podani, J. (2007). Quantifying positional importance in food webs: a comparison of centrality indices. *Ecological Modelling*, *205*, 270–275. doi:10.1016/j.ecolmodel.2007.02.032

Jordán, F., Liu, W. C., & Mike, Á. (2009). Trophic field overlap: a new approach to quantify keystone species. *Ecological Modelling*, *220*, 2899–2907. doi:10.1016/j.ecolmodel.2008.12.003

Jordán, F., Liu, W. C., & van Veen, F. J. F. (2003). Quantifying the importance of species and their interactions in a host-parasitoid community. *Community Ecology*, *4*, 79–88. doi:10.1556/ComEc.4.2003.1.12

Jordán, F., Okey, T. A., Bauer, B., & Libralato, S. (2008). Identifying important species: a comparison of structural and functional indices. *Ecological Modelling*, *216*, 75–80.

Jordán, F., & Scheuring, I. (2004). Network Ecology: topological constraints on ecosystems dynamics. *Physics of Life Reviews*, *1*, 139–172. doi:10.1016/j.plrev.2004.08.001

Jordán, F., Scheuring, I., & Molnár, I. (2003). Persistence and flow reliability in simple food webs. *Ecological Modelling*, *161*, 117–124. doi:10.1016/S0304-3800(02)00296-X

Jordán, F., Scheuring, I., & Vida, G. (2002). Species positions and extinction dynamics in simple food webs. *Journal of Theoretical Biology*, *215*, 441–448. doi:10.1006/jtbi.2001.2523

Jordán, F. (2009). Keystone species and food webs. *Philosophical Transactions of the Royal Society of London. Series B, Biological Sciences*, *364*(1524), 1733–1741. doi:10.1098/rstb.2008.0335

Jordán, F., Liu, W., & Davis, A. J. (2006). Topological keystone species: measures of positional importance in food webs. *Oikos*, *112*, 535–546. doi:10.1111/j.0030-1299.2006.13724.x

Jordán, F., & Scheuring, I. (2002). Searching for keystones in ecological networks. *Oikos*, *99*, 607–612. doi:10.1034/j.1600-0706.2002.11889.x

Jordán, F., Takács-Sánta, A., & Molnár, I. (1999). A reliability theoretical quest for keystones. *Oikos*, *86*, 453–462. doi:10.2307/3546650

Joshi-Tope, G., Gillespie, M., Vastrik, I., D'Eustachio, P., Schmidt, E., & de Bono, B. (2005). Reactome: a knowledgebase of biological pathways. *Nucleic Acids Research*, *33*(Database issue), D428–D432. doi:10.1093/nar/gki072

Jourdren, L., Duclos, A., Brion, C., Portnoy, T., Mathis, H., Margeot, A., & Le Crom, S. (2010). Teolenn: an efficient and customizable workflow to design high-quality probes for microarray experiments. *Nucleic Acids Research*, *38*(10), e117. doi:10.1093/nar/gkq110

Judson, O. P. (1994). The rise of the individual-based model in ecology. *Trends in Ecology & Evolution, 9*, 9–14. doi:10.1016/0169-5347(94)90225-9

Kaddurah-Daouk, R., Kristal, B. S., & Weinshilboum, R. M. (2008). Metabolomics: a global biochemical approach to drug response and disease. *Annual Review of Pharmacology and Toxicology, 48*, 653–683. doi:10.1146/annurev.pharmtox.48.113006.094715

Kaderali, L., & Schliep, A. (2002). Selecting signature oligonucleotides to identify organisms using DNA arrays. *Bioinformatics (Oxford, England), 18*(10), 1340–1349. doi:10.1093/bioinformatics/18.10.1340

Kahramanoğulları, O., & Cardelli, L. (2011). (in press). An intuitive modelling interface for systems biology. *International Journal of Software and Informatics*.

Kahramanoğulları, O., Cardelli, L., & Caron, E. (2009). An intuitive automated modelling interface for systems biology. *Electronic Proceedings in Theoretical Computer Science, 9*, 73–86. doi:10.4204/EPTCS.9.9

Kai, Z., Linqiang, P., & Jin, X. (2007). A global heuristically search algorithm for DNA encoding. *Progress in Natural Science, 17*(6). doi:10.1080/10002007088537469

Kaitala, V., Ranta, E., & Lindstroem, J. (1996). Cyclic population dynamics and random perturbations. *Journal of Animal Ecology, 65*, 249–251. doi:10.2307/5728

Kalendar, R., Lee, D., & Schulman, A. H. (2009). FastPCR Software for PCR Primer and Probe Design and Repeat Search. *Genes. Genomes and Genomics, 3*(1), 1–14.

Kamel, M., & Wanas, N. (2003). Data dependence in combining classifiers. In *proceedings of the Fourth International Workshop on MCS*, No. 2709 Lecture Notes in Computer Science, (pp. 1-14).

Kanehisa, M., Araki, M., Goto, S., Hattori, M., Hirakawa, M., & Itoh, M. (2008). KEGG for linking genomes to life and the environment. *Nucleic Acids Research, 36*(Database issue), D480–D484. doi:10.1093/nar/gkm882

Kao, M.-Y., Sanghi, M., & Schweller, R. (2009). Randomized fast design of short DNA words. *ACS Transactions on Algorithms, 5*(4), 43.

Kapur, K., Jiang, H., Xing, Y., & Wong, W. H. (2008). Cross-hybridization modeling on Affymetrix exon arrays. *Bioinformatics (Oxford, England), 24*(24), 2887–2893. doi:10.1093/bioinformatics/btn571

Karp, P. D., Paley, S., Krieger, C. J., & Zhang, P. (2004). An evidence ontology for use in pathway/genome databases. *Pacific Symposium on Biocomputing. Pacific Symposium on Biocomputing*, 190–201.

Kazanci, C. (2009). Cycling in ecosystems: an individual based approach. *Ecological Modelling, 220*, 2908–2914. doi:10.1016/j.ecolmodel.2008.09.013

Keerthi, S. S., & Shevade, S. K. (2003). SMO algorithm for least-squares SVM formulations. *Neural Computation, 15*(2), 487–507. doi:10.1162/089976603762553013

Keller, J. M., Gader, P., Tahani, H., Chiang, J. H., & Mohamed, M. (1994). Advances in fuzzy integration for pattern recognition. *Fuzzy Sets and Systems, 65*, 273–283. doi:10.1016/0165-0114(94)90024-8

Kenny, D., & Loehle, C. (1991). Are food webs randomly connected? *Ecology, 72*, 1794–1799. doi:10.2307/1940978

Kent, W. J. (2002). BLAT--the BLAST-like alignment tool. *Genome Research, 12*(4), 656–664.

Kercher, J. R., & Shugart, H. H. (1975). Trophic structure, effective trophic position, and connectivity in food webs. *American Naturalist, 109*, 191–206. doi:10.1086/282986

Khalid, N. K., Ibrahim, Z., Kurniawan, T. B., Khalid, M., & Enggelbrecht, A. P. (2009). Implementation of binary particle swarm optimization for DNA sequence design. *Lecture Notes in Computer Science, 5518*, 450–457. doi:10.1007/978-3-642-02481-8_64

KInfer. (2009). Tratto da. Retrieved from http://www.cosbi.eu/index.php/research/prototypes/kinfer.

King, O. D. (2003). Bounds for DNA codes with constant GC-content. *Electronic Journal of Combinatorics, 10*, R33.

Kitano, H., Funahashi, A., Matsuoka, Y., & Oda, K. (2005). Using process diagrams for the graphical representation of biological networks. *Nature Biotechnology, 23*(8), 961–966. doi:10.1038/nbt1111

Kitano, H. (2002). Systems biology: A brief overview. *Science, 295*, 1662–1666. doi:10.1126/science.1069492

Kleinberg, J. M. (1998). Authoritative sources in a hyperlinked environment. In *Proceedings of the ninth ACM-SIAM symposium on Discrete algorithms*, San Francisco, USA.

Kobayashi, S., Kondo, T., & Arita, M. (2003). On Template Method for DNA Sequence Design. *Lecture Notes in Computer Science, 2568*, 205–214. doi:10.1007/3-540-36440-4_18

Kohonen, T. (1982). Self-organized formation of topologically correct feature maps. *Biological Cybernetics, 43*, 59–69. doi:10.1007/BF00337288

Kokkoris, G. D., Troumbis, A. Y., & Lawton, J. H. (1999). Patterns of species interaction strength in assembled theoretical competition communities. *Ecology Letters, 2*, 70–74. doi:10.1046/j.1461-0248.1999.22058.x

Kolasa, J. (2005). Complexity, system integration, and susceptibility to change: biodiversity connection. *Ecological Complexity, 2*, 431–442. doi:10.1016/j.ecocom.2005.05.002

Koul, N. (2010). *Metaheuristics for DNA codes design.* Master thesis. Università della Svizzera Italiana, Switzerland.

Kouskoumvekaki, I., Yang, Z., & Jonsdottir, S. O. (2008). Identification of biomarkers for genotyping Aspergilli using non-linear methods for clustering and classification. *BMC Bioinformatics, 9*, 59. doi:10.1186/1471-2105-9-59

Kozak, M. (1987). An analysis of 5'-noncoding sequences from 699 vertebrates messenger RNA. *Nucleic Acids Research, 15*, 8125–8148. doi:10.1093/nar/15.20.8125

Kreil, D. P., Russell, R. R., & Russell, S. (2006). Microarray oligonucleotide probes. *Methods in Enzymology, 410*, 73–98. doi:10.1016/S0076-6879(06)10004-X

Krooshof, P. W., Ustun, B., Postma, G. J., & Buydens, L. M. (2010). Visualization and recovery of the (bio)chemical interesting variables in data analysis with support vector machine classification. *Analytical Chemistry, 82*(16), 7000–7007. doi:10.1021/ac101338y

Kuncheva, L. (Ed.). (2005). Diversity in multiple classifier systems. *Information Fusion, 6*(1). doi:10.1016/j.inffus.2004.04.009

Kuncheva, L., Bezdek, J., & Duin, R. (2001). Decision templates for multiple classifier fusion: An experimental comparison. *Pattern Recognition, 34*, 299–314. doi:10.1016/S0031-3203(99)00223-X

Kuncheva, L. I. (2004). *Combining pattern classifiers: Methods and algorithms*. New York, NY: Wiley. doi:10.1002/0471660264

Kuncheva, L. I., Bezdek, J. C., & Sutton, M. A. (1998). On combining multiple classifiers by fuzzy templates. *Proc. NAFIPS Conf. EDS, *193-197.

Kurniawan, T. B., Khalid, N. K., Ibrahim, Z., Khalid, M., & Middendorf, M. (2008). An ant colony system for DNA sequence design based on thermodynamics. *Proceedings of the Fourth IASTED International Conference on Advances in Computer Science and Technology*, 144-149.

Lage, K., Karlberg, E. O., Storling, Z. M., Olason, P. I., Pedersen, A. G., & Rigina, O. (2007). A human phenome-interactome network of protein complexes implicated in genetic disorders. *Nature Biotechnology, 25*, 309. doi:10.1038/nbt1295

Lam, L. (2000). *Classifier combinations: Implementations and theoretical issues. Multiple Classifier Systems, No. 1857 of Lecture Notes in Computer Science* (pp. 78–86). Cagliari, Italy: Springer.

Land, W. H. Jr, & Verheggen, E. A. (2009). Multiclass primal support vector machines for breast density classification. *Int J Comput Biol Drug Des, 2*(1), 21–57. doi:10.1504/IJCBDD.2009.027583

Lande, R., Engen, S., & Swether, B.-E. (2003). *Stochastic population dynamics in ecology and conservation*. Oxford, UK: Oxford University Press. doi:10.1093/acprof:oso/9780198525257.001.0001

Lawrence, N. D., Girolami, M., Rattray, M., & Sanguinetti, G. (2010). *Learning and Inference in Computational and Systenms Biology*. Cambridge, MA: The MIT Press.

Lawton, J. H., & Brown, V. K. (1994). Redundancy in ecosystems. In Schulze, E. D., & Mooney, H. A. (Eds.), *Biodiversity and Ecosystem Function* (pp. 255–270). Berlin: Springer Verlag.

Lecca, P., Palmisano, A., Ihekwaba, A. E., & Priami, C. (2010). Calibration of dynamic models of biological systems with KInfer. *European Journal of Biophysics, 39*(6), 1019. doi:10.1007/s00249-009-0520-3

Lecca, P., Nguyen, P., Priami, C., & Quaglia, P. (2010). Network inference from Time-Dependent Omics Data. In B. Mayer. Humana Press Springer Science+Businnes Media, LLC.

Lecca, P., Palmisano, P., & Ihekwaba, A. E. (2010). Correlation-based network inference and modelling in systems biology: the NF-κB signalling network case study. *Int. Conf. on Intelligent Systems, Modelling and Simulation* (p. 170-175). Liverpool: IEEE Computer Society.

Lee, D.S., Park, J., Kay, K.A., Christakis, N.A., & Oltvai, Z.N. & Barabä¡Si, A.L. (2008). The implications of human metabolic network topology for disease comorbidity. *Proceedings of the National Academy of Sciences of the United States of America, 105,* 9880–9885. doi:10.1073/pnas.0802208105

Lemoine, S., Combes, F., & Le Crom, S. (2009). An evaluation of custom microarray applications: the oligonucleotide design challenge. *Nucleic Acids Research, 37*(6), 1726–1739. doi:10.1093/nar/gkp053

Lengauer, T., & Tarjan, R. E. (1979). A fast algorithm for finding dominators in a flowgraph. *ACM Transactions on Programming Languages Systems, 1,* 121–141. doi:10.1145/357062.357071

Lenz, E. M., & Wilson, I. D. (2007). Analytical strategies in metabonomics. *Journal of Proteome Research, 6*(2), 443–458. doi:10.1021/pr0605217

Lettice, L. A., & Hill, R. E. (2005). Preaxial polydactyly: a model for defective long-range regulation in congenital abnormalities. *Current Opinion in Genetics & Development, 15,* 294–300. doi:10.1016/j.gde.2005.04.002

Leung, Y., & Hung, Y. (2010). A multiple-filter-multiple-wrapper approach to gene selection and microarray data classification. *IEEE/ACM Transactions on Computational Biology and Bioinformatics, 7*(1), 108–117. doi:10.1109/TCBB.2008.46

Levin, S. A. (1997). Mathematical and computational challenges in population biology and ecosystems science. *Science, 275,* 334–343. doi:10.1126/science.275.5298.334

Levin, S. A. (1998). Ecosystems and the biosphere as complex adaptive systems. *Ecosystems (New York, N.Y.), 1,* 431–436. doi:10.1007/s100219900037

Levy, Y., Gilgun-Sherki, Y., Melamed, E., & Offen, D. (2005). Therapeutic potential of neurotrophic factors in neurodegenerative diseases. *BioDrugs, 19,* 97–127. doi:10.2165/00063030-200519020-00003

Li, X., Lu, X., & Tian, J. (2009). Application of Fuzzy c-means clustering in data analysis of metabolomics. *Analytical Chemistry, 81,* 4468–4475. doi:10.1021/ac900353t

Li, C., & Wong, W. H. (2001). Model-based analysis of oligonucleotide arrays: expression index computation and outlier detection. *Proceedings of the National Academy of Sciences of the United States of America, 98*(1), 31–36. doi:10.1073/pnas.011404098

Li, F., & Stormo, G. D. (2001). Selection of optimal DNA oligos for gene expression arrays. *Bioinformatics (Oxford, England), 17,* 1067–1076. doi:10.1093/bioinformatics/17.11.1067

Li, M., Lee, H. J., Condon, A. E., & Corn, R. M. (2002). DNA word design strategy for creating sets of non-interacting oligonucleotides for DNA microarrays. *Langmuir, 18,* 805–812. doi:10.1021/la0112209

Li, X., Hel, Z., & Zhou, J. (2005). Selection of optimal oligonucleotide probes for microarrays using multiple criteria, global alignment and parameter estimation. *Nucleic Acids Research, 33*(19), 6114–6123. doi:10.1093/nar/gki914

Li G, L &Leong, T.Y. (2005). Feature Selection for the Prediction of Translation Initiation Sites. *Genomics Proteomics Bioinformatics. May, 3*(2), 73-83.

Li G, Leong TY, & Zhang L (2004). Translation Initiation Sites Prediction wit Mixture Gaussian Models. *Algorithms in Bioinformatics (2004),* 338-349.

Libralato, S., Christensen, V., & Pauly, D. (2006). A method for identifying keystone species in food web models. *Ecological Modelling, 195,* 153–171. doi:10.1016/j.ecolmodel.2005.11.029

Lindeman, R. (1942). The trophic-dynamic aspect of ecology. *Ecology, 23,* 399–418. doi:10.2307/1930126

Liu, H., & Wong, L. (2003). Data Mining Tools for Biological Sequences. *Journal of Bioinformatics and Computational Biology, 1*(1), 139–167. doi:10.1142/S0219720003000216

Livi, C. M., Jordán, F., Lecca, P., & Okey, T. A. (in press). Identifying key species in ecosystems with stochastic sensitivity analysis. *Ecological Modelling.*

Livi, C. M. (2009). *Modelling and simulating ecological networks with BlenX. The food web of Prince William Sound: a case study.* Unpublished doctoral dissertation, Universita di Bologna, Bologna, Italy.

Lotka, A. J. (1927). Fluctuations in the abundance of a species considered mathematically. *Nature, 119,* 12.

Lu, X., Bennet, B., & Mu, E. (2010). Metabolomic changes accompanying transformation and acquisition of metastatic potential in a syngeneic mouse mammary tumour model. *The Journal of Biological Chemistry, 285,* 9317–9321. doi:10.1074/jbc.C110.104448

Lu, Z. J., Turner, D. H., & Mathews, D. H. (2006). A set of nearest neighbor parameters for predicting the enthalpy change of RNA secondary structure formation. *Nucleic Acids Research, 34,* 4912–4924. doi:10.1093/nar/gkl472

Luczkovich, J. J., Borgatti, S. P., Johnson, J. C., & Everett, M. G. (2003). Defining and measuring trophic role similarity in food webs using regular equivalence. *Journal of Theoretical Biology, 220,* 303–321. doi:10.1006/jtbi.2003.3147

Ludwig, C., Ward, D. G., Martin, A., Viant, M. R., Ismail, T., & Johnson, P. J. (2009). Fast targeted multidimensional NMR metabolomics of colorectal cancer. *Magnetic Resonance in Chemistry, 47*(Suppl 1), S68–S73. doi:10.1002/mrc.2519

Ludwig, W., Strunk, O., Westram, R., Richter, L., & Meier, H., Yadhukumar, *et al.* (2004). ARB: a software environment for sequence data. *Nucleic Acids Research, 32*(4), 1363–1371. doi:10.1093/nar/gkh293

Lundberg, P., Ranta, E., & Kaitala, V. (2000). Species loss leads to community closure. *Ecology Letters, 3,* 465–468. doi:10.1046/j.1461-0248.2000.00170.x

Luts, J., Ojeda, F., Van de Plas, R., De Moor, B., Van Huffel, S., & Suykens, J. A. (2010). A tutorial on support vector machine-based methods for classification problems in chemometrics. *Analytica Chimica Acta, 665*(2), 129–145. doi:10.1016/j.aca.2010.03.030

Ma, C., Zhou, D., & Zhou, Y. (2006). *Feature Mining Integration for Improving the Prediction Accuracy of Translation Initiation Sites in Eukaryotic mRNAs.* gccw, 349-356. Fifth International Conference on Grid and Cooperative Computing Workshops.

Ma'ayan, A., Jenkins, S. L., Goldfarb, J., & Iyengar, R. (2007). Network analysis of FDA approved drugs and their targets. *The Mount Sinai Journal of Medicine, New York, 74,* 27–32. doi:10.1002/msj.20002

MacAlpine, D. M., & Bell, S. P. (2005). A genomic view of eukaryotic DNA replication. *Chromosome Research, 13,* 309–326. doi:10.1007/s10577-005-1508-1

MacArthur, R. H. (1955). Fluctuations of animal populations and a measure of community stability. *Ecology, 36,* 533–536. doi:10.2307/1929601

Mace, G. M., & Collar, N. J. (2002). Priority-setting in species conservation. In Norris, K., & Pain, D. J. (Eds.), *Conserving bird biodiversity* (pp. 61–73). Cambridge, UK: Cambridge University Press. doi:10.1017/CBO9780511606304.005

Madsen, R., Lundstedt, T., & Trygg, J. (2010). Chemometrics in metabolomics – A review in human disease diagnosis. *Analytica Chimica Acta, 659,* 23–33. doi:10.1016/j.aca.2009.11.042

Mahadevan, S., Shah, S. L., Marrie, T. J., & Slupsky, C. M. (2008). Analysis of metabolomic data using support vector machines. *Analytical Chemistry, 80*(19), 7562–7570. doi:10.1021/ac800954c

Mahner, M., & Kary, M. (1997, May 7). What exactly are genomes, genotypes and phenotypes? And what about phenomes? *Journal of Theoretical Biology, 186*(1), 55–63. doi:10.1006/jtbi.1996.0335

Mäkinen, V. P., Soininen, P., & Forsblom, C. (2008). 1H NMR metabonomics approach to the disease continuum of diabetic complications and premature death. *Molecular Systems Biology, 4,* 167. doi:10.1038/msb4100205

Mapelli, V., Olsson, L., & Nielsen, J. (2008). Metabolic footprinting in microbiology: methods and applications in functional genomics and biotechnology. *Trends in Biotechnology, 26*(9), 490–497. doi:10.1016/j.tibtech.2008.05.008

Marathe, A., Condon, A. E., & Corn, R. M. (2001). On combinatorial DNA word design. *Journal of Computational Biology, 8*(3), 201–219. doi:10.1089/10665270152530818

Margalef, R. (1968). *Perspectives in ecological theory*. University of Chicago Press.

Margalef, R. (1991). Networks in ecology. In Higashi, M., & Burns, T. P. (Eds.), *Theoretical Studies of Ecosystems - the Network Perspective* (pp. 288–351). Cambridge: Cambridge University Press.

Markowitz, S. D., & Bertagnolli, M. M. (2009). Molecular Basis of Colorectal Cancer. *The New England Journal of Medicine, 361*, 2449–2460. doi:10.1056/NEJMra0804588

Martinez, N. D. (1991). Artifacts or attributes? Effects of resolution on the Little Rock Lake food web. *Ecological Monographs, 61*, 367–392. doi:10.2307/2937047

Martinez, N. D., Hawkins, B. A., Dawah, H. A., & Feifarek, B. P. (1999). Effects of sampling effort on characterization of food-web structure. *Ecology, 80*, 1044–1055. doi:10.1890/0012-9658(1999)080[1044:EOSEOC]2.0.CO;2

May, R. M., Beddington, J. R., Clark, C. W., Holt, S. J., & Laws, R. M. (1979). Management of multispecies fisheries. *Science, 205*, 267–277. doi:10.1126/science.205.4403.267

May, R. M. (1983). The structure of foodwebs. *Nature, 301*, 566–568. doi:10.1038/301566a0

McCaig, C. (2009). From individuals to populations: a symbolic process algebra approach to epidemiology. *Mathematics in Computer Science, 2*, 535–556. doi:10.1007/s11786-008-0066-2

McCann, K., Hastings, A., & Huxel, G. R. (1998). Weak trophic interactions and the balance of nature. *Nature, 395*, 794–798. doi:10.1038/27427

Mehra, A., Lee, K. H., & Hatzimanikatis, V. (2003). Insights into the relation between mRNA and protein expression patterns: I. Theoretical considerations. *Biotechnology and Bioengineering, 84*(7), 822–833. doi:10.1002/bit.10860

Mehta, M. (2007). *Classification of hereditary and genetic disorders*. Retrieved March 21, 2011, from http://pharmaxchange.info/notes/clinical/genetic_disorders.html.

Meier, S., Gehring, C., MacPherson, C. R., Kaur, M., Maqungo, M., & Reuben, S. (2008). The promoter signatures in rice LEA genes can be used to build a co-expressing LEA gene network. *RICE, 1*(2), 177. doi:10.1007/s12284-008-9017-4

Meinicke, P., Lingner, T., & Kaever, A. (2008). Metabolite-based clustering and visualization of mass spectrometry data using one-dimensional self-organized maps. *Algorithms for Molecular Biology; AMB, 3*, 9. doi:10.1186/1748-7188-3-9

Mendes, P. (1993). GEPASI: a software package for modelling the dynamics, steady states and control of biochemical and other systems. *Computer Applications in the Biosciences, 9*(5), 563–571.

Michopoulos, F., Lai, L., Gika, H., Theodoridis, G., & Wilson, I. (2009). UPLC-MS-based analysis of human plasma for metabonomics using solvent precipitation or solid phase extraction. *Journal of Proteome Research, 8*(4), 2114–2121. doi:10.1021/pr801045q

Mills, L. S., Soulé, M. L., & Doak, D. F. (1993). The keystone-species concept in ecology and conservation. *Bioscience, 43*, 219–224. doi:10.2307/1312122

Milner, R. (1999). *Communicating and mobile systems: the pi-calculus*. Cambridge, UK: Cambridge University Press.

Mitchell, T. (1997). *Machine Learning* (*International Edition*). New York: McGraw Hill.

Mogilevskaya, E., Bagrova, N., Plyusnina, T., Gizzatkulov, N., Metelkin, E., & Goryacheva, E. (2009). Kinetic modeling as a tool to integrate multilevel dynamic experimental data. *Methods in Molecular Biology (Clifton, N.J.), 563*, 197–218. doi:10.1007/978-1-60761-175-2_11

Mogilner, A., & Oster, G. (2003). Force generation by actin polymerization II: The elastic ratchet and tethered filaments. *Biophysical Journal, 84,* 1591–1605. doi:10.1016/S0006-3495(03)74969-8

Mogilner, A., & Oster, G. (2008). Cell motility driven by actin polymerization. *Biophysical Journal, 71,* 3030–3045. doi:10.1016/S0006-3495(96)79496-1

Mohanty, B., Krishnan, S. P., Swarup, S., & Bajic, V. B. (2005). Detection and Preliminary Analysis of Motifs in Promoters of Anaerobically Induced Genes of Different Plant Species. *Annals of Botany, 96*(4), 669–681. doi:10.1093/aob/mci219

Moles, G. C., Mendes, P., & Banga, J. R. (2003). parameter estimation in biochemical pathways: a comparison of global optimiztion methods. *Genome Research, 13,* 2467–2474. doi:10.1101/gr.1262503

Monaco, M. E., & Ulanowicz, R. E. (1997). Comparative ecosystem trophic structure of three U.S. mid-Atlantic estuaries. *Marine Ecology Progress Series, 161,* 239–254. doi:10.3354/meps161239

Montemanni, R., & Smith, D. H. (2008). Construction of constant GC-content DNA codes via a Variable Neighbourhood Search algorithm. *Journal of Mathematical Modelling and Algorithms, 7,* 311–326. doi:10.1007/s10852-008-9087-8

Montemanni, R., & Smith, D. H. (2009). Heuristic algorithms for constructing binary constant weight codes. *IEEE Transactions on Information Theory, 55*(10), 4651–4656. doi:10.1109/TIT.2009.2027491

Montemanni, R., Smith, D.H., & Koul, N. Three meta-heuristics for the construction of constant GC-content DNA codes. *Springer volume on metaheuristic algorithms,* S. Voβ and M. Caserta eds., to appear.

Montoliu, I., Martin, F. J., & Collino, S. (2008). Multivariate modeling strantegy for intercompartmental analysis of tissue and plasma 1H NMR spectrotypes. *Journal of Proteome Research, 8,* 2397–2406. doi:10.1021/pr8010205

Montoya, J. M., Woodward, G., Emmerson, M. C., & Solé, R. V. (2009). Press perturbations and indirect effects in real food webs. *Ecology, 90,* 2426–2433. doi:10.1890/08-0657.1

Montoya, J. M., & Solé, R. V. (2002). Small world patterns in food webs. *Journal of Theoretical Biology, 214,* 405–412. doi:10.1006/jtbi.2001.2460

Montoya, J. M., & Solé, R. V. (2003). Topological properties of food webs: from real data to community assembly models. *Oikos, 102,* 614–622. doi:10.1034/j.1600-0706.2003.12031.x

Morgenthal, K., Weckwerth, W., & Steuer, R. (2006). Metabolomic networks in plants: Transitions from pattern recognition to biological interpretation. *Bio Systems, 83*(2-3), 108–117. doi:10.1016/j.biosystems.2005.05.017

Morgenthal, K., Wienkoop, S., Wolschin, F., & Weckwerth, W. (2007). Integrative profiling of metabolites and proteins: improving pattern recognition and biomarker selection for systems level approaches. *Methods in Molecular Biology (Clifton, N.J.), 358,* 57–75. doi:10.1007/978-1-59745-244-1_4

Moskovitch, R. (2007). A Comparative Evaluation of Full-text, Concept-based, and Context-sensitive Search. *Journal of the American Medical Informatics Association, 14,* 164–174. doi:10.1197/jamia.M1953

Mrowka, R., Schuchhardt, J., & Gille, C. (2002). Oligodb--interactive design of oligo DNA for transcription profiling of human genes. *Bioinformatics (Oxford, England), 18*(12), 1686–1687. doi:10.1093/bioinformatics/18.12.1686

Mukherjea, S. (2005). Information retrieval and knowledge discovery utilising a biomedical Semantic Web. *Briefings in Bioinformatics, 6,* 252–262. doi:10.1093/bib/6.3.252

Muller-Felber, W., Ansevin, C. F., Ricker, K., Muller-Jenssen, A., Töpfer, M., Goebel, H. H., & Pongratz, D. E. (1999). Immunosuppressive treatment of rippling muscles in patients with myasthenia gravis. *Neuromuscular Disorders, 9,* 604–607. doi:10.1016/S0960-8966(99)00065-6

Nayer, M, Wanas, Rozita A. Dara, Mohamed S. Kamel. (2006). Adaptive fusion and co-operative training for classifier ensembles Pattern Recognition. *Pattern Recognition, 39*(9), 1781–1794. doi:10.1016/j.patcog.2006.02.003

Neumanna, N. F., & Galvez, F. (2002). DNA microarrays and toxicogenomics: applications for ecotoxicology? *Biotechnology Advances*, *20*(5-6), 391–419. doi:10.1016/S0734-9750(02)00025-3

Nicholson, J. K. (1999). 'Metabonomics' understanding the metabolic responses of living systems to pathophysiological stimuli via multivariate statistical analysis of biological NMR spectroscopic data. *Xenobiotica*, *29*, 1181–1189. doi:10.1080/004982599238047

Nicholson, J. K., Connelly, J., Lindon, J. C., & Holmes, E. (2002). Metabonomics: a platform for studying drug toxicity and gene function. *Nature Reviews. Drug Discovery*, *1*, 153–161. doi:10.1038/nrd728

Nicolaidoua, P., Papadopouloua, A., Matsinosb, Y. G., Georgoulic, H., Fretzayasa, A., & Papadimitrioua, A. (2007). Vitamin D Receptor Polymorphisms in Hypocalcemic Vitamin D-Resistant Rickets Carriers. *Hormone Research*, *67*, 179–183. doi:10.1159/000097014

Nie, L., Wu, G., Culley, D. E., Scholten, J. C., & Zhang, W. (2007). Integrative analysis of transcriptomic and proteomic data: challenges, solutions and applications. *Critical Reviews in Biotechnology*, *27*(2), 63–75. doi:10.1080/07388550701334212

Nie, L., Wu, G., & Zhang, W. (2006). Correlation of mRNA expression and protein abundance affected by multiple sequence features related to translational efficiency in Desulfovibrio vulgaris: a quantitative analysis. *Genetics*, *174*(4), 2229–2243. doi:10.1534/genetics.106.065862

Nielsen, H. B., & Knudsen, S. (2002). Avoiding cross hybridization by choosing nonredundant targets on cDNA arrays. *Bioinformatics (Oxford, England)*, *18*, 321–322. doi:10.1093/bioinformatics/18.2.321

Nielsen, H. B., Wernersson, R., & Knudsen, S. (2003). Design of oligonucleotides for microarrays and perspectives for design of multi-transcriptome arrays. *Nucleic Acids Research*, *31*(13), 3491–3496. doi:10.1093/nar/gkg622

Nisbet, R. M., & Gurney, W. S. C. (1982). *Modelling fluctuating populations*. New York: John Wiley & Sons.

Noble, D. (1960). Cardiac action and pacemaker potentials based on the Hodgkin-Huxley equations. *Nature*, *188*, 495–497. doi:10.1038/188495b0

Noble, D. (2002). The rise of computational biology. *Nat. Rev. Mol. Biol.* (3), 459-463.

Nordberg, E. K. (2005). YODA: selecting signature oligonucleotides. *Bioinformatics (Oxford, England)*, *21*, 1365–1370. doi:10.1093/bioinformatics/bti182

Norman, R., & Shankland, C. (2004). Developing the use of process algebra in the derivation and analysis of mathematical models of infectious disease. *Lecture Notes in Computer Science*, *280*, 404–414.

NSF. (1999). *Decision-making and Valuation for Environmental Policy. NSF Bulletin 99-14*. Ballston, VA: National Science Foundation.

Odum, E. P. (1969). The strategy of ecosystem development. *Science*, *164*, 262–270. doi:10.1126/science.164.3877.262

Okey, T. A., & Wright, B. A. (2004). Toward ecosystem-based extraction policies for Prince William Sound, Alaska: Integrating conflicting objectives and rebuilding pinnipeds. *Bulletin of Marine Science*, *74*, 727–747.

Okey, T. A., Banks, S., Born, A. R., Bustamante, R. H., Calvopina, M., & Edgar, G. J. (2004). A trophic model of a Galápagos subtidal rocky reef for evaluating fisheries and conservation strategies. *Ecological Modelling*, *172*, 383–401. doi:10.1016/j.ecolmodel.2003.09.019

Okey, T. A. (2004). *Shifted community states in four marine ecosystems: some potential mechanisms*. Unpublished doctoral dissertation, University of British Columbia, Vancouver.

Okey, T. A., & Pauly, D. (Eds.). (1999). *A trophic mass-balance model of Alaska's Prince William Sound ecosystem, for the post-spill period 1994-1996*. 2nd edition, Vol. Fisheries Centre Research Report 7(4), Vancouver, BC: University of British Columbia.

Okoniewski, M. J., & Miller, C. J. (2006). Hybridization interactions between probesets in short oligo microarrays lead to spurious correlations. *BMC Bioinformatics*, *7*, 276. doi:10.1186/1471-2105-7-276

Okuyama, T. (2009). Local interactions between predators and prey call into question commonly used functional responses. *Ecological Modelling*, *220*, 1182–1188. doi:10.1016/j.ecolmodel.2009.02.010

Oldiges, M., Lutz, S., Pflug, S., Schroer, K., Stein, N., & Wiendahl, C. (2007). Metabolomics: current state and evolving methodologies and tools. *Applied Microbiology and Biotechnology*, *76*(3), 495–511. doi:10.1007/s00253-007-1029-2

Olff, H., et al. (2009). Parallel ecological networks in ecosystems. *Philosophical Transactions of the Royal Society, London, series B*, 364, 1755-1779.

Oliver, S. G., Winson, M. K., & Kell, D. B. (1998). Systematic functional analysis of the yeast genome. *Trends in Biotechnology*, *16*, 373–378. doi:10.1016/S0167-7799(98)01214-1

Oltvai, Z. N., & Barabási, A.-L. (2002). Life's complexity pyramid. *Science*, *298*, 763–764. doi:10.1126/science.1078563

Orlov, Y. L., Zhou, J. T., Lipovich, L., Yong, H. C., Li, Y., Shahab, A., & Kuznetsov, V. A. (2006). A comprehensive quality assessment of the Affymetrix U133A&B probesets by an integrative genomic and clinical data analysis approach. *Proceedings of the Fifth International Conference on Bioinformatics of Genome Regulation and Structure*, Novosibirsk, Inst. of Cytology & Genetics, 1, 126-129.

Östergård, P. R. J. (2002). A fast algorithm for the maximum clique problem. *Discrete Applied Mathematics*, *120*, 197–207. doi:10.1016/S0166-218X(01)00290-6

Ozdinler, P. H., & Erzurumlu, R. S. (2002). Slit2, a Branching-Arborization Factor for Sensory Axons in the Mammalian CNS. *The Journal of Neuroscience*, *22*, 4540–4549.

Paine, R. T. (1966). Food web complexity and species diversity. *American Naturalist*, *100*, 65–75. doi:10.1086/282400

Paine, R. T. (1992). Food-web analysis through field measurement of per capita interaction strength. *Nature*, *355*, 73–75. doi:10.1038/355073a0

Paley, S. M., & Karp, P. D. (2006). The Pathway Tools cellular overview diagram and Omics Viewer. *Nucleic Acids Research*, *34*(13), 3771–3778. doi:10.1093/nar/gkl334

Palsson, B. (2006). *Systems biology. Properties of reconstructed networks*. Cambridge, UK: Cambridge University Press. doi:10.1017/CBO9780511790515

Pardalos, P. M., & Xue, J. (1994). The maximum clique problem. *Journal of Global Optimization*, *4*, 301–328. doi:10.1007/BF01098364

Park, M. R., Yun, K. Y., Mohanty, B., Herath, V., Xu, F., & Wijaya, E. (2010). Supra-optimal expression of the cold-regulated OsMyb4 transcription factor in transgenic rice changes the complexity of transcriptional network with major effects on stress tolerance and panicle development. [Epub ahead of print]. *Plant, Cell & Environment*, *2010*(Aug), 27. doi:.doi:10.1111/j.1365-3040.2010.02221.x

Pascual, M. (2005). Computational ecology: from the complex to the simple and back. *PLoS Computational Biology*, *1*, e18. doi:10.1371/journal.pcbi.0010018

Pascual, M., & Dunne, J. A. (Eds.). (2006). *Ecological Networks: Linking Structure to Dynamics in Food Webs*. Oxford: Oxford University Press.

Pasquer, F., Pelludat, C., Duffy, B., & Frey, J. E. (2010). Broad spectrum microarray for fingerprint-based bacterial species identification. *BMC Biotechnology*, *10*, 13. doi:10.1186/1472-6750-10-13

Patel, J. C., Hall, A., & Caron, E. (2002). Vav regulates activation of Rac but not Cdc42 during FcγR -mediated phagocytosis. *Molecular Biology of the Cell*, *13*, 1215–1226. doi:10.1091/mbc.02-01-0002

Patel, S., Thakkar, T., Swaminarayan, P., & Sajja, P. (2010). Development of Agent-Based Knowledge Discovery Framework to Access Data Resource Grid. *Advances in Computational Sciences and Technology*, *3*, 23–31.

Patrício, J., Ulanowicz, R. E., Pardal, M. A., & Marques, J. C. (2004). Ascendency as an ecological indicator: a case study of estuarine pulse eutrophication. *Estuarine, Coastal and Shelf Science*, *60*, 23–35. doi:10.1016/j.ecss.2003.11.017

Patten, B. C. (1981). Environs: the superniches of ecosystems. *American Zoologist*, *21*, 845–852.

Patten, B. C. (1991). Concluding remarks. Network ecology: indirect determination of the life-environment relationship in ecosystems. In Higashi, M., & Burns, T. P. (Eds.), *Theoretical Studies of Ecosystems - the Network Perspective* (pp. 288–351). Cambridge: Cambridge University Press.

Patterson, A. D., Li, H., & Eichler, G. S. (2008). UPLC-ESI-TOFMS-based metabolomics and gene expression dynamics inspector self-organizing metabolomic maps as tools for understanding the cellular response to ionizing radiation. *Analytical Chemistry, 80*, 665–674. doi:10.1021/ac701807v

Pavlidis, T. (1977). *Structural pattern recognition.* New York, NY: Springer-Verlag.

Pedersen, A. G., & Nielsen, H. (1997). *Neural network prediction of translation initiation sites in eukaryotes: Perspectives for EST and genome analysis.*Proc. 5th International Conference on Intelligent Systems for Molecular Biology, 226–233.

Pedrycz, W., Bezdek, J. C., Hathaway, R. J., & Rogers, G. W. (1998). Two nonparametric models for fusing heterogenous fuzzy data. *IEEE Transactions on Fuzzy Systems, 6*(3), 411–425. doi:10.1109/91.705509

Peng, Y., Li, W., & Liu, Y. (2007). A hybrid approach for biomarker discovery from microarray gene expression data for cancer classification. *Cancer Informatics, 2*, 301–311.

Perner, P., Wang, P., and& Rosenfeld. (Eds.). (1996). *Advances in structural and syntactical pattern recognition.* New York, NY: Springer-Verlag.

Pers, T. H., Albrechtsen, A., Holst, C., Sorensen, T. I., & Gerds, T. A. (2009). The validation and assessment of machine learning: a game of prediction from high-dimensional data. *PLoS ONE, 4*(8), e6287. doi:10.1371/journal.pone.0006287

Pertea, M., & Salzberg, S. (2002). A Method to Improve the Performance of Translation Start Site Detection and Its Application for Gene Finding. InR. Guigo&D. Gusfield (Eds.) *WABI 2002, LNCS 2452.*pp. 210–219, (2002). Springer-Verlag Berlin Heidelberg.

Pfaff, D. A., Clarke, K. M., Parr, T. A., Cole, J. M., Geierstanger, B. H., Tahmassebi, D. C., & Dwyer, T. J. (2008). Solution structure of a DNA duplex containing a guanine-difluorotoluene pair: a wobble pair without hydrogen bonding? *Journal of the American Chemical Society, 130*(14), 4869–4878. doi:10.1021/ja7103608

Philip, P. (2002). Letter from the Dean. In *Standford Medicine Magazine.*

Phillips, A., Cardelli, L., & Castagna, G. (2006). A graphical representation for biological processes in the stochastic pi-calculus. *Transactions in Computational Systems Biology, 4230*, 123–152.

Phillips, A., & Cardelli, L. (2007). Efficient, correct simulation of biological processes in the stochastic pi-calculus. In Calder, M. & Gilmore, S. (Eds.), *Computational Methods in Systems Biology, International Conference, CMSB 2007*, Proceedings. Lecture Notes in Computer Science 4695, (pp. 184-199), Springer.

Pimm, S. L. (1991). *The Balance of Nature?*Chicago, IL: University of Chicago Press.

Pimm, S. L. (1980). Food web design and the effect of species deletion. *Oikos, 35*, 139–149. doi:10.2307/3544422

Pimm, S. L., Lawton, J. H., & Cohen, J. E. (1991). Food web patterns and their consequences. *Nature, 350*, 669–674. doi:10.1038/350669a0

Pinkel, D., & Albertson, D. G. (2005). Comparative genomic hybridization. *Annual Review of Genomics and Human Genetics, 6*, 331–354. doi:10.1146/annurev.genom.6.080604.162140

Pitkin, R. M. (2007). Folate and neural tube defects. *The American Journal of Clinical Nutrition, 85*, 285–288.

Planells-Cases, R., Lerma, J., & Ferrer-Montiel, A. (2006). Pharmacological intervention at ionotropic glutamate receptor complexes. *Current Pharmaceutical Design, 12*, 3583–3596. doi:10.2174/138161206778522092

Platt, T. C., Mann, K. H., & Ulanowicz, R. E. (1981). *Mathematical Models in Biological Oceanography.* Paris, France: UNESCO Press.

Polis, G., & Winemiller, K. (1995). *Food Webs: Integration of Patterns and Dynamics.* New York: Chapman and Hall.

Polis, G. A., & Strong, D. R. (1996). Food web complexity and community dynamics. *American Naturalist, 147*, 813–846. doi:10.1086/285880

Polisetty, P. K., Voit, E. O., & Gatzke, E. P. (2006). Identification of metabolic system parameters usign global optimization methods. *Theoretical Biology & Medical Modelling, 3*(4).

Pollard, T. D. (2007). Regulation of actin filament assembly by Arp2/3 complex and formins. *Annual Review of Biophysics and Biomolecular Structure, 36*, 451–477. doi:10.1146/annurev.biophys.35.040405.101936

Pope, G. A., MacKenzie, D. A., Defernez, M., Aroso, M. A., Fuller, L. J., & Mellon, F. A. (2007). Metabolic footprinting as a tool for discriminating between brewing yeasts. *Yeast (Chichester, England), 24*(8), 667–679. doi:10.1002/yea.1499

Pope, G. A., MacKenzie, D. A., Defernez, M., & Roberts, I. N. (2009). Metabolic footprinting for the study of microbial biodiversity. *Cold Spring Harb Protoc, 2009*(5), pdb prot5222.

Powell, C. R., & Boland, R. P. (2009). The effects of stochastic population dynamics on food web structure. *Journal of Theoretical Biology, 257*, 170–180. doi:10.1016/j.jtbi.2008.11.006

Power, M. E. (1996). Challenges in the quest for keystones. *Bioscience, 46*, 609–620. doi:10.2307/1312990

Pozhitkov, A. E., Tautz, D., & Noble, P. A. (2007). Oligonucleotide microarrays: widely applied--poorly understood. *Briefings in Functional Genomics & Proteomics, 6*(2), 141–148. doi:10.1093/bfgp/elm014

Prechelt, L. (1998). Early stopping – but when? InG.B. Orr, K.–R. Müller (Eds.),*Neural Networks: Tricks of the Trade.* LNCS 1524, pp. 55–69, 1998. Ó Springer–Verlag Berlin Heidelberg (1998)

Preiss, T., & Hentze, M. (2003). Starting the protein synthesis machine: eukaryotic translation initiation. *BioEssays, 25*(12), 1201–1211. doi:10.1002/bies.10362

Premier Biosoft. Array Designer v4.25. (1994-2011). Retrieved from http://www.premierbiosoft.com/dnamicroarray/index.html, (Retrieved September 20, 2010).

Priami, C. (2009). Algorithmic Systems Biology. An opportunity for computer science. *Communications of the ACM, ACM, 52*(5), 80–88. doi:10.1145/1506409.1506427

Priami, C. (1995). Stochastic pi-calculus. *The Computer Journal, 38*(7), 578–589. doi:10.1093/comjnl/38.7.578

Priami, C. (2009). Algorithmic systems biology. *Communications of the ACM, 52*(5), 80–88. doi:10.1145/1506409.1506427

Priami, C., Regev, A., Shapiro, E., & Silverman, W. (2001). Application of a stochastic name-passing calculus to representation and simulation of molecular processes. *Information Processing Letters, 80*(1), 25–31. doi:10.1016/S0020-0190(01)00214-9

Priami, C., Ballarini, P., & Quaglia, P. (2009). BlenX4Bio - BlenX for Biologists. Degano, P. & Gorrieri, R. (Eds.), *Computational Methods in Systems Biology, 7th International Conference, CMSB 2009,* Proceedings. Lecture Notes in Computer Science, 5688, (pp. 26-51), Springer.

Priami, C., Guerriero, M. L., & Heath, J. K. (2007). An automated translation from a narrative language for biological modelling into process algebra. In Calder, M. & Gilmore S. (Eds.). *Computational Methods in Systems Biology, International Conference, CMSB 2007,* Proceedings. Lecture Notes in Computer Science 4695, (pp 136–151), Springer.

ProbePicker. (n.d.). Retrieved from http://sourceforge.net/projects/probepicker/, (Retrieved September 2010).

Proulx, S. R., Promislow, D. E. L., & Phillips, P. C. (2005). Network thinking in ecology and evolution. *Trends in Ecology & Evolution, 20*, 345–353. doi:10.1016/j.tree.2005.04.004

Purcell, J. E. (2000). Aggregations of the jellyfish Aurelia labiata: abundance, distribution, association with age-0 walleye pollock, and behaviors promoting aggregation in Prince William Sound, Alaska, USA. *Marine Ecology Progress Series, 195*, 145–158. doi:10.3354/meps195145

Qu, X., Gudivada, R. C., Jegga, A., Neumann, E., & Aronow, B. (2007). Semantic Web-based Data Representation and Reasoning Applied to Disease Mechanism and Pharmacology. In *IEEE International Conference on Bioinformatics & Biomedicine,* Freemont, USA, 131-143.

Quackenbush, J. (2002). Microarray data normalization and transformation. *Nature Genetics, 32*, 496–501. doi:10.1038/ng1032

Quince, C., Higgs, P. G., & McKane, A. J. (2005). Deleting species from model food webs. *Oikos, 110*, 283–296. doi:10.1111/j.0030-1299.2005.13493.x

Raddatz, G., Dehio, M., Meyer, T. F., & Dehio, C. (2001). PrimeArray: genome-scale primer design for DNA-microarray construction. *Bioinformatics (Oxford, England)*, *17*, 98–99. doi:10.1093/bioinformatics/17.1.98

Radhakrishna, U., Blouin, J. L., Solanki, J. V., Dhoriani, G. M., & Antonarakis, S. E. (1996). An autosomal dominant triphalangeal thumb: polysyndactyly syndrome with variable expression in a large Indian family maps to 7q36. *American Journal of Medical Genetics*, *66*, 209–215. doi:10.1002/(SICI)1096-8628(19961211)66:2<209::AID-AJMG17>3.0.CO;2-X

Rahmann, S. (2003). Fast large scale oligonucleotide selection using the longest common actor approach. *Journal of Bioinformatics and Computational Biology*, *1*(2), 343–361. doi:10.1142/S0219720003000125

Rajapakse, J. C., & Ho, L. S. (2005, Apr-Jun). Markov encoding for detecting signals in genomic sequences. *IEEE/ACM Transactions on Computational Biology and Bioinformatics*, *2*(2), 131–142. doi:10.1109/TCBB.2005.27

Random House Unabridged Dictionary. (n.d.). Retrieved from http://www.dictionary.com (accessed in Feb. 2009).

Rasmussen, P. E., Goulding, K. W. T., Brown, J. R., Grace, P. R., Janzen, H. H., & Körschens, M. (1998). Long-term agroecosystem experiments: assessing agricultural sustainability and global change. *Science*, *282*, 893–896. doi:10.1126/science.282.5390.893

Ray, J. G., Wyatt, P. R., Thompson, M. D., Vermeulen, M. J., Meier, C., & Wong, P.-Y. (2007). Vitamin B12 and the Risk of Neural Tube Defects in a Folic-Acid-Fortified Population. *Epidemiology (Cambridge, Mass.)*, *18*, 362–366. doi:10.1097/01.ede.0000257063.77411.e9

Refolo, L., Pappolla, M., Lafrancois, J., Malester, B., Schmidt, S., & Thomas-Bryant, T. (2001). A cholesterol-lowering drug reduces beta-amyloid pathology in a transgenic mouse model of Alzheimer's disease. *Neurobiology of Disease*, *8*, 890–899. doi:10.1006/nbdi.2001.0422

Regev, A., & Shapiro, E. (2002). Cells as computations. *Nature*, *419*, 343. doi:10.1038/419343a

Regev, A., & Shapiro, E. (2002). Cellular abstractions: Cells as computation. *Nature*, *419*, 343. doi:10.1038/419343a

Reif, J. H., Labean, T. H., & Seeman, N. C. (2001). Challenges and applications for self-assembled DNA nanostructures. *Lecture Notes in Computer Science*, *2054*, 173. doi:10.1007/3-540-44992-2_12

Reinker, S., Altman, R. M., & Timmer, J. (2006). Parameter estimation in stochastic biochemical reactions. *153* (4), 168-178.

Renshaw, E. (1993). *Modelling biological populations in space and time*. Cambridge, UK: Cambridge University Press.

Reymond, N., Charles, H., Duret, L., Calevro, F., Beslon, G., & Fayard, J.-M. (2004). ROSO: Optimizing Oligonucleotide Probes for Microarrays. *Bioinformatics (Oxford, England)*, *20*, 271–273. doi:10.1093/bioinformatics/btg401

Rimour, S., Hill, D., Militon, C., & Peyret, P. (2005). GoArrays: highly dynamic and efficient microarray probe design. *Bioinformatics (Oxford, England)*, *21*(7), 1094–1103. doi:10.1093/bioinformatics/bti112

Ripa, J., & Ives, A. R. (2003). Food web dynamics in correlated and autocorrelated environments. *Theoretical Population Biology*, *64*, 369–384. doi:10.1016/S0040-5809(03)00089-3

Robert Molidor As, M. M. A. Z. T. (2003). New trends in bioinformatics: from genome sequence to personalized medicine. *Experimental Gerontology*, *38*, 4.

Robu, I., Robu, V., & Thirion, B. (2006). An introduction to the Semantic Web for health sciences librarians. *Journal of the Medical Library Association*, *94*, 198–205.

Rodrigez-Fernandez, M., Mendes, P., & Banga, J. (2006). A hybrid apporach for efficient and robust parameter estimation in biochemical pathways. *Bio Systems*, *83*, 248–265. doi:10.1016/j.biosystems.2005.06.016

Roessner, U., Luedemann, A., Brust, D., Fiehn, O., Linke, T., Willmitzer, L., & Fernie, A. R. (2001). Metabolic profiling allows comprehensive phenotyping of genetically or environmentally modified plant systems. *The Plant Cell*, *13*, 11–29.

Roff, D. A. (1997). *Evolutionary Quantitative Genetics*. New York, NY: Chapman and Hall. doi:10.1007/978-1-4615-4080-9

Rogers, S., Khanin, R., & Girolami, M. (2007). Bayesian model-based inference of transcription factor activity. *BMC Bioinformatics*, *8*, 52. doi:10.1186/1471-2105-8-S2-S2

Romanel, A. (2010). *Dynamic Biological Modelling: a language-based approach.* Unpublished doctoral dissertation, University of Trento, Italy.

Ross, D. T., Scherf, U., Eisen, M. B., Perou, C. M., Rees, C., & Spellman, P. (2000). Systematic variation in gene expression patterns in human cancer cell lines. *Nature Genetics*, *24*, 227–235. doi:10.1038/73432

Rouchka, E. C., Khalyfa, A., & Cooper, N. G. F. (2005). MPrime: efficient large scale multiple primer and oligonucleotide design for customized gene microarrays. *BMC Bioinformatics*, *6*, 175. doi:10.1186/1471-2105-6-175

Rouillard, J.-M., Herbert, C. J., & Zuker, M. (2002)... *Bioinformatics (Oxford, England)*, *18*(3), 486–487. doi:10.1093/bioinformatics/18.3.486

Rouillard, J.-M., Zuker, M., & Gulari, E. (2003). OligoArray 2.0: design of oligonucleotide probes for DNA microarrays using a thermodynamic approach. *Nucleic Acids Research*, *31*, 3057–3062. doi:10.1093/nar/gkg426

Rouillard, J.-M., Lee, W., Truan, G., Gao, X., Zhou, X., & Gulari, E. (2004). Gene2Oligo: Oligonucleotide design for in vitro gene synthesis. *Nucleic Acids Research*, *32*, W176-80. doi:10.1093/nar/gkh401

Royall, D. R., Lauterbach, E. C., Cummings, J. L., Reeve, A., Rummans, T. A., & Kaufer, D. I. (2002). Executive Control Function: A Review of Its Promise and Challenges for Clinical Research. A Report From the Committee on Research of the American Neuropsychiatric Association. *The Journal of Neuropsychiatry and Clinical Neurosciences*, *14*, 377–405. doi:10.1176/appi.neuropsych.14.4.377

Rozen, S., & Skaletsky, H. J. (2000). Primer3 on the WWW for general users and for biologist programmers. In Krawetz, S., & Misener, S. (Eds.), *Bioinformatics Methods and Protocols: Methods in Molecular Biology* (pp. 365–386). Totowa, NJ: Humana Press.

Ruppin, E., Papin, J. A., de Figueiredo, L. F., & Schuster, S. (2010). Metabolic reconstruction, constraint-based analysis and game theory to probe genome-scale metabolic networks. *Current Opinion in Biotechnology*, *21*(4), 502–510. doi:10.1016/j.copbio.2010.07.002

Russell, S., & Norvig, P. (2003). *Artificial Intelligence A Modern Approach* (2nd ed.). New York: Prentice Hall.

Ruta, D., & Gabrys, B. (2000). An overview of classifier fusion method. *Computing and Information Systems*, *7*, 1–10.

Rutledge, R. W., Basorre, B. L., & Mulholland, R. J. (1976). Ecological stability: an information theory viewpoint. *Journal of Theoretical Biology*, *57*, 355–371. doi:10.1016/0022-5193(76)90007-2

Ruttenberg, A., Clark, T., Bug, W., Samwald, M., Bodenreider, O., & Chen, H. (2007). Advancing translational research with the Semantic Web. *BMC Bioinformatics*, *8*, 1–2. doi:10.1186/1471-2105-8-S3-S2

Ryan, D., & Robards, K. (2006). Metabolomics: the greatest omics of them all? *Analytical Chemistry*, *78*, 7954–7958. doi:10.1021/ac0614341

Saeys, Y., Abeel, T., Degroeve, S., & Van de Peer, Y. (2007). Translation Initiation Site Prediction on a Genomic Scale: Beauty of Simplicity. *Bioinformatics (Oxford, England)*, *23*, i418–i423. doi:10.1093/bioinformatics/btm177

Saeys, Y., Inza, I. & Larrañaga, P. (2007). A review of feature selection techniques in bioinformatics. *Bioinformatics.* Oct 1;*23*(19), 2507-17. Epub 2007 Aug 24.

Sagarin, R. D., & Taylor, T. (2008). *Natural Security: a Darwinian Approach to a Dangerous World.* Berkeley: University of California Press.

Sala, E., & Graham, M. H. (2002). Community-wide distribution of predator-prey interaction strength in kelp forests. *Proceedings of the National Academy of Sciences of the United States of America*, *99*, 3678–3683. doi:10.1073/pnas.052028499

Samoilov, M., Arkin, A., & Ross, J. (2001). On the deduction of chemical reaction pathways from measurements of time series of concentrations. *Chaos (Woodbury, N.Y.)*, *11*(1), 108. doi:10.1063/1.1336499

Sansone, S. A., Fan, T., Goodacre, R., Griffin, J. L., Hardy, N. W., & Kaddurah-Daouk, R. (2007). The metabolomics standards initiative. *Nature Biotechnology*, *25*(8), 846–848. doi:10.1038/nbt0807-846b

SantaLucia, J., Allawi, H. T., & Seneviratne, P. A. (1996). Improved nearest-neighbor parameters for predicting DNA duplex stability. *Biochemistry*, *35*(11), 3555–3562. doi:10.1021/bi951907q

SantaLucia, J. (1998). A unified view of polymer, dumbbell, and oligonucleotide DNA nearest-neighbor thermodynamics. *Proceedings of the National Academy of Sciences of the United States of America*, *95*(4), 1460–1465. doi:10.1073/pnas.95.4.1460

SantaLucia, J., & Hicks, D. (2004). The thermodynamics of DNA structural motifs. *Annual Review of Biophysics and Biomolecular Structure*, *3*, 415–440. doi:10.1146/annurev.biophys.32.110601.141800

Sarwal, M. M. (2009). Deconvoluting the 'omics' for organ transplantation. *Current Opinion in Organ Transplantation*, *14*(5), 544–551. doi:10.1097/MOT.0b013e32833068fb

Sato, S., Arita, M., & Soga, T. (2008). Time-resolved metabolomics reveals metabolic modulation in rice foliage. *BMS Syst Biol*, *2*, 51. doi:10.1186/1752-0509-2-51

Sauer, S. W., Okun, J. G., Schwab, M. A., Crnic, L. R., Hoffmann, G. F., & Goodman, S. I. (2005). Bioenergetics in Glutaryl-Coenzyme A Dehydrogenase Deficiency: A Role For Glutaryl-Coenzyme A. *The Journal of Biological Chemistry*, *280*, 21830–21836. doi:10.1074/jbc.M502845200

Scardoni, G., & Laudanna, C. (2009). Analyzing biological network parameters with CentiScaPe. *Bioinformatics (Oxford, England)*, *25*, 2857–2859. doi:10.1093/bioinformatics/btp517

Scheffer, M. (1995). Super-individuals a simple solution for modelling large populations on an individual basis. *Ecological Modelling*, *80*, 161–170. doi:10.1016/0304-3800(94)00055-M

Schena, M., Shalon, D., Davis, R. W., & Brown, P. O. (1995). Quantitative monitoring of gene expression patterns with a complementary DNA microarray. *Science*, *270*, 467–470. doi:10.1126/science.270.5235.467

Schmitt, W. A., Raab, R. M., & Stephanopoulos, G. (2004). Elucidation of gene interaction networks through time-lagged correlation analysis of transcriptional data. *Genome Research*, *14*, 1654–1663. doi:10.1101/gr.2439804

Schretter, C., & Milinkovitch, M. C. (2006). OligoFaktory: a visual tool for interactive oligonucleotide design. *Bioinformatics (Oxford, England)*, *22*(1), 115–116. doi:10.1093/bioinformatics/bti728

Scotti, M., Allesina, S., Bondavalli, C., Bodini, A., & Abarca-Arenas, L. G. (2006). Effective trophic positions in ecological acyclic networks. *Ecological Modelling*, *198*, 495–505. doi:10.1016/j.ecolmodel.2006.06.005

Sellick, C. A., Hansen, R., Maqsood, A. R., Dunn, W. B., Stephens, G. M., & Goodacre, R. (2009). Effective quenching processes for physiologically valid metabolite profiling of suspension cultured Mammalian cells. *Analytical Chemistry*, *81*(1), 174–183. doi:10.1021/ac8016899

Serkova, N. J., Spratlin, J. L., & Eckhardt, S. G. (2007). NMR-based metabolomics: translational application and treatment of cancer. *Current Opinion in Molecular Therapeutics*, *9*(6), 572–585.

Seth, A. K. (2007). The ecology of action selection: insights from artificial life. *Philosophical Transactions of the Royal Society, London, series B*, *362*, 1545-1558.

Shahrezaei, V., & Swain, P. S. (2008). The stochastic nature of biochemical networks. *Current Opinion in Biotechnology*, *19*(4), 369–374. doi:10.1016/j.copbio.2008.06.011

Sharkey, A. J. C. (1999). *Combining artificial neural nets: Ensemble and modular multi-net systems. London*. London: Springer-Verlag.

Shirvan, A., Reshef, A., Yogev-Falach, M., & Ziv, I. (2009). Molecular imaging of neurodegeneration by a novel cross-disease biomarker. *Experimental Neurology*, *219*, 274–283. doi:10.1016/j.expneurol.2009.05.032

Shlens, J. (2003). *A tutorial on PCA*. Retrieved from http://www.snl.salk.edu/~shlens/pca.pdf

Simberloff, D. (1980). A succession of paradigms in ecology: essentialism to materialism and probabilism. *Synthese*, *43*, 3–39. doi:10.1007/BF00413854

Simberloff, D. (1998). Flagships, umbrellas, and keystones: is single-species management passé in the landscape area? *Biological Conservation*, *83*, 247–257. doi:10.1016/S0006-3207(97)00081-5

Simberloff, D. (2003). Community and ecosystem impacts of single-species extinctions. In Kareiva, P., & Levin, S. A. (Eds.), *The Importance of Species* (pp. 221–233). Princeton, NJ: Princeton University Press.

Sleator, R. D. (2010, Aug 1). An overview of the current status of eukaryote gene prediction strategies. *Gene*, *461*(1-2), 1–4. Epub 2010 Apr 27. doi:10.1016/j.gene.2010.04.008

Smart, K. F., Aggio, R. B., Van Houtte, J. R., & Villas-Boas, S. G. (2010). Analytical platform for metabolome analysis of microbial cells using methyl chloroformate derivatization followed by gas chromatography-mass spectrometry. *Nature Protocols*, *5*(10), 1709–1729. doi:10.1038/nprot.2010.108

Smith, L. M., Maher, A. D., & Cloarec, O. (2007). Statistical correlation and projection methods for improved information recovery from diffusion-edited NMR spectra of biological samples. *Analytical Chemistry*, *79*, 5682–5689. doi:10.1021/ac0703754

Smith, D. H., Aboluion, N., Montemanni, R., & Perkins, S. (to appear). Linear and nonlinear constructions of DNA codes with constant GC-content. *Discrete Mathematics*.

Soininen, P., Kangas, A. J., & Wurtz, P. (2009). High throughput serum NMR metabonimics for cost-effective holistic studies on systemic metabolism. *Analyst (London)*, *134*, 1781–1785. doi:10.1039/b910205a

Solberg, R., Enot, D., & Deigner, H.-P. (2010). Metabolomic Analyses of Plasma Reveals New Insights into Asphyxia and Resuscitation in Pigs. *PLoS ONE*, *5*, e9606. doi:10.1371/journal.pone.0009606

Solé, R. V., & Montoya, J. M. (2001). Complexity and fragility in ecological networks. *Proceedings. Biological Sciences*, *268*, 2039–2045. doi:10.1098/rspb.2001.1767

Solow, A. R., & Beet, A. R. (1998). On lumping species in food webs. *Ecology*, *79*, 2013–2018. doi:10.1890/0012-9658(1998)079[2013:OLSIFW]2.0.CO;2

Somorjai, R. L., Alexander, M., & Baumgartner, S. (2004). A data-driven, flexible machine learning strategy for the classification of biomedical data. In Dubitzky, W., & Azuaje, F. (Eds.), *Artificial Intelligence Methods and Tools for Systems Biology* (pp. 67–85). Dordrecht: Springer.

Sparks, D. L., Sabbagh, M. N., Connor, D. J., Jean Lopezn, C., Launer, L. J., & Browne, P. (2005). Atorvastatin for the Treatment of Mild to Moderate Alzheimer Disease. *Archives of Neurology*, *62*, 753–757. doi:10.1001/archneur.62.5.753

Sparks, M.E. & Brendel, V. (2008). MetWAMer: eukaryotic translation initiation site prediction. *BMC Bioinformatics*. Sep 18(9),381.

Spratlin, J. L., Serkova, N. J., & Eckhardt, S. G. (2009). Clinical applications of metabolomics in oncology: a review. *Clinical Cancer Research*, *15*(2), 431–440. doi:10.1158/1078-0432.CCR-08-1059

Sprite, P., Glymour, C., & Scheines, R. (2000). *Causation, Prediction and Search Adaptive Computation and Machine Learning*. MIT Press.

Sreekuman, A., Poisson, L. M., & Rajendiran, T. M. (2009). Metabolomic profiles delineate potential role for sarcosine in prostate cancer progression. *Nature*, *457*, 910–915. doi:10.1038/nature07762

Srivastava, G. P., Guo, J., Shi, H., & Xu, D. (2008). PRIMEGENS-v2: genome-wide primer design for analyzing DNA methylation pattern of CpG island. *Bioinformatics (Oxford, England)*, *24*(17), 1837–1842. doi:10.1093/bioinformatics/btn320

Stein, L. D. (2004). Using the Reactome database. *Curr Protoc Bioinformatics, Chapter 8*, Unit 8 7.

Stenberg, J., Nilsson, M., & Landegren, U. (2005). ProbeMaker: an extensible framework for design of sets of oligonucleotide probes. *BMC Bioinformatics*, *6*, 229. doi:10.1186/1471-2105-6-229

Steven, A. G. (2004). Acquired rippling muscle disease with myasthenia gravis. *Muscle & Nerve*, *29*, 143–146. doi:10.1002/mus.10494

Stevens, J. D. (2000). The effects of fishing on sharks, rays, and chimaeras (chondrichthyans), and the implications for marine ecosystems. *Journal of Marine Science*, *57*, 476–494.

Stibor, H. (2004). Copepods act as a switch between alternative trophic cascades in marine pelagic food webs. *Ecology Letters, 7*, 321–325. doi:10.1111/j.1461-0248.2004.00580.x

Stouffer, D. B., Camacho, J., & Amaral, L. A. N. (2006). A robust measure of food web intervality. *Proceedings of the National Academy of Sciences of the United States of America, 103*, 19015–19020. doi:10.1073/pnas.0603844103

Sugimoto, N., Nakano, S., Yoneyama, M., & Honda, K. (1996). Improved thermodynamic parameters and helix initiation factor to predict stability of DNA duplexes. *Nucleic Acids Research, 24*(22), 4501–4505. doi:10.1093/nar/24.22.4501

Sugimoto, M., Kikuchi, S., & Tomita, M. (2005). Reverse engineering of biochemical equations from time-course data by means of genetic programming. *Bio Systems, 80*, 155–164. doi:10.1016/j.biosystems.2004.11.003

Suna, T., Salminen, A., & Soininen, P. (2007). 1H NMR metabonomics of plasma lipoprotein subclasses – elucidation of metabolic clustering by SOM. *NMR in Biomedicine, 20*, 658–672. doi:10.1002/nbm.1123

Swan, M. (2009). Emerging Patient-Driven Health Care Models: An Examination of Health Social Networks, Consumer Personalized Medicine and Quantified Self-Tracking. *International Journal of Environmental Research and Public Health, 6*, 492–525. doi:10.3390/ijerph6020492

Swanson, J. A., & Hoppe, A. D. (2004). The coordination of signaling during Fc receptor-mediated phagocytosis. *Journal of Leukocyte Biology, 76*, 1093–1103. doi:10.1189/jlb.0804439

Tahani, H., & Keller, J. M. (1990). Information fusion in computer vision using fuzzy integral. *IEEE Transactions on Systems, Man, and Cybernetics, 20*(3), 733–741. doi:10.1109/21.57289

Takagi, A., Kojima, S., Watanabe, T., Ida, M., & Kawagoe, S. (2002). Rippling Muscle Syndrome Preceding Malignant Lymphoma. *Internal Medicine (Tokyo, Japan), 41*, 147–150. doi:10.2169/internalmedicine.41.147

Talcott, C. L. (2008). Pathway Logic. Bernardo, M. & Degano, P. & Zavattaro G. (Eds.). *Formal Methods for Computational Systems Biology, 8th International School on Formal Methods for the Design of Computer, Communication, and Software Systems, SFM 2008*, Advanced Lectures. Lecture Notes in Computer Science 5016, (pp. 21-53), Springer.

Talla, E., Tekaia, F., Brino, L., & Dujon, B. (2003). A novel design of whole-genome microarray probes for Saccharomyces cerevisiae which minimizes cross-hybridization. *BMC Genomics, 4*, 38. doi:10.1186/1471-2164-4-38

Tang, H., Xiao, C., & Wang, Y. (2009). Important roles of the hyphenated HPLC-DAD-MS-SPE-NMR technique in metabonomics. *Magnetic Resonance in Chemistry, 47*(Suppl 1), S157–S162. doi:10.1002/mrc.2513

Tax, D., Van Breukelen, M., Duin, R., & Kittler, J. (2000). Combining multiple classifiers by averaging or by multiplying? *Pattern Recognition, 33*, 1475–1485. doi:10.1016/S0031-3203(99)00138-7

Teletchea1, F., Bernillon, J., Duffraisse, M., Laudet, V., & Hänni, C. (2008). Molecular identification of vertebrate species by oligonucleotide microarray in food and forensic samples. *Journal of Applied Ecology, 45*(3), 967–975.

Temtamy, S. A., Aglan, M. S., & Nemat, A. & M., E. (2003). Expanding the phenotypic spectrum of the Baller-Gerold syndrome. *Genetic Counseling (Geneva, Switzerland), 14*, 299–312.

The FANTOM Consortium. (2005, Sep 2). The transcriptional landscape of the mammalian genome. [*Erratum in: Science. 2006 Mar 24,311*] [5768] [:1713; www.sciencemag.org/content/309/5740/1559.long]. *Science, 309*(5740), 1559–1563. doi:10.1126/science.1112014

Thompson, J. N. (1982). *Interaction and Coevolution*. New York, NY: Wiley and Sons.

Thompson, J. N. (1988). Variation in interspecific interactions. *Annual Review of Ecology and Systematics, 19*, 65–87. doi:10.1146/annurev.es.19.110188.000433

Tian, T., Xu, S., & Burrage, K. (2007). Simulated maximum likelihood method for estimating kinetic rates in gene expression. *Bioinformatics (Oxford, England), 23*(1), 84–91. doi:10.1093/bioinformatics/btl552

Tikole, S. & Sankararamakrishnan, R. (2008). Prediction of Translation Initiation Sites in Human mRNA sequences with AUG Start Codon. *Weak Kozak Context: A Neural Network Approach, BBRC*, 1166-1168.

Tiziani, S., Lodi, A., & Khanim, F. L. (2009). Metabolic profiling of drug response in acute myeloid leukemia cell lines. *PLoS ONE*, *4*, e4251. doi:10.1371/journal.pone.0004251

Tofts, C. (1993). Algorithms for task allocation in ants (A study on temporal polyethism: Theory). *Bulletin of Mathematical Biology*, *55*, 891–918.

Tofts, C. (1993). Describing social insect behavior using process algebra. *Transactions on Social Computing Simulation*, *10*, 227–283.

Tolstrup, N., Nielsen, P. S., Kolberg, J. G., Frankel, A. M., Vissing, H., & Kauppinen, S. (2003). OligoDesign: Optimal design of LNA (locked nucleic acid) oligonucleotide capture probes for gene expression profiling. *Nucleic Acids Research*, *31*(13), 3758–3762. doi:10.1093/nar/gkg580

Torralba, A. S., Yu, K., Shen, P. D., Oefner, P. J., & Ross, J. (2003). Experimental test of a method for determining causal connectivity of species in reactions. *Proceedings of the National Academy of Sciences of the United States of America*, *100*, 1494–1498. doi:10.1073/pnas.262790699

Torres-Garcia, W., Zhang, W., Runger, G. C., Johnson, R. H., & Meldrum, D. R. (2009). Integrative analysis of transcriptomic and proteomic data of Desulfovibrio vulgaris: a non-linear model to predict abundance of undetected proteins. *Bioinformatics (Oxford, England)*, *25*(15), 1905–1914. doi:10.1093/bioinformatics/btp325

Trauger, S. A., Kalisak, E., Kalisiak, J., Morita, H., Weinberg, M. V., & Menon, A. L. (2008). Correlating the transcriptome, proteome, and metabolome in the environmental adaptation of a hyperthermophile. *Journal of Proteome Research*, *7*(3), 1027–1035. doi:10.1021/pr700609j

Trygg, J., Holmes, E., & Lundstedt, T. (2007). Chemometrics in metabonomics. *Journal of Proteome Research*, *6*(2), 469–479. doi:10.1021/pr060594q

Tsang, T. M., Haselden, J. N., & Holmes, E. (2009). Metabonomic characterization of the 3-nitropropionic acid rat model of Huntington's disease. *Neurochemical Research*, *34*(7), 1261–1271. doi:10.1007/s11064-008-9904-5

Tsukurov, O., Boehmer, A., Flynn, J., Nicolai, J.-P., Hamel, B. C. J., & Traill, S. (1994). A complex bilateral polysyndactyly disease locus maps to chromosome 7q36. *Nature Genetics*, *6*, 282–286. doi:10.1038/ng0394-282

Tukiainen, T., Tynkkynen, T., & Makinen, V.-P. (2008). A multi-metabolite analysis of serum by 1H NMR spectroscopy: early systemic signs of Alzheimer's disease. *Biochemical and Biophysical Research Communications*, *375*, 356–361. doi:10.1016/j.bbrc.2008.08.007

Tulpan, D., Andronescu, M., Chang, S. B., Shortreed, M. R., Condon, A., Hoos, H. H., & Smith, L. M. (2005). Thermodynamically based DNA strand design. *Nucleic Acids Research*, *33*(15), 4951–4964. doi:10.1093/nar/gki773

Tulpan, D., Andronescu, M., & Leger, S. (2010). Free energy estimation of short DNA duplex hybridizations. *BMC Bioinformatics*, *11*(1), 105. doi:10.1186/1471-2105-11-105

Tulpan, D. C. (2006). Effective Heuristic Methods of DNA Strand Design. *Ph.D. thesis*, University of British Columbia, BC, Canada.

Tulpan, D. C., & Hoos, H. H. (2003). Hybrid randomised neighbourhoods improve stochastic local search for DNA code design. *Lectures Notes in Computer Science*, Springer, Berlin, 2671, 418–433.

Tulpan, D. C., Hoos, H. H., & Condon, A. E. (2002). Stochastic local search algorithms for DNA word design. *Lectures Notes in Computer Science*, Springer, Berlin, 2568, 229–241, 2002.

Tylianakis, J. M., Tscharntke, T., & Lewis, O. T. (2007). Habitat modification alters the structure of tropical host-parasitoid food webs. *Nature*, *455*, 202–205. doi:10.1038/nature05429

Tzanis, G., & Vlahavas, I. (2006). *Prediction of Translation Initiation Sites Using Classifier Selection*. Chapter in Advances in Artificial Intelligence. [Springer-Verlag]. *Lecture Notes in Computer Science*, *3955*, 367–377. doi:10.1007/11752912_37

Ueda, N. (2000). Optimal linear combination of neural networks for improving classification performance. *IEEE Transactions on Pattern Analysis and Machine Intelligence*, 22(2), 207–215. doi:10.1109/34.825759

Ueda, N., Nakano, R., Ghahramani, Z. and & Hinton, G. E. (2000). SMEM algorithm for mixture models., to appear in *Neural Computations, 12* (9), 2109-2128.

Ulanowicz, R. E. (1986). *Growth and Development -ecosystems phenomenology*. Berlin: Springer Verlag.

Ulanowicz, R. E. (2004). Quantitative methods for ecological network analysis. *Computational Biology and Chemistry*, 28(5-6), 321–339. doi:10.1016/j.compbiolchem.2004.09.001

Ulanowicz, R. E., & Kemp, W. M. (1979). Toward canonical trophic aggregations. *American Naturalist, 114*, 871–883. doi:10.1086/283534

Ulanowicz, R. E., & Wolff, W. F. (1991). Ecosystem flow networks: loaded dice? *Mathematical Biosciences, 103*, 45–68. doi:10.1016/0025-5564(91)90090-6

Ulanowicz, R.E., Bondavalli, C., & Egnotovich, M.S. (1997). *Network Analysis of Trophic Dynamics in South Florida Ecosystems, FY 96: The Cypress Wetland Ecosystem.* - Tech. Rep. [UMCES] CBL 97-075, Chesapeake Biological Laboratory, Solomons.

Ulanowicz, R.E., Bondavalli, C., & Egnotovich, M.S. (1998). *Network Analysis of Trophic Dynamics in South Florida Ecosystems, FY 97: The Florida Bay Ecosystem.* - Tech. Rep. [UMCES] CBL 98-123, Chesapeake Biological Laboratory, Solomons.

Ulanowicz, R.E., Bondavalli, C., Heymans, J.J., & Egnotovich, M.S. (1999). *Network Analysis of Trophic Dynamics in South Florida Ecosystem, FY 98: The Mangrove Ecosystem.* - Tech. Rep. [UMCES] CBL 99-0073, Chesapeake Biological Laboratory, Solomons.

Ulanowicz, R.E., Heymans, J.J., & Egnotovich, M.S. (2000). *Network Analysis of Trophic Dynamics in South Florida Ecosystems FY 99: The Graminoid Ecosystem.* - Tech. Rep. [UMCES] CBL 00-0176, Chesapeake Biological Laboratory, Solomons.

Ultsch, A. (1999). Data mining and knowledge discovery with emergent self-organizing feature maps for multivariate time series. In Oja, E., & Kaski, S. (Eds.), *Kohonen Maps* (pp. 33–45). Elsevier. doi:10.1016/B978-044450270-4/50003-6

Valentini, R., & Jordán, F. (2010). CoSBiLab Graph: the network analysis module of CoSBiLab. *Environmental Modelling & Software, 25*, 886–888. doi:10.1016/j.envsoft.2010.02.001

Valentini, G. and & Masulli, F. (2002). Ensembles of learning machines. *Neural Nets*, No. 2486 of Lecture Notes in Computer Science, 3-19.

van der Zanden, M. J., Cabana, G., & Rasmussen, J. B. (1997). Comparing trophic position of freshwater littoral fish species using stable nitrogen isotopes (d15N) and literature dietary data. *Canadian Journal of Fisheries and Aquatic Sciences, 54*, 1142–1158. doi:10.1139/f97-016

van Velzen, E. J., Westerhuis, J. A., van Duynhoven, J. P., van Dorsten, F. A., Hoefsloot, H. C., & Jacobs, D. M. (2008). Multilevel data analysis of a crossover designed human nutritional intervention study. *Journal of Proteome Research, 7*(10), 4483–4491. doi:10.1021/pr800145j

Vance, W., Arkin, A., & Ross, J. (2002). Determination of causal connectivities of species in reaction network. *Proceedings of the National Academy of Sciences of the United States of America, 99*, 5816–5821. doi:10.1073/pnas.022049699

Viant, M. R. (2003). Improved methods for the acquisition and interpretation of NMR metabolomic data. *Biochemical and Biophysical Research Communications, 310*(3), 943–948. doi:10.1016/j.bbrc.2003.09.092

Viant, M. R. (2007). Revealing the metabolome of animal tissues using 1H nuclear magnetic resonance spectroscopy. *Methods in Molecular Biology (Clifton, N.J.), 358*, 229–246. doi:10.1007/978-1-59745-244-1_13

Villas-Boas, S. G., & Bruheim, P. (2007). The potential of metabolomics tools in bioremediation studies. *OMICS: A Journal of Integrative Biology, 11*(3), 305–313. doi:10.1089/omi.2007.0005

Villas-Boas, S. G., Hojer-Pedersen, J., Akesson, M., Smedsgaard, J., & Nielsen, J. (2005). Global metabolite analysis of yeast: evaluation of sample preparation methods. *Yeast (Chichester, England), 22*(14), 1155–1169. doi:10.1002/yea.1308

Vittorio, C., Jill, S., Melvyn, J. B., Ricardo Palacios, P., Nicolas, G. B., & Walter, J. L. (2002). Gene expression profiling of 12633 genes in Alzheimer hippocampal CA1: Transcription and neurotrophic factor down-regulation and up-regulation of apoptotic and pro-inflammatory signaling. *Journal of Neuroscience Research, 70*, 462–473. doi:10.1002/jnr.10351

Vologodskii, A. V., Amirikyan, B. R., Lyubchenko, Y. L., & Frank-Kamenetskii, M. D. (1984). Allowance for heterogeneous stacking in the DNA helix-coil transition theory. *Journal of Biomolecular Structure & Dynamics, 2*, 131–148.

Volterra, V. (1926). Fluctuations in the abundance of species considered mathematically. *Nature, 118*, 558–560. doi:10.1038/118558a0

Walczak, S. (2009). Managing personal medical knowledge: agent-based knowledge acquisition. *International Journal of Technology Management, 47*, 22–36. doi:10.1504/IJTM.2009.024112

Walters, C., Christensen, V., & Pauly, D. (1997). Structuring dynamic models of exploited ecosystems from trophic mass-balance assessments. *Reviews in Fish Biology and Fisheries, 7*, 139–172. doi:10.1023/A:1018479526149

Wang, D., & Bodovitz, S. (2010). Single cell analysis: the new frontier in 'omics'. *Trends in Biotechnology, 28*(6), 281–290. doi:10.1016/j.tibtech.2010.03.002

Wang, X., & Seed, B. (2003). Selection of Oligonucleotide Probes for Protein Coding Sequences. *Bioinformatics (Oxford, England), 19*(7), 796–802. doi:10.1093/bioinformatics/btg086

Wang, Y., Miao, Z.-H., Pommier, Y., Kawasaki, E. S., & Player, A. (2007). Characterization of mismatch and high-signal intensity probes associated with Affymetrix genechips. *Bioinformatics (Oxford, England), 23*(16), 2088–2095. doi:10.1093/bioinformatics/btm306

Wang, Y., Scott, C., Mjolsness, E., & Xie, X. (2010). Parameter inference for discretely observed stochastic kinetic models using stochastic gradient descendent. *BMC Systems Biology, 4*(99).

Wang, D., Keller, J. M., Carson, C. A., McAdoo-Edwards, K. K., & Bailey, C. W. (1998). Use of fuzzy-logic-inspired features to improve bacterial recognition through classifier fusion. *IEEE Transactions on Systems, Man, and Cybernetics, 28*(4), 583–591. doi:10.1109/3477.704297

Want, E. J., O'Maille, G., Smith, C. A., Brandon, T. R., Uritboonthai, W., & Qin, C. (2006). Solvent-dependent metabolite distribution, clustering, and protein extraction for serum profiling with mass spectrometry. *Analytical Chemistry, 78*(3), 743–752. doi:10.1021/ac051312t

Want, E. J., Wilson, I. D., Gika, H., Theodoridis, G., Plumb, R. S., & Shockcor, J. (2010). Global metabolic profiling procedures for urine using UPLC-MS. *Nature Protocols, 5*(6), 1005–1018. doi:10.1038/nprot.2010.50

Webb Cp, P. H. (2004). Translation research: from accurate diagnosis to appropriate treatment. *Journal of Translational Medicine, 2*, 35. doi:10.1186/1479-5876-2-35

Webster, Y., Gudivada, R., Dow, E., Koehler, J., & Palakal, M. (2010). A Framework for Cross-Disciplinary Hypothesis Generation. In *ACM 25th Symposium on Applied Computing*, Sierre, Switzerland.

Weckwerth, W., & Morgenthal, K. (2005). Metabolomics: from pattern recognition to biological interpretation. *Drug Discovery Today, 10*(22), 1551–1558. doi:10.1016/S1359-6446(05)03609-3

Weeds, A., & Yeoh, S. (2001). Action at the Y-branch. *Science, 294*, 1660–1661. doi:10.1126/science.1067619

Weljie, A. M., Newton, J., Mercier, P., Carlson, E., & Slupsky, C. M. (2006). Targeted profiling: quantitative analysis of 1H NMR metabolomics data. *Analytical Chemistry, 78*(13), 4430–4442. doi:10.1021/ac060209g

Werth, M. T., Halouska, S., Shortridge, M. D., Zhang, B., & Powers, R. (n.d.). Analysis of metabolomic PCA data using tree diagrams. *Analytical Biochemistry, 399*(1), 58–63. doi:10.1016/j.ab.2009.12.022

Westerhuis, J. A., van Velzen, E. J., Hoefsloot, H. C., & Smilde, A. K. (2010). Multivariate paired data analysis: multilevel PLSDA versus OPLSDA. *Metabolomics*, *6*(1), 119–128. doi:10.1007/s11306-009-0185-z

Whipple, S. J. (1998). Path-based network unfolding: A solution for the problem of mixed trophic and non-trophic processes in trophic dynamic analysis. *Journal of Theoretical Biology*, *190*, 263–276. doi:10.1006/jtbi.1997.0551

White, S., & Smyth, P. (2003). Algorithms for estimating relative importance in networks. In *Proceedings of the ninth ACM SIGKDD international conference on Knowledge discovery and data mining*, Washington, D.C., USA.

Wilkinson, D. J. (2006). *Stochastic modelling for systems biology*. London: Chapman and Hall/CRC Taylor & Francis Group.

Wilkinson, D. J. (2007). Bayesian methods in bioinformatics and computational systems biology. *Briefings in Bioinformatics*, *2*(8), 109–116.

Williams, T. M. (2008). Killer appetites: assessing the role of predators in ecological communities. *Ecology*, *85*, 3373–3384. doi:10.1890/03-0696

Williams, R. J., & Martinez, N. D. (2000). Simple rules yield complex food webs. *Nature*, *404*, 180–183. doi:10.1038/35004572

Wilson, E. O. (1987). The little things that run the world. *Conservation Biology*, *1*, 344–346. doi:10.1111/j.1523-1739.1987.tb00055.x

Winder, C. L., Dunn, W. B., Schuler, S., Broadhurst, D., Jarvis, R., & Stephens, G. M. (2008). Global metabolic profiling of Escherichia coli cultures: an evaluation of methods for quenching and extraction of intracellular metabolites. *Analytical Chemistry*, *80*(8), 2939–2948. doi:10.1021/ac7023409

Wishart, D. S. (2005). Metabolomics: the principles and potential applications to transplantation. *American Journal of Transplantation*, *5*(12), 2814–2820. doi:10.1111/j.1600-6143.2005.01119.x

Wishart, D. S. (2007). Current progress in computational metabolomics. *Briefings in Bioinformatics*, *8*(5), 279–293. doi:10.1093/bib/bbm030

Wishart, D. S. (2010). Computational approaches to metabolomics. *Methods in Molecular Biology (Clifton, N.J.)*, *593*, 283–313. doi:10.1007/978-1-60327-194-3_14

Wishart, D. S., Knox, C., Guo, A. C., Eisner, R., Young, N., & Gautam, B. (2009). HMDB: a knowledgebase for the human metabolome. *Nucleic Acids Research*, *37*(Database issue), D603–D610. doi:10.1093/nar/gkn810

Witten, I. H., & Frank, E. (2000). *Data Mining: Practical Machine Learning Tools with Java Implementations*. San Francisco: Morgan Kaufmann.

Wittkopp, P. J. (2010). Variable Transcription Factor Binding: A Mechanism of Evolutionary Change. *PLoS Biology*, *8*(3), e1000342. doi:10.1371/journal.pbio.1000342

Wolkenhauer, O., Ullah, M., Kolch, W., & Cho, K. H. (2004). Modeling and simulation of intracellular dynamics: Choosing an appropriate framework. *IEEE Transactions on Nanobioscience*, *3*, 200–207. doi:10.1109/TNB.2004.833694

Wolpert, D. (1992). Stacked generalization. *Neural Networks*, 5241–5259.

Woods, K., Kegelmeyer, W. P., & Bowyer, K. (1997). Combination of multiple classifiers using local accuracy estimates. *IEEE Transactions on Pattern Analysis and Machine Intelligence*, *19*(4), 405–410. doi:10.1109/34.588027

Woods, K., Philip Kegelmeyer Jr, W., & Bowyer, K. (1997). Combination of multiple classifiers using local accuracy estimates. *IEEE Transactions on Pattern Analysis and Machine Intelligence*, *19*(4), 405–410. doi:10.1109/34.588027

Woodward, G., & Hildrew, A. G. (2001). Invasion of a stream food web by a new top predator. *Journal of Animal Ecology*, *70*, 273–288. doi:10.1046/j.1365-2656.2001.00497.x

Woolf, P. J., Prudhomme, W., Daheron, W., Daley, G. Q., & Lauffebberger, D. A. (2005). Bayesian analysis of signaling networks governing embryonic stem cell fate decisions. *Bioinfromatics*, *21*, 741–753. doi:10.1093/bioinformatics/bti056

Wray, G. A., Hahn, M. W., Abouheif, E., Balhoff, J. P., Pizer, M., Rockman, M. V., & Romano, L. A. (2003, Sep). The evolution of transcriptional regulation in eukaryotes. *Molecular Biology and Evolution, 20*(9), 1377–1419. doi:10.1093/molbev/msg140

Wu Ch, A.R., & Bairoch, A, Natale Da, Barker Wc, Boeckmann B, Ferro S, Gasteiger E, Huang H, Lopez R, Magrane M, Martin Mj, Mazumder R, O'donovan C, Redaschi N & Suzek B. (2006). The Universal Protein Resource (UniProt): an expanding universe of protein information. *Nucleic Acids Research, 34*, D187–D191. doi:10.1093/nar/gkj161

Wulff, F., & Ulanowicz, R. E. (1989). A comparative anatomy of the Baltic Sea and Chesapeake Bay ecosystems. In Wulff, F., Field, J., & Mann, K. (Eds.), *Network analysis in marine ecology - methods and applications. Vol. 32 of Coastal and Estuarine Studies.* Springer-Verlag, New York.

Xia, J., Wu, X., & Yuan, Y. (2007). Integration of wavelet transform with PCA and ANN for metabolomics data-mining. *Metabolmics, 3*, 531–537. doi:10.1007/s11306-007-0090-2

Xia, J., Bjorndahl, T. C., Tang, P., & Wishart, D. S. (2008). MetaboMiner--semi-automated identification of metabolites from 2D NMR spectra of complex biofluids. *BMC Bioinformatics, 9*, 507. doi:10.1186/1471-2105-9-507

Xia, Y., Yu, H., Jansen, R., Seringhaus, M., Baxter, S., & Greenbaum, D. (2004). Analyzing cellular biochemistry in temrs of molecualr networks. *Annual Review of Biochemistry, 73*, 1051–1087. doi:10.1146/annurev.biochem.73.011303.073950

Xia, J., Psychogios, N., Young, N., & Wishart, D. S. (2009). MetaboAnalyst: a web server for metabolomic data analysis and interpretation. *Nucleic Acids Res, 37*(Web Server issue), W652-660.

Xiong, Z.-Q., Qian, W., Suzuki, K., & Mcnamara, J. O. (2003). Formation of Complement Membrane Attack Complex in Mammalian Cerebral Cortex Evokes Seizures and Neurodegeneration. *The Journal of Neuroscience, 23*, 955–956.

Xu, R., & Wunsch, D. (2005). Survey of Clustering Algorithms. *IEEE Transactions on Neural Networks, 16*(3), 645–678. doi:10.1109/TNN.2005.845141

Xu, L., Krzyzak, A., & Suen, C. Y. (1992). Methods of combining multiple classifiers and their applications to handwriting recognition. *IEEE Transactions on Systems, Man, and Cybernetics, 22*(3), 418–435. doi:10.1109/21.155943

Xu, H., Yuan, X., Guan, C., Duan, S., Wu, C., & Feng, L. (2004). Calcium signaling in chemorepellant Slit2-dependent regulation of neuronal migration. *Proceedings of the National Academy of Sciences of the United States of America, 101*, 4296–4301. doi:10.1073/pnas.0303893101

Xu, J., & Li, Y. (2006). Discovering disease-genes by topological features in human protein-protein interaction network. *Bioinformatics (Oxford, England), 22*, 2800–2805. doi:10.1093/bioinformatics/btl467

Yang, Y. H., Dudoit, S., Luu, P., Lin, D. M., & Peng, V. (2002). Normalization for cDNA microarray data: a robust composite method addressing single and multiple systemic variation. *Nucleic Acids Research, 30*, e15. doi:10.1093/nar/30.4.e15

Yang, C., Richardson, A. D., Smith, J. W., & Osterman, A. (2007) Comparative metabolomics of breast cancer. *Pacif Symp Biocomp 12*, 181-192.

Yano, K., Imai, K., Shimizu, A., & Hanashita, T. (2006)... *Nucleic Acids Research, 34*(5), 1532–1539. doi:10.1093/nar/gkl058

Yee, J. C., Wlaschin, K. F., Chuah, S. H., Nissom, P. M., & Hu, W. S. (2008). Quality assessment of cross-species hybridization of CHO transcriptome on a mouse DNA oligo microarray. *Biotechnology and Bioengineering, 101*(6), 1359–1365. doi:10.1002/bit.21984

Yeo, S.-Y., Miyashita, T., Fricke, C., Little, M. H., Yamada, T., & Kuwada, J. Y. (2004). Involvement of Islet-2 in the Slit signaling for axonal branching and defasciculation of the sensory neurons in embryonic zebrafish. *Mechanisms of Development, 121*, 315–324. doi:10.1016/j.mod.2004.03.006

Yildirim, M. A., Goh, K. I., Cusick, M. E., Barabasi, A. L., & Vidal, M. (2007). Drug-target network. *Nature Biotechnology, 25*, 1119–1126. doi:10.1038/nbt1338

Yodzis, P. (2000). Diffuse effects in food webs. *Ecology, 81*, 261–266. doi:10.1890/0012-9658(2000)081[0261:DEIFW]2.0.CO;2

Yodzis, P. (2001). Must top predators be culled for the sake of fisheries? *Trends in Ecology & Evolution*, *16*, 78–84. doi:10.1016/S0169-5347(00)02062-0

Yodzis, P., & Winemiller, K. O. (1999). In search of operational trophospecies in a tropical aquatic food web. *Oikos*, *87*, 327–340. doi:10.2307/3546748

Yodzis, P. (1989). Patterns in food webs. *Trends in Ecology & Evolution*, *4*(2), 49–50. doi:10.1016/0169-5347(89)90140-7

Yodzis, P. (2001). Must top predators be culled for the sake of fisheries? *Trends in Ecology & Evolution*, *16*, 78–84. doi:10.1016/S0169-5347(00)02062-0

Yodzis, P., & Winemiller, K. O. (1999). In search of operational trophospecies in a tropical aquatic food web. *Oikos*, *87*, 327–340. doi:10.2307/3546748

Yoo, S. M., Choi, J. H., Lee, S. Y., & Yoo, N. C. (2009). Applications of DNA microarray in disease diagnostics. *Journal of Microbiology and Biotechnology*, *19*(7), 635–646.

Yu, J., Smith, V. A., Wang, P. P., Hartemink, A. J., & Jarvis, E. D. (2004). Advances to Bayesian network inference for generating causal networks from observational data. *Bioinformatics (Oxford, England)*, *20*(18), 3594–3603. doi:10.1093/bioinformatics/bth448

Yun, K. Y., Park, M. R., Mohanty, B., Herath, V., Xu, F., & Mauleon, R. (2010). Transcriptional regulatory network triggered by oxidative signals configures the early response mechanisms of japonica rice to chilling stress. *BMC Plant Biology*, *10*(1), 16. doi:10.1186/1471-2229-10-16

Yurke, B., Turberfield, A. J., Mills, A. P., Simmel, F. C., & Neumann, J. L. (2000). A DNA-fuelled molecular machine made of DNA. *Nature*, *406*(6796), 605–608. doi:10.1038/35020524

Zelena, E., Dunn, W. B., Broadhurst, D., Francis-McIntyre, S., Carroll, K. M., & Begley, P. (2009). Development of a robust and repeatable UPLC-MS method for the long-term metabolomic study of human serum. *Analytical Chemistry*, *81*(4), 1357–1364. doi:10.1021/ac8019366

Zeng, F., Yap, R. H., & Wong, L. (2002). Using feature generation and feature selection for accurate prediction of translation initiation sites. *Genome Inform.*, *13*, 192–200.

Zeng, J., & Alhajj, R. (2008). Predicting translation initiation sites using a multi-agent architecture empowered with reinforcement learning. *CIBCB*, *2008*, 241–248.

Zetina-Rejon, M. J., Arreguin-Sanchez, F., & Chavez, E. A. (2004). Exploration of harvesting strategies for the management of a Mexican coastal lagoon fishery. *Ecological Modelling*, *172*, 361–372. doi:10.1016/j.ecolmodel.2003.09.017

Zguricas, J., Heus, H., Morales-Peralta, E., Breedveld, G., Kuyt, B., & Mumcu, E. F. (1999). Clinical and genetic studies on 12 preaxial polydactyly families and refinement of the localisation of the gene responsible to a 1.9 cM region on chromosome 7q36. *Journal of Medical Genetics*, *36*, 33–40.

Zhang, H., Holford, T., & Bracken, M. B. (1996). A tree-based method of analysis for prospective studies. *Statistics in Medicine*, *15*(1), 37–49. doi:10.1002/(SICI)1097-0258(19960115)15:1<37::AID-SIM144>3.0.CO;2-0

Zhang, W., Li, F., & Nie, L. (2010). Integrating multiple 'omics' analysis for microbial biology: application and methodologies. *Microbiology*, *156*(Pt 2), 287–301. doi:10.1099/mic.0.034793-0

Zhang, X., Liu, H., Wu, J., Zhang, X., Liu, M., & Wang, Y. (2009). Metabonomic alterations in hippocampus, temporal and prefrontal cortex with age in rats. *Neurochemistry International*, *54*(8), 481–487. doi:10.1016/j.neuint.2009.02.004

Zhang, B.-T., & Shin, S.-Y. (1998). Molecular algorithms for efficient and reliable DNA computing. *Proceedings of the Third Annual Conference in Genetic Programming* (University of Wisconsin, Madison, Wiscon- sin, USA, 22-25 1998), J. R. Koza, W. Banzhaf, K. Chellapilla, K. Deb, M. Dorigo, D. B. Fogel, M. H. Garzon, D. E. Goldberg, H. Iba, and R. Ri- olo, Eds., Morgan Kaufmann, 735–744.

Zhao, Q., Stoyanova, R., Du, S., Sajda, P., & Brown, T. R. (2006). HiRes--a tool for comprehensive assessment and interpretation of metabolomic data. *Bioinformatics (Oxford, England)*, *22*(20), 2562–2564. doi:10.1093/bioinformatics/btl428

Zhao, Y., Li, M.-C., & Simon, R. (2005). An adaptive method for cDNA microarray normalization. *BMC Bioinformatics*, *6*, 28. doi:10.1186/1471-2105-6-28

Zheng, J., Svensson, J. T., Madishetty, K., Close, T. J., Jiang, T., & Lonardi, S. (2006). OligoSpawn: a software tool for the design of overgo probes from large unigene datasets. *BMC Bioinformatics*, *7*, 7. doi:10.1186/1471-2105-7-7

Zou, W., & Tolstikov, W. (2008). Probing genetic algorithms for feature selection in comprehensive metabolic profiling approach. *Rapid Communications in Mass Spectrometry*, *22*, 1312–1324. doi:10.1002/rcm.3507

Zou, Y. Y., Yang, J., & Zhu, J. (2006). A robust statistical procedure to discover expression biomarkers using microarray genomic expression data. *Journal of Zhejiang University. Science*, *7*(8), 603–607. doi:10.1631/jzus.2006.B0603

Zwolak, J. (2007). *PET- Parameter Estimation toolkit*. Retrieved from http://mpf.biol.vt.edu/pet/contact.php.

About the Contributors

Paola Lecca received a Master Degree in Theoretical Physics from the University of Trento (Italy) and a PhD in Computer Science from the International Doctorate School in Information and Communication Technologies at the University of Trento (Italy). Currently Paola Lecca is the Principal Investigator of the Inference and Data manipulation research group at The Microsoft Research – University of Trento Centre for Computational and Systems Biology (Trento,, Italy). Dr. Paola Lecca's research interests include stochastic biochemical kinetic, biological networks inference, optimal experimental design in biochemistry, and computational cell biology. She designed prototypes for biological model calibration and for the simulation of diffusion pathways in cells and tissues. She has published articles in leading medical, biological and bioinformatics Journals and Conferences. She received a best paper prize at Brain, Vision and Artificial Intelligence (Naples, Italy 2007) presenting a kinetic model of cerebral glucose metabolism in astrocytes. Paola Lecca is carrying on an intense editorial activity, editing books and as editorial member of CSC bioinformatics journals. She is a member of the Italian Society of Pure and Applied Biophysics. Paola Lecca has experience in organizing international conferences and as PC member of many international conferences as well (SAC ACM, ISB, ICCB, ICCMB). More information, such as the complete list of publications and prototypes, the editorial activity, and the research interests of Paola Lecca are available at: http://www.cosbi.eu/index.php/people/people-research/16-paola-lecca.

Dan Tulpan received a BSc/B.eng. Degree (2000) from POLITEHNICA University of Bucharest (Romania) and a PhD Degree in Computer Science (2006) from the University of British Columbia (Canada). Dan is a research officer in the Knowledge Discovery Group at the Institute for Information Technology, National Research Council Canada and lead of the NRC-IIT Bioinformatics Laboratory. Dan is also appointed as Adjunct Professor (2010) in the Department of Biology, University of Moncton, Honorary Research Associate (2009) in the Department of Computer Science, University of New Brunswick and Research Associate (2009) at the Atlantic Cancer Research Institute in Moncton. Dan's research interests include the development of algorithms and technologies in biotechnology (microarray probe design), bioinformatics (comparative genomics, metabolomics) and data analysis and visualization.

Rajaraman Kanagasabai is currently a Principal Investigator at the Data Mining Department, Institute for Infocomm Research (I2R), Singapore, and leads the Semantic Technology Group. He has widely published in top peer-reviewed journals and conferences, and served in the Programme Committees of many international conferences. He has also chaired or co-chaired several international events related to Bioinformatics, Bio Ontologies and Analytics. He was part of the core research team behind the multiple-award winning iAgent – the first multilingual search engine, WebWatch - the key technology behind the successful startup BuzzCity (www.buzzcity.com), and the KnowleSuite technology that has been spunoff as Knorex (www.knorex.com). He was also the leader of the team that won the Tan Kah Kee Young InventorÂ's Award for Web Data Extraction technology in 2006. His research interests include Semantic technologies, Bio Ontologies, SOA & Web services, text/web mining. He is on the web at: http://datam.i2r.a-star.edu.sg/~kanagasa/.

* * *

Bernadetta Kwintiana Ane is a research fellow at the Institute of Computer-aided Product Development Systems, Universität Stuttgart, Germany. She has been 16 years working experiences in industry and academy. She published more than 40 scientific papers in the referred international journals and conferences, as well as book chapters, white papers, scientific oratio, and owned international patent. Presently, as a Humboldtian as well as an IEEE member she serves internationally as a research fellow at several research centers in Japan and Austria. Meantime, she also contributes as an associate editor for the Journal of Intelligent Automation and Soft Computing in USA, as well as research grant assessor for the Czech Science Foundation and reviewers for IEEE and several well-known referred international journals.

John Archer, on completion of his PhD in 1986 in molecular genetics of plasmids in Escherichia coli with Prof. David Sherratt at the department of Genetics, University of Glasgow, Scotland, Dr. Archer moved to the Massachusetts Institute of Technology, Cambridge, USA, for his postdoctoral studies where he studied metabolic engineering of primary metabolism of Corynebacterium glutamicum under the supervision of Prof. Tony Sinskey. In 1992, Dr. Archer joined the department of Genetics, Cambridge University, setting up molecular genetics and genomics in nocardioform actinomycetes. In 2009, Dr. Archer joined the Computational Bioscience Research Center at King Abdullah University of Science and Technology where his research concentrates on computational analysis of genomic data and metabolic engineering of heterotrophic and phototrophic microorganisms.

Haitham Ashoor is a Master student at Computational Bioscience Research Center (CBRC) at King Abdullah University of Science and Technology (KAUST). He received his bachelor degree in Computer Engineering from University of Jordan in Amman. Before joining CBRC Haitham worked in several areas including: high performance computing, computer networking, and text to speech conversion for Arabic language. Haitham's current research interests include discovery and identification of biological signals, text mining, and machine learning.

Karim Awara is currently a Ph.D student at KAUST University in Saudi Arabia. Prior to his PhD study, he acquired his bachelor degree in Science majoring in Computer Science from the American University in Cairo (AUC) in Egypt. Mr. Awara's research interest involves topics about data management and high performance computing. Mr. Awara has done research in diverse areas of computer science. He has worked on high-performance computing at IBM Thomas J. Watson Research Center in New York. He was a team leader at Microsoft Egypt in addition to other diverse internships at major companies and research centers. The above quote is his favorite and he enjoys playing tennis and squash. "Success is the ability to go from one failure to another with no loss of enthusiasm." (Winston Churchill).

Vladimir Bajic is Director of Computational Bioscience Research Center and Professor at King Abdullah University of Science and Technology, Saudi Arabia. He was a Professor of Bioinformatics, Acting and Deputy Director of the South African National Bioinformatics Institute (SANBI) at the University of the Western Cape. He worked in industry and academia. Vladimir is an elected member of the Academy of Nonlinear Sciences (Russia), was a registered Professional Engineer in South Africa, was awarded the first South African National Research Chair in Bioinformatics and Human Health and was an elected role model of the Institute for Infocomm Research, Singapore, in 2002. He earned graduate and master's degrees in Electrical Engineering from the University of Belgrade, Serbia, and a doctorate of Engineering Sciences in Electrical Engineering from the University of Zagreb, Croatia. His current interest is in modeling, artificial intelligence and knowledge discovery platforms in life sciences.

Rajesh Chowdhary is Associate Research Scientist in Bioinformatics and Computational Biology at Marshfield Clinic, USA. He received his Bachelor's degree in Engineering from the Indian Institute of Technology, Bombay, MSc in Bioengineering from Imperial College, London and PhD in Computer Science from National University of Singapore. He completed his post-doctoral fellowship from Harvard University. His research interests include Machine learning, Bayesian networks, Biological textmining, Biomedical informatics, Gene regulation, and Systems biology.

Miroslava Cuperlovic-Culf obtained PhD in Biophysical Chemistry in 1997 at University of California, Santa Barbara under direction of Dr.'s W. Palke and J.T. Gerig. Following post-doc in Biophysics with Prof. Myer Bloom at University of British Columbia Miroslava has worked as Research Scientist at Atlantic Cancer Research Institute in Moncton, Canada. Since 2007 she has been a Research Officer at National Research Council of Canada, Institute for Information Technology as well as Adjunct Professor of Chemistry in the department of Chemistry & Biochemistry at Mount Allison University. Miroslava is particularly interested in bioinformatics and computational biology and biochemistry applied to medical research and development.

Ernst Dow is a Sr. Research Scientist in the Discovery Informatics department of Eli Lilly & Company. He is also an Adjunct professor at School of Informatics, Indiana University Purdue University Indianapolis. Dr. Dow is an Associate Member of Center for Computational Biology and Bioinformatics at Indiana University School of Medicine Dr. Dow received his PhD in Biophysics and Computational Biology from University of Illinois at Urbana-Champaign. He has been worldwide leader of Eli Lilly's Bioinformatics Expression Group (DNA microarray, proteomics, and metabonomics).

Jose M. Garcia Manteiga studied Biochemistry (Barcelona, 1998) and obtained a PhD in Biochemistry and Molecular Biology (Biochemistry and Molecular Biololgy Dept., University of Barcelona, Barcelona, 2004). During his PhD, he contributed to expand the knowledge about the regulation of expression of nucleoside transporters in macrophages and lymphocytes and their contribution to chemotherapy resistance to nucleoside analogues in pancreatic cancer cells. He was post doctoral fellow in the division of Molecular Oncology at the San Raffaele Scientific Institute (Milan, 2005) where he characterized a new protein tyrosine phosphatase involved in the recycling of the EGFR and cell migration. In 2008 he moved to the Protein Transport and Secretion Unit of the San Raffaele Scientific Institute and held a post doctoral fellowship studying the metabolomics of the plasma cell phenotype. He holds collaboration with the centre for systems biology, CosBi (Trento, Italy), where he is modelling the metabolism of the differentiation of a B cell into a plasma cell through high-throughput omics approaches. He is also now interested in the redox metabolism of B lymphocytes and the signalling role of hydrogen peroxide.

Athos Ghiggi received a Bsc Degree in Computer Science from the Scuola Universitaria Professionale della Svizzera Italiana (SUPSI), Manno, Switzerland in 2008 and Msc Degree in Intelligent systems from the University of Lugano, Switzerland in 2010. He is currently a member of the R and D at Saphyrion Sagl, a young company oriented to space bourn and GNSS applications. His research interests include the development algorithms for GPS and global position applications.

Boris Jankovic is a member of the Computational Bioscience Research Center (CBRC) team at King Abdullah University of Science and Technology, Saudi Arabia. His primary interests are in mathematical modelling, stochastic processes, machine learning and biological networks. Prior to joining CBRC, he was technology consultant at Dimension Data, where he was working on modelling of internet traffic dynamics as well as on scalability, robustness and performances of communication networks. He was also the Chief Architect for Network Services Solutions at Cplane, a Sunnyvale, CA, based company, where he worked on algorithms for discovery and provisioning of virtual services in service-enabled networks. Dr. Jankovic holds a D.Tec. degree from Technikon Natal in Durban, South Africa and Graduate Electrical Engineer degree from School of Electrical Engineering at the University of Belgrade, Serbia.

Ferenc Jordán was born in Budapest, Hungary, on 11 June 1973. He studied Biology (MSc 1996) and received his PhD in Genetics (1999) from the Eotvos University, Budapest. Ferenc was an Assisant Professor at the Department of Genetics, Eotvos University (1999-2002); Postdoc Researcher at the Department of Ecology and Plant Taxonomy (2002-2003); Associate Professor at the Institute of Ecology and Botany of the Hungarian Academy of Sciences (2003-2006) and Research Professor at the Animal Ecology Research Group of HAS (2007-2008). He was also a Junior Fellow (2000/2001) and Branco Weiss Fellow (2003-2008) at the Collegium Budapest, Institute for Advanced Study. The latter was supported by the Society in Science foundation, ETH, Zurich, Switzerland. Ferenc has given a number of talks in different countries (from India to Taiwan and from the US to South Africa) and maintains a rich network of collaborators in 8-10 countries. He was a participant in the Darwinian Homeland Security workshop organized at NCEAS, Santa Barbara, CA (2005), and is an editor for Ecology Letters.

Ozan Kahramanoğulları obtained his Bachelor of Science degree in mathematics in Ankara, Turkey. During his Masters studies in artificial intelligence and computer science at the TU Dresden, and exchange studies at the University of Amsterdam, he developed an increasing interest in theoretical aspects of computer science. In his PhD work at the TU Dresden, with a grant from German Research Foundation, he has applied ideas from proof theory to proof search and language design. Between 2006 and 2009, he has worked as a research associate at the Imperial College London, Department of Computing, in a joint project with the Centre for Integrative Systems Biology at the Imperial College, on computational modeling of biological processes. Since 2009, he is working at the Microsoft Research – University of Trento, Centre for Computational and System Biology. His main research interests include formal methods in computer science, proof theory, concurrency theory, language design, and their applications to modeling of biological systems.

Marimuthu Krishnaveniis a researcher in the Naval Research Board of Defense Research Development Organisation in the Indian Ministry of Defense. She has been a consultant for some military related application projects. She has published 33 papers in both national and international conferences and journals. She focuses on research and experimental processes on the use of digital technologies such as: MATLAB, Computer Science, Biological Computation, along with Machine Intelligence and Real-Pime physical Computation. Presently, she acts as a resource person for a project related to the University grants Commission (India).

Carmen M. Livi received her MSc degree in Bioinformatics from the University of Bologna, Italy, in 2009. Currently she is a PhD student at the Department of Information Engineering and Computer Science of the University of Trento, Italy. Her research interests are in the prediction of protein-RNA binding with machine learning methods.

Roberto Montemanni received a Laurea Degree in Computer Science from the Università di Bologna, Italy in 1999 and a PhD Degree in Applied Mathematics from the University of Glamorgan, Wales, United Kingdom in 2002. He is currently a Senior Researcher at Istituto Dalle Molle di Studi sull'Intelligenza Artificiale (IDSIA), Lugano, Switzerland. His research interests include the development of exact, heuristic and matheuristic algorithms for optimization problems mainly arising in transportation, telecommunication and bioinformatics. He is a lecturer at the Department of Innovative Technology (DTI) of Scuola Universitaria Professionale della Svizzera Italiana (SUPSI), Lugano, Switzerland, and at the Faculty of Informatics of Università della Svizzera Italiana (USI), Lugano, Switzerland.

Arturo Magana Mora was born in Mexico City. He studied Computer Engineering at the Universidad Autónoma de San Luis Potosí and graduated in 2009 with the first class honor. During his studies, Arturo has been the recipient of five scholarships for computer engineering, including the General Electric Scholar-Leader Program and the French-Mexican Exchange Program. The latter allowed him to study one year at the Institut National des Sciences Appliquées de Lyon, France. Always interested in Artificial Intelligence and biology disciplines, Arturo followed a supplementary training at the University of Nottingham, UK. He is now finishing his Masters degree at King Abdullah University of Science and Technology (KAUST), Saudi Arabia, in computer science specialized in Artificial Intelligence and Bioinformatics. Arturo has as an objective to develop and research topics that could enhance or solve problems to improve human life.

Mathew Palakal is the Associate Dean of Research & Graduate Programs and the Director of Informatics Research Institute at School of Informatics, Indiana University Purdue University Indianapolis. He is also the Director of TiMAP, as well as a professor in the Department of Computer Science at Indiana University Purdue University Indianapolis. His Laboratory for Text information Mining, Analysis, and Discovery, focuses on extracting knowledge from published literature documents in the areas of Health and Life Sciences. Dr. Palakal's team has also developed a text mining system called BioMAP - Biomedical Associations and Pathways.

Alida Palmisano obtained her PhD in December 2010, carrying on researches in Computational Systems Biology at The Microsoft Research – University of Trento Centre for Computational and Systems Biology (CoSBi). The title of her thesis is "Modelling and inference strategies for Biological Systems". She attended the Faculty of Science at the University of Trento, where she obtained a Bachelor's degree (2005) and a Master's degree (2007) in Computer Science. The Master thesis, "Formal models of examples of biological synthesis and signal transduction pathways" focused on building models of real biological systems using Beta-binders formalism and some specific extensions. In 2004 she worked at ITC-irst (Center for Scientific and Technological Research) in Trento. The main goal of her work was the analysis of service-oriented architectures for the development of softwares able to manage the automation of domotic devices.

Dieter Roller holds the position of director of the Institute of Computer-aided Product Development at the University of Stuttgart. He is full professor and chair of computer science fundamentals. Additionally he has been awarded the distinction as a honorary professor of the University of Kaiserslautern and also serves as member of the board of trustees of the Technische Akademie Esslingen. He is chairman of several national and international working groups, and also the leader of the experts group "Computer Graphics in Engineering - GRIB" of the German computer science society "Gesellschaft für Informatik e.V.". Professor Roller serves as reviewer for several scientific organizations and the Baden-Württemberg Ministry of Science and Research for project grants, as well as for well-known scientific journals and several national and international programme committees. As former R&D manager with world-wide responsibility for CAD-technology within an international computer company, he gathered a comprehensive industrial experience. He is the inventor of several patents and is well-known through numerous technical talks in countries all over the world, 71 published books and over 180 contributions to journals and proceedings books. With his wealth of experience, he also serves as a technology consultant to various high-tech companies.

Ulf Schaefer received his bachelor's degree in Computer Science from the University of Applied Science in Karlsruhe, Germany in 2005. After that he completed his Master of Science degree in Computer Science at St. Cross College at the University of Oxford, UK. Subsequently he studied for his doctoral degree in Bioinformatics at the University of the Western Cape in Cape Town, South Africa. His dissertation dealt with transcriptional regulation in mammals. He graduated from there in 2009. Since then he conducts research in Computational Biology at the Computational Bioscience Research Center at King Abdullah University of Science and Technology in Saudi Arabia.

Marco Scotti was born in Codogno, Italy, on 20 April 1978. He graduated in Environmental Sciences (2004) and received his PhD in Ecology (2007) from the University of Parma. He worked as postdoctoral fellow at the Central European University, Center for Network Science (2008-2009), and joined COSBI in January 2010. His main research interests are the study of complex systems, network theory and the development of computational models for systems biology. He started working on food webs and ecological networks, extending the focus of his analyses to other fields as social science, energy policy and bioinformatics. His studies aim at understanding the mechanisms linking network structure to system dynamics. Beside the application of network theory, he recently started to work on analysis and simulation of stochastic systems. He maintains a rich network of collaborators in different countries (Hungary, Mexico, US and France).

Parthasarathy Subashini is currently an Associate Professor at the Department of Computer Science in the Avinashilingam University for Women (AUFW), in Tamil Nadu, India. She has also held short-term appointments at several institutions around the state. Her research has spanned a large number of disciplines like Image Analysis, Pattern Recognition, Neural Networks, and applications to Digital Image processing. Simultaneously, she also contributes to researches in mathematics, especially in Biology-inspired Computing and Fuzzy Logic. She has authored and co-authored 61 papers, including IEEE, Springer's and various international journals. To date, she has won five research projects from various funding agencies, like the Indian Defense Research and Development Organization as well as the University Grants Commission (India).

Yue Webster works in the Discovery Informatics department of Eli Lilly & Company as a Research Scientist. She has received a Master's degree in Electrical & Computer Engineering and a PhD degree in Health Informatics from School of Informatics, Indiana University Purdue University Indianapolis. She has worked with multi-disciplinary teams in large-scale discovery and translational research projects and developed algorithms and applications to fill drug discovery informatics need. Dr. Webster is most interested in the development of novel methods and approaches for translational research.

Index